IARC MONOGRAPHS
ON THE
EVALUATION OF THE CARCINOGENIC RISK
OF CHEMICALS TO MAN:

Some aromatic azo compounds

Volume 8

This publication represents the views of an
IARC Working Group on the
Evaluation of the Carcinogenic Risk of Chemicals to Man
which met in Lyon,
26 November - 2 December 1974

IARC WORKING GROUP ON THE EVALUATION OF THE CARCINOGENIC RISK OF CHEMICALS TO MAN: SOME AROMATIC AZO COMPOUNDS

Lyon, 26 November - 2 December 1974

Members[1]

Dr E. Arrhenius, Department of Environmental Toxicology, Stockholms Universitet, Wallenberglaboratoriet, Lilla Frescati, S 10405 Stockholm 50, Sweden

Professor E. Boyland, Visiting Professor of Environmental Toxicology, London School of Hygiene and Tropical Medicine, Keppel Street, London WC1E 7HT, UK

Dr D.B. Douglas, Department of Employment, Employment Medical Advisory Service, London and South Eastern Region, Atlantic House, Holborn Viaduct, London EC4A 4BA, UK

Dr E.G. Knox, Health Services Research Centre, Department of Social Medicine, The Medical School, Edgbaston, Birmingham B15 2TJ, UK

Dr N. Loprieno, Laboratorio di Mutagenesi e Differenziamento - C.N.R., Via Cisanello 147, 56100 Pisa, Italy

Dr S. Odashima, Chief, Department of Chemical Pathology, National Institute of Hygienic Sciences, 1-18-1 Kami Yooga, Setagaya-Ku, Tokyo 158, Japan (*Vice-Chairman*)

Professor R. Preussmann, Deutsches Krebsforschungszentrum, Institut für Toxikologie und Chemotherapie, Kirschnerstrasse 6, Postfach 449, D-6900 Heidelberg 1, FRG

Dr B. Teichmann, Akademie der Wissenschaften der DDR, Zentralinstitut für Krebsforschung, Lindenberger Weg 80, 1115 Berlin Buch, DDR

Dr B. Terracini, Istituto di Anatomia e Istologia Patologica, Università di Torino, via Santena 7, 10126 Torino, Italy

---

[1]Unable to attend: Dr D.B. Clayson, Department of Experimental Pathology and Cancer Research, University of Leeds, 171 Woodhouse Lane, Leeds LS1 3AR, UK; Dr G. Gortalum, Chief, Laboratory of Carcinogenic Substances, Nutrition Institute of the Academy of Medical Science, Ustinsky pr. 2/14, Moscow 109240, USSR; Dr C. Ramel, Department of Environmental Toxicology, Stockholms Universitet, Wallenberglaboratoriet, Lilla Frescati, S 10405 Stockholm 50, Sweden; Dr G.J. Van Esch, Head of the Laboratory for Toxicology, Rijks Instituut voor de Volksgezondheid, Sterrenbos 1, Utrecht, The Netherlands

Professor R. Truhaut, Laboratoire de Toxicologie et d'Hygiène industrielles, 4 Avenue de l'Observatoire, 75006 Paris, France (*Chairman*)

Dr Elizabeth Weisburger, Carcinogen Metabolism Toxicology Branch, Building 37, National Cancer Institute, Bethesda, Maryland 20014, USA

Invited Guests

Dr G. Eisenbrand, Deutsches Krebsforschungszentrum, Institut für Toxikologie und Chemotherapie, Kirschnerstrasse 6, Postfach 449, D-6900 Heidelberg 1, FRG

Dr P.S. Elias, Principal Medical Officer, Department of Health and Social Security, Alexander Fleming House, Elephant and Castle, London SE1 6BY, UK

Mr D.E. Schendel, Industrial Economist, Chemical Information Services, Stanford Research Institute, Menlo Park, California 94025, USA (*Rapporteur sections 2.1 and 2.2*)

Representative from the National Cancer Institute

Dr J. Cooper, Office of the Associate Director, Carcinogenesis, National Cancer Institute, Bethesda, Maryland 20014, USA

Secretariat

    Dr C. Agthe, Unit of Chemical Carcinogenesis (*Secretary*)

    Dr H. Bartsch, Unit of Chemical Carcinogenesis (*Rapporteur section 3.2*)

    Dr. L. Griciute, Chief, Unit of Environmental Carcinogens

    Dr O.M. Jensen, Unit of Epidemiology and Biostatistics

    Dr J.E. Korneev, Environmental Pollution Unit, WHO

    Dr R. Montesano, Unit of Chemical Carcinogenesis (*Rapporteur section 3.1*)

    Mrs C. Partensky, Unit of Chemical Carcinogenesis (*Technical editor*)

    Mrs I. Peterschmitt, Unit of Chemical Carcinogenesis, Geneva (*Bibliographic researcher*)

    Dr V. Ponomarkov, Unit of Chemical Carcinogenesis

    Professor T. Schramm, Akademie der Wissenschaften der DDR, Zentralinstitut fur Krebsforschung, Lindenberger Weg 80, 1115 Berlin-Buch, DDR (*Temporary advisor*)

    Dr L. Tomatis, Chief, Unit of Chemical Carcinogenesis (*Head of the Programme*)

    Dr A. Tuyns, Unit of Epidemiology and Biostatistics (*Rapporteur section 3.3*)

Mr E.A. Walker, Unit of Environmental Carcinogens (*Rapporteur sections 1 and 2.3*)

Mrs E. Ward, Montignac, France (*Editor*)

Mr J.D. Wilbourn, Unit of Chemical Carcinogenesis (*Co-secretary*)

Note to the reader

Every effort is made to present the monographs as accurately as possible without unduly delaying their publication. Nevertheless, mistakes have occurred and are still likely to occur. In the interest of all users of these monographs, readers are requested to communicate any errors observed to the Unit of Chemical Carcinogenesis of the International Agency for Research on Cancer, Lyon, France, in order that these can be included in corrigenda which will appear in subsequent volumes.

As stated in the preamble, great efforts are made to cover the whole literature, but some studies may have been inadvertently overlooked. Since the monographs are not intended to be a review of the literature and contain only data considered relevant by the Working Group, it is not possible for the reader to determine whether a certain study was considered or not. However, research workers who are aware of important published data which may change the evaluation are requested to make them available to the above-mentioned address, in order that they can be considered for a possible re-evaluation by a future Working Group.

CONTENTS

	Page
BACKGROUND AND PURPOSE OF THE IARC PROGRAMME ON THE EVALUATION OF THE CARCINOGENIC RISK OF CHEMICALS TO MAN	11
SCOPE OF THE MONOGRAPHS	11
MECHANISM FOR PRODUCING THE MONOGRAPHS	12
Priority for the preparation of monographs	12
Data on which the evaluation is based	13
The Working Group	13
GENERAL PRINCIPLES FOR THE EVALUATION	13
Terminology	14
Response to carcinogens	14
Purity of the compounds tested	14
Qualitative aspects	14
Quantitative aspects	15
Animal data in relation to the evaluation of risk to man	15
Evidence of human carcinogenicity	15
EXPLANATORY NOTES ON THE MONOGRAPHS	16
GENERAL REMARKS ON THE SUBSTANCES CONSIDERED	27
THE MONOGRAPHS	
Amaranth	41
para-Aminoazobenzene	53
ortho-Aminoazotoluene	61
Azobenzene	75
Carmoisine	83
Chrysoidine	91
C.I. Disperse Yellow 3	97
Citrus red No. 2	101
D & C Red No. 9	107
Diacetylaminoazotoluene	113
2,6-Diamino-3-(phenylazo)pyridine (hydrochloride)	117

para-Dimethylaminoazobenzene	125
para-Dimethylaminobenzenediazo sodium sulphonate	147
Evans blue	151
4-Hydroxyazobenzene	157
Methyl red	161
Oil orange SS	165
Orange I	173
Orange G	181
Ponceau MX	189
Ponceau 3R	199
Ponceau SX	207
Scarlet red	217
Sudan I	225
Sudan II	233
Sudan III	241
Sudan brown RR	249
Sudan red 7B	253
Sunset yellow FCF	257
Trypan blue	267
Yellow AB	279
Yellow OB	287
INDEX	297
SUPPLEMENTARY CORRIGENDA TO VOLUMES 1 - 7	349
CUMULATIVE INDEX TO MONOGRAPHS	351

BACKGROUND AND PURPOSE OF THE IARC PROGRAMME ON THE
EVALUATION OF THE CARCINOGENIC RISK OF CHEMICALS TO MAN

The International Agency for Research on Cancer (IARC) initiated in 1971 a programme on the evaluation of the carcinogenic risk of chemicals to man. This programme was supported by a Resolution of the Governing Council at its Ninth Session concerning the role of IARC in providing government authorities with expert, independent scientific opinion on environmental carcinogenesis. As one means to this end, the Governing Council recommended that IARC should continue to prepare monographs on the carcinogenic risk of individual chemicals to man.

In view of the importance of this programme and in order to expedite the production of monographs, the National Cancer Institute of the United States has provided IARC with additional funds for this purpose.

The objective of this programme is to elaborate and publish in the form of monographs a critical review of carcinogenicity and related data in the light of the present state of knowledge, with the final aim of evaluating the data in terms of possible human risk, and at the same time to indicate where additional research efforts are needed.

SCOPE OF THE MONOGRAPHS

The monographs summarize the evidence for the carcinogenicity of individual chemicals and other relevant information. The data are compiled, reviewed and evaluated by a Working Group of experts. No recommendations are given concerning preventive measures or legislation, since these matters depend on risk-benefit evaluation, which seems best made by individual governments and/or international agencies such as WHO and ILO.

Since 1973, when the programme was started, seven volumes have been published[1,2,3,4,5,6,7].

As new data on chemicals for which monographs have already been written and new principles for evaluation become available, re-evaluations will be made at future meetings, and revised monographs will be published as necessary. The monographs are being distributed to international and governmental agencies and will be available to industries and scientists dealing with these chemicals. They also form the basis of advice from IARC on carcinogenesis from these substances.

MECHANISM FOR PRODUCING THE MONOGRAPHS

As a first step, a list of chemicals for possible consideration by the Working Group is established. IARC then collects pertinent references regarding physico-chemical characteristics, production and use[*], occurrence and analysis, and biological data[**] on these compounds. The material is summarized by an expert consultant or an IARC staff member, who prepares the first draft, which in some cases is sent to another expert for comments. The drafts are circulated to all members of the Working Group about one month before the meeting. During the meeting further additions to and deletions from the data are agreed upon, and a final version of comments and evaluation on each compound is adopted.

Priority for the Preparation of Monographs

Priority is given mainly to chemicals belonging to groups for which at least some suggestion of carcinogenicity exists from observations in animals and/or man and for which there is evidence of human exposure. However, neither human exposure nor potential carcinogenicity can be judged until all the relevant data have been collected and examined in detail, and the inclusion of a particular compound in a monograph does not necessarily mean

---

[*] Data provided by Chemical Information Services, Stanford Research Institute, Menlo Park, California, USA

[**] In the collection of original data reference was made to the publications "Survey of compounds which have been tested for carcinogenic activity"[8,9,10,11,12,13] and to a bibliography provided by the Franklin Institute Research Laboratory, Philadelphia, USA

that the substance is considered to be carcinogenic. Equally, the fact that a substance has not yet been considered does not imply that it is without carcinogenic hazard.

Data on which the Evaluation is Based

With regard to the biological data, only published articles and papers already accepted for publication are reviewed. Every effort is made to cover the whole literature, but some studies may have been inadvertently overlooked. The monographs are not intended to be a full review of the literature, and they contain only data considered relevant by the Committee. Research workers who are aware of important data (published or accepted for publication) which may influence the evaluation are invited to make them available to the Unit of Chemical Carcinogenesis of the International Agency for Research on Cancer, Lyon, France.

The Working Group

The tasks of the Working Group are five-fold: (1) to verify that as far as feasible all data have been collected; (2) to select the data relevant for the evaluation; (3) to determine whether the data, as summarized, will enable the reader to follow the reasoning of the committee; (4) to judge the significance of the experimental results; and (5) to make an evaluation.

The members of the Working Group who participated in the consideration of particular substances are listed at the beginning of each publication. The members of the Working Group serve in their individual capacities as scientists, and not as representatives of their governments or of any organization with which they are affiliated.

GENERAL PRINCIPLES FOR THE EVALUATION

The general principles for the evaluation which are listed below were elaborated by previous Working Groups and were also applied to the substances listed in this volume.

Terminology

The term "chemical carcinogenesis" in its widely accepted sense is used to indicate the induction or enhancement of neoplasia by chemicals. It is recognized that, in the strict etymological sense, this term means the induction of cancer; however, common usage has led to its employment to denote the induction of various types of neoplasms. The terms "tumourigen", "oncogen" and "blastomogen" have all been used synonymously with "carcinogen", although occasionally "tumourigen" has been used specifically to denote the induction of benign tumours.

Response to Carcinogens

For present purposes, in general, no distinction is made between the induction of tumours and the enhancement of tumour incidence, although it is noted that there may be fundamental differences in mechanisms that will eventually be elucidated.

The response in experimental animals to a carcinogen may take several forms:

(1) a significant increase in the incidence of one or more of the same types of neoplasms as found in control animals;

(2) the occurrence of types of neoplasms not observed in control animals;

(3) a decreased latent period as compared with control animals.

Purity of the Compounds Tested

In any evaluation of biological data with respect to a possible carcinogenic risk, particular attention must be paid to the purity of the chemicals tested and to their stability under conditions of storage or administration. Information on purity and stability is given, when available, in the monographs.

Qualitative Aspects

The qualitative nature of neoplasia has been much discussed. In many instances, both benign and malignant tumours are induced by chemical carcinogens. There are so far few recorded instances in which only benign tumours are induced by chemicals that have been studied extensively. Their occurrence in experimental systems has been taken to indicate the possibility of an increased risk of malignant tumours also.

In experimental carcinogenesis, the type of cancer seen can be the same as that recorded in human studies (e.g., bladder cancer in man, monkeys, dogs and hamsters after administration of 2-naphthylamine). In other instances, however, a chemical can induce other types of neoplasms or neoplasms at different sites in various species (e.g., benzidine induces hepatic carcinoma in the rat, but bladder carcinoma in man).

Quantitative Aspects

Dose-response studies are important in the evaluation of human and animal carcinogenesis. The confidence with which a carcinogenic effect can be established is strengthened by the observation of an increasing incidence of neoplasms with increasing exposure. Such studies are the only ones on which a minimal effective dose can be established. The determination of such a dose allows a comparison with reliable data on human exposure.

Comparison of potency between compounds can only be made if and when substances have been tested simultaneously.

Animal Data in Relation to the Evaluation of Risk to Man

At the present time no attempt can be made to interpret the animal data directly in terms of human risk since no objective criteria are available to do so. The critical assessment of the validity of the animal data given in these monographs is intended to assist national and/or international authorities to make decisions concerning preventive measures or legislation. In this connection attention is drawn to WHO recommendations in relation to food additives[14], drugs[15] and occupational carcinogens[16].

Evidence of Human Carcinogenicity

Evaluation of the carcinogenic risk to man of suspected environmental agents rests on purely observational studies. Such studies require sufficient variation in the levels of human exposure to allow a meaningful relationship between cancer incidence and exposure to a given chemical to be established. Difficulties in isolating the effects of individual agents arise, however, since populations are exposed to multiple carcinogens.

The initial suggestion of a relationship between an agent and disease often comes from case reports of patients who have had similar exposures. Variations and time trends in regional or national cancer incidence, or their correlation with regional or national 'exposure' levels, may also provide valuable insights. Such observations by themselves, however, cannot in most circumstances be regarded as conclusive evidence of carcinogenicity. The most satisfactory epidemiological method is to compare the cancer risk (adjusted for age, sex and other confounding variables) among groups or cohorts, or among individuals exposed to various levels of the agent in question and among control groups not so exposed. Ideally this is accomplished directly, by following such groups forward in time (prospectively) to determine time relationships, dose-response relationships and other aspects of cancer induction. Large cohorts and long observation periods are required to provide sufficient cases for a statistically valid comparison.

An alternative to prospective investigation is to assemble cohorts from past records and to evaluate their subsequent morbidity or mortality by means of medical histories and death certificates. Such occupational carcinogens as nickel, β-naphthylamine, asbestos and benzidine have been confirmed by this method. Another method is to compare the past exposures of a defined group of cancer cases with those of control samples from the hospital or general population. This does not provide an absolute measure of carcinogenic risk but can indicate the relative risks associated with different levels of exposure. The indirect means (e.g., interviews or tissue residues) used to measure exposures which may have commenced many years before can constitute a major source of error. Nevertheless such "case-control" studies can often isolate one factor from several suspected agents. The carcinogenic effect of this substance could then be confirmed by cohort studies.

EXPLANATORY NOTES ON THE MONOGRAPHS

In sections 1, 2 and 3 of each monograph, except for minor remarks, the data are recorded as given by the author, whereas the comments by the Working Group are given in section 4, headed "Comments on Data Reported and Evaluation".

Chemical and Physical Data (section 1)

The Colour Index Number, Colour Index Name, Chemical Abstracts Registry Serial Number and the latest Chemical Abstracts Name are recorded in this section. Other synonyms and trade names are listed separately in an index appended to this volume.

Chemical and physical properties include data that might be relevant to carcinogenicity (for example, lipid solubility) and those that concern identification. Where applicable, data on solubility, volatility and stability are indicated. All chemical data in this section refer to the pure substance.

Production, Use, Occurrence and Analysis (section 2)

The ultimate purpose of this section is to give an idea of the extent of possible human exposure, and therefore data on production, use and occurrence are given when available. With regard to these data, IARC has collaborated with the Stanford Research Institute, USA, with the support of the National Cancer Institute of the USA, in order to obtain production figures of chemicals and their patterns of use.

Since the United States, Western Europe and Japan are reasonably representative industrialized areas, and since Stanford Research Institute has regional offices in these areas, such data are commonly acquired from these countries. It should *not* be inferred that these nations are the sole sources or even the major sources of any individual chemical.

Production data are obtained from both governmental and trade publications in the three geographic areas. Information on use and occurrence is obtained by a comprehensive review of published data, complemented by direct contact with manufacturers of the chemicals in question.

Since cancer is a delayed toxic effect, past use and production data are also of importance. With respect to past and present use and production, regulatory actions in some countries are mentioned as examples only. However, statements concerning regulations may not reflect the most recent situation, since such legislation is in a constant state of change; nor should it be taken to imply that other countries do not have similar regulations. In the cases of drugs, mention of the therapeutic uses of such chemicals does not necessarily represent presently accepted therapeutic indications, nor does it imply judgement as to their clinical efficacy.

It is hoped that in further revisions of these monographs more information on production and use can be made available to IARC from other countries.

Biological Data Relevant to the Evaluation of Carcinogenic Risk to Man (section 3)

As pointed out earlier in this introduction, the monographs are not intended to consider all reported studies. Although every effort was made to review the whole literature, some studies were purposely omitted (a) because of their inadequacy, as judged from previously described criteria[17,18,19,20] (e.g., too short a duration, too few animals, poor survival or too small a dose); (b) because they only confirmed findings which have already been fully described; or (c) because they were judged irrelevant for the purpose of the evaluation. However, in certain cases, reference is made to studies which did not meet established criteria of adequacy, particularly when this information was considered a useful supplement to other reports or when it may have been the only data available. This does not, however, imply acceptance of the adequacy of experimental designs in these cases.

In general, the data recorded in this section are summarized as given by the author; however, certain shortcomings of reporting or of experimental design are also mentioned, and minor comments by the Working Group are given in square brackets.

The essential comments by the Working Group are made in section 4, "Comments on Data Reported and Evaluation".

Carcinogenicity and related studies in animals: Mention is usually made of all routes of administration by which the compound has been tested and of all species in which relevant tests have been carried out. In most cases the animal strains are given; general characteristics of mouse strains have been reported in a recent review[21]. Quantitative data are given in so far as they will enable the reader to realize the order of magnitude of the effective doses. In general, the doses are indicated as they appear in the original paper; sometimes conversions have been made for better comparison, and these are given in parentheses.

Other relevant biological data: The reporting of metabolic data is restricted to studies showing the metabolic fate of the chemical in animals and man. Comparison of animal and human data is made when possible. Other metabolic information (e.g., absorption, storage and excretion) is given when the Working Group considered that it would enable the reader to have a better understanding of the fate of the compound in the body. When the carcinogenicity of known metabolites has been tested, this also is reported.

Some LD_{50}'s are given, and other data on toxicity are included occasionally, if considered relevant.

Mutagenicity data are included for the first time, and the reasons for including such data and the principles adopted by the Working Group for selection of the data are outlined below.

Most of the chemical carcinogens which have so far been studied have been shown to require metabolic activation in order to produce their biological effects. This metabolic activation is in many cases associated with binding to nucleophilic sites in nucleic acids and proteins. The growing experimental evidence linking the carcinogenic activity of numerous chemicals to their capacity to be converted into electrophilic derivatives that may also exert a mutagenic effect has led to the suggestion that a relationship between chemical carcinogenesis and mutagenesis may exist. Such a correlation has so far been limited to those changes of the genotype which appear as a consequence of structural or functional alterations of nucleic acids.

Although not all chemical mutagens have been shown to be carcinogenic, most chemical carcinogens, several of which cause cancer in man, have now been found to be mutagens when tested in one of the mutagenicity test procedures that combine microbial, mammalian or other animal-cell systems as genetic targets with an *in vitro* or *in vivo* metabolic activation system. The results of appropriate mutagenicity tests, which are relatively rapid and inexpensive, may help to pre-screen chemicals and may also aid in the selection of the most relevant animal species in which to carry out long-term carcinogenicity tests on these chemicals. The use of human tissues in such *in vitro* testing procedures allows correlations between experimental animals and humans to be made. For all these reasons, the Working Group decided to consider data on mutagenicity as relevant biological information to be included in the monographs.

There are many genetic indicators and metabolic activation systems available for detecting mutagenic activity; they all, however, have individual advantages and limitations. Ideally, an appropriate mutagenicity test system would include the full metabolic competency of the intact human. Since the development or application of such a system appears to be impossible, the conclusion has been reached that a battery of test systems is needed in order to detect the mutagenic potential of chemicals.

In many cases, reactive metabolites with a limited life-span may fail to reach or to react with the genetic indicator, either because they are further metabolized to inactive compounds or because they react with other cellular constituents. For this reason mutagenicity assays in intact animals may give false-negative results, and appropriate *in vitro* techniques involving organ perfusion, tissue slices, cultured cell lines or tissue fractions should be included in screening programmes. Useful information may also be provided by investigation of other biological functions relevant to carcinogenesis in humans, such as enzymes involved in the metabolic conversion of chemicals, DNA repair in human cells and immunological surveillance mechanisms.

Metabolism in mammals is affected by exogenous and endogenous factors, such as chemicals causing enzyme induction and inhibition, diet and gastrointestinal flora. Other factors should also be considered in the experimental design, e.g., age, sex and strain of animals, diurnal and seasonal rhythms, differences between the foetal and adult states, mode of administration, cellular uptake, and distribution and excretion of the chemical. Differences in the metabolism of foreign compounds by *in vitro* preparations and by intact animals should also be taken into account. In view of all these factors, an incomplete picture of the mutagenic effects of chemical carcinogens *in vivo* may be obtained by *in vitro* techniques.

It is difficult in the present state of knowledge to select specific mutagenicity tests as being the most appropriate for the pre-screening of substances for possible carcinogenic activity. In deciding which mutagenicity test procedures should be used, preference should be given to systems that are genetically and metabolically reasonably well defined and/or that provide data shown to be valid for the prediction of the carcinogenicity of chemicals. Consideration of the results (positive or negative) of mutagenicity tests using chemicals and their identified metabolites should be of great value in assessing the reliability of the correlation between carcinogenic and mutagenic activities of chemicals.

For more detailed information see references 22-27.

<u>Observations in man</u>: Epidemiological studies are summarized. Clinical and other observations in man have been reviewed, when relevant.

<u>Comments on Data Reported and Evaluation</u> (section 4)

This section gives the critical view of the Working Group on the data reported. It should be read in conjunction with the "General Remarks on Substances Considered".

<u>Animal data</u>: The animal species mentioned are those in which the carcinogenicity of the substances was clearly demonstrated, irrespective of the route of adminsitration. In the case of inadequate studies, when mentioned, comments to that effect are included. The route of administration used in experimental animals that is similar to the possible human exposure (ingestion, inhalation and skin exposure) is given particular mention. In most cases tumour sites are also indicated. Experiments involving a possible action of the vehicle or a physical effect of the agent, such as in subcutaneous injection or bladder implantation studies, are also mentioned; however, the results of such tests require careful consideration, particularly if they are the only ones raising a suspicion of carcinogenicity. If the substance has produced tumours on pre-natal exposure or in single-dose experiments, this is also indicated. This sub-section should be read in the light of comments made in the section, "Animal Data in Relation to the Evaluation of Risk to Man" of this introduction.

Human data: In some cases, a brief statement is made on the possible exposure of man. The significance of epidemiological studies and case reports is discussed, and the data are interpreted in terms of possible human risk.

References

1. IARC (1972) *IARC Monographs on the Evaluation of Carcinogenic Risk of Chemicals to Man, 1*, Lyon

2. IARC (1973) *IARC Monographs on the Evaluation of Carcinogenic Risk of Chemicals to Man, 2, Some Inorganic and Organometallic Compounds*, Lyon

3. IARC (1973) *IARC Monographs on the Evaluation of Carcinogenic Risk of Chemicals to Man, 3, Certain Polycyclic Aromatic Hydrocarbons and Heterocyclic Compounds*, Lyon

4. IARC (1974) *IARC Monographs on the Evaluation of Carcinogenic Risk of Chemicals to Man, 4, Some Aromatic Amines, Hydrazine and Related Substances, N-Nitroso Compounds and Miscellaneous Alkylating Agents*, Lyon

5. IARC (1974) *IARC Monographs on the Evaluation of Carcinogenic Risk of Chemicals to Man, 5, Some Organochlorine Pesticides*, Lyon

6. IARC (1974) *IARC Monographs on the Evaluation of Carcinogenic Risk of Chemicals to Man, 6, Sex Hormones*, Lyon

7. IARC (1974) *IARC Monographs on the Evaluation of Carcinogenic Risk of Chemicals to Man, 7, Some Anti-thyroid and Related Substances, Nitrofurans and Industrial Chemicals*, Lyon

8. Hartwell, J.L. (1951) *Survey of compounds which have been tested for carcinogenic activity*, Washington DC, US Government Printing Office (Public Health Service Publication No. 149)

9. Shubik, P. & Hartwell, J.L. (1957) *Survey of compounds which have been tested for carcinogenic activity*, Washington DC, US Government Printing Office (Public Health Service Publication No. 149: Supplement 1)

10. Shubik, P. & Hartwell, J.L. (1969) *Survey of compounds which have been tested for carcinogenic activity*, Washington DC, US Government Printing Office (Public Health Service Publication No. 149: Supplement 2)

11. Carcinogenesis Program National Cancer Institute (1971) *Survey of compounds which have been tested for carcinogenic activity*, Washington DC, US Government Printing Office (Public Health Service Publication No. 149: 1968-1969)

12. Carcinogenesis Program National Cancer Institute (1973) *Survey of compounds which have been tested for carcinogenic activity*, Washington DC, US Government Printing Office (Public Health Service Publication No. 149: 1961-1967)

13. Carcinogenesis Program National Cancer Institute (1974) <u>Survey of compounds which have been tested for carcinogenic activity</u>, Washington DC, US Government Printing Office (Public Health Service Publication No. 149: 1970-1971)

14. WHO (1961) Fifth Report of the Joint FAO/WHO Expert Committee on Food Additives. Evaluation of carcinogenic hazard of food additives. <u>Wld Hlth Org. techn. Rep. Ser.</u>, <u>No. 220</u>, pp. 5, 18, 19

15. WHO (1969) Report of a WHO Scientific Group. Principles for the testing and evaluation of drugs for carcinogenicity. <u>Wld Hlth Org. techn. Rep. Ser.</u>, <u>No. 426</u>, pp. 19, 21, 22

16. WHO (1964) Report of a WHO Expert Committee. Prevention of cancer. <u>Wld Hlth Org. techn. Rep. Ser.</u>, <u>No. 276</u>, pp. 29, 30

17. WHO (1958) Second Report of the Joint FAO/WHO Expert Committee on Food Additives. Procedures for the testing of intentional food additives to establish their safety for use. <u>Wld Hlth Org. techn. Rep. Ser., No. 144</u>

18. WHO (1961) Fifth Report of the Joint FAO/WHO Expert Committee on Food Additives. Evaluation of carcinogenic hazard of food additives. <u>Wld Hlth Org. techn. Rep. Ser., No. 200</u>

19. WHO (1967) Scientific Group. Procedures for investigating intentional and unintentional food additives. <u>Wld Hlth Org. techn. Rep. Ser., No. 348</u>

20. UICC (1969) Carcinogenicity testing. <u>UICC techn. Rep. Ser.</u>, <u>2</u>

21. Committee on Standardized Genetic Nomenclature for Mice (1972) Standardized nomenclature for inbred strains of mice. Fifth listing. <u>Cancer Res.</u>, <u>32</u>, 1609-1646

22. Bartsch, H. & Grover, P.L. (1974) Chemical carcinogenesis and mutagenesis. In: Symington, T. & Carter, R.L., eds, <u>Scientific Foundations of Oncology</u>, Vol. IX, <u>Chemical Carcinogenesis</u>, London, Heinemann Medical Books Ltd

23. Holländer, A., ed. (1971) <u>Chemical Mutagens. Principles and methods for their detection</u>, Vols 1-3, New York, Plenum Press

24. Montesano, R. & Tomatis, L., eds (1974) Chemical Carcinogenesis Essays, <u>IARC Scientific Publications</u>, <u>No. 10</u>, Lyon

25. Ramel, C., ed. (1973) <u>Evaluation of genetic risks of environmental chemicals</u>, Report of a symposium held at Skokloster, Sweden, 1972, <u>Ambio Special Report No. 3</u>

26. Stoltz, D.R., Poirier, L.A., Irving, C.C., Stich, H.F., Weisburger, J.H. & Grice, H.C. (1974) Evaluation of short-term tests for carcinogenicity. Toxicol. appl. Pharmacol., 29, 157-180

27. WHO (1974) Report of a WHO Scientific Group. Assessment of the carcinogenicity and mutagenicity of chemicals. Wld Hlth Org. techn. Rep. Ser., No. 546

GENERAL REMARKS ON THE SUBSTANCES CONSIDERED

This volume of monographs is devoted to some aromatic azo colours, selected on the bases of evidence of human exposure and the availability of experimental studies suggesting carcinogenicity.

These aromatic azo compounds are manufactured on a wide scale and have extensive uses. Both industrial workers and the general population are exposed, since the compounds are used to colour fabrics, paper, food, drugs, cosmetics, lubricants and other products.

The simplest of the aromatic azo compounds, azobenzene, was first prepared by Mitscherlich in 1834, by partial reduction of nitrobenzene. Other azo compounds have usually been made by the reaction of diazonium compounds, first prepared by Griess in 1862, with aromatic amines or phenols. This reaction, known as coupling, has been used for the synthesis of thousands of compounds, many of which have been used commercially. One review on azo compounds contains over 2500 references (Zollinger, 1958, 1961).

Aromatic azo colours are generally fairly stable under environmental conditions, although definitive studies in this area are often lacking. A particular difficulty with aromatic azo and other colours is that the commercial products are often mixtures. Rigid specifications to exclude toxic materials, including carcinogenic aromatic amines, are therefore necessary.

Depending on the substituent groups, some of the aromatic azo colours are water-soluble; but many are lipid-soluble.

Synthesis of azo colours

In many cases it is not possible to specify the synthetic process by which the dyes or colours are produced, since manufacturers consider this information to be proprietary. In general, the starting materials and overall reaction pathways described are the ones used commercially; but details of the reaction conditions, which could alter the impurities present, were not available to the Working Group.

It should also be kept in mind when assessing the biological effects of these compounds that the starting materials for their synthesis are frequently technical grade chemicals which may produce a relatively large number of reaction products, including free aromatic amines and other materials. No rigid chemical specifications are applied to batches of colours, except when they are used in certain food, drug or cosmetic applications; as a result, they are frequently produced in such a way as to meet customer shade and intensity requirements.

Analytical methods

Analytical methods used for the isolation, identification and quantitative determination of aromatic azo colours can be divided into those applicable for lipid-soluble and those for water-soluble compounds.

(a) Identification

(i) Lipid-soluble compounds

The identification of lipid-soluble colours is usually carried out by chromatographic methods, and several different systems have been developed. Earlier methods relied on paper chromatography: Bastianutti (1963) used Whatman No. 1 with the solvent system ethanol:dimethylformamide (9:1); Szokolay (1963) recommended reversed-phase chromatography on paraffin-impregnated paper; while Ciglar et al. (1962) used cetyl alcohol-impregnated paper and an alkaline solvent system to identify basic lipid-soluble colours.

More recent work involves thin-layer chromatography. A survey (Stahl, 1967) of the separation characteristics of various sorbents, such as silica gel, alumina, 1:1 mixtures of silica gel and alumina, starch, cellulose and polyamide powder, used with a wide variety of solvents indicates the techniques capable of separating most lipid-soluble azo colours. Hoodless et al. (1971) obtained good separation of ten lipid-soluble food colours by reversed phase thin-layer chromatography.

Lehmann et al. (1973) describe a method for the isolation of lipid-soluble colours from fats and chocolate by liquid/liquid partition and adsorption chromatography followed by identification by thin-layer chromatography.

(ii) <u>Water-soluble compounds</u>

As with lipid-soluble colours, separation and identification are carried out almost exclusively by chromatographic methods. Earlier methods relied mainly on paper chromatography, using alkaline and acidic aqueous/organic solvent systems (British Food Manufacturing Industries Research Association, 1963; Pla Delfina, 1962; Thaler & Sommer, 1953a,b). The Deutsche Forschungsgemeinschaft (DFG, 1956) provided standard samples and paper chromatograms of food colours permitted in the Federal Republic of Germany.

Today, paper chromatography has largely been displaced by thin-layer chromatography (TLC), which is more rapid, sensitive and reproducible. Separations have been carried out on a large variety of sorbents, including silica gel, alumina, Kieselgur, cellulose and polyamide, and mixtures of these, using various solvent systems. An extensive review of chromatographic methods for a great variety of water-soluble azo colours can be found in Stahl (1967). All food colours permitted in the Federal Republic of Germany in 1962 could be identified by TLC on cellulose with a single solvent sytem (Wollenweber, 1962).

Isolation of water-soluble azo colours from the food matrix has been carried out by the so-called wool-thread method (Thaler & Sommer, 1953a,b), by adsorption on alumina columns (Illi, 1963), by liquid-liquid extraction using quinoline (Mottier, 1956), by quarternary ammonium compounds (Sohár & Sohár, 1963) and by liquid ion exchangers (Dolinsky & Stein, 1962). Lehmann *et al.* (1970) claim that polyamide is a relatively more selective adsorbent for water-soluble acidic dyes and carboxymethylcellulose for basic dyes.

(b) <u>Examination of purity and quantitative determination</u>

For some azo compounds the percentage of colour is easily determined by titration of a suitably buffered solution with titanous chloride, using the sample as its own indicator (Horwitz, 1970). Cerma (1960) described the qualitative and quantitative determination of different classes of colours by polarography; but, according to Nagy & Sohár (1962a,b), the polarographic half-wave potentials of food colours are so similar that they cannot be differentiated by classical, direct-current polarographic methods. Oscillopolarography, however, may be used for the quantitative determination of these compounds, even in mixtures.

Matrka *et al.* (1971) describe an analytical method for the quantitative determination of several azo colours, which is based on potentiometric titration with sodium nitrite in acid solution.

The most widely-used method for the quantitative determination of azo colours, however, is spectrophotometry. A detailed list of references giving spectrophotometric data for azo colours is provided by Woidich (1967). Spectra of food colours permitted in the Federal Republic of Germany have been issued by the Deutsche Forschungsgemeinschaft (DFG, 1955, 1957). A list of all food colours permitted in the UK was published by the Association of Public Analysts (1957).

Przybylski & McKeown (1960a,b) quantitatively determined two lipid-soluble azo compounds in mixtures by taking advantage of their different absorption wave lengths. A similar procedure for the quantitative determination of mixtures of red, orange, yellow and blue colours has been worked out by Koether (1960).

Sasaki & Iwata (1972) scanned the separated spots of four lipid-soluble and 12 water-soluble azo colours on paper chromatograms with a photoelectric densitometer.

IR-spectrometry has also been applied to quantitative measurements; it has been shown to give satisfactory results even when mixtures of two compounds were analyzed (Oi & Inaba, 1967).

Many methods have also been developed for the determination of by-products, intermediates and subsidiary colours; a list of references is given by Woidich (1967).

A recent development is reported by Singh (1974), who used high-pressure liquid chromatography on a strong anion exchange column for the detection and quantitative determination of unreacted starting materials (referred to as "intermediates") in sunset yellow FCF. He found that this method gave accurate results with substantial saving of time when compared with a column chromatographic procedure used formerly.

Finally, nuclear magnetic resonance (NMR) has also been applied as an analytical tool for the study of food colours (Marmion, 1974). It has been found useful for identifying and differentiating between single colours and mixtures, identifying and semiquantitating them in secondary mixtures, establishing the presence of excipients such as sucrose and detecting the adulteration of a colour additive by forbidden colouring materials. NMR also shows promise as a method for determining the purity of food colours and for studying process conditions.

Specifications for identity and purity of food colours and standard methods for their analysis have been issued by a number of national and international bodies, e.g., British Standards Institution (1960), DFG (1962, 1964), FAO (1963), Fujii *et al.* (1965), AOAC (Horwitz, 1970), Inoue *et al.* (1967, 1968), Japan Food Hygiene Association (1974) and US Code of Federal Regulations (1974).

General remarks on biological data

Evaluation of data on aromatic azo compounds was difficult because of uncertainty over the exact composition of the materials tested. In addition, many of the early studies, although representing pioneering work in this field, could not be cited because of their relative inadequacy for purposes of evaluation; however, references to these studies may be found in several extensive reviews on amino azo compounds (Miller & Miller, 1953; Terayama, 1967; Truhaut, 1955), which also cover such topics as structure-activity relationships, nutritional effects and interactions of the compounds with cellular constituents. A review on the toxicology of food colours, including several aromatic azo compounds, has also been published (Radomski, 1974).

Mutagenicity data

The majority of the data on mutagenicity for the series of aromatic azo compounds considered by the Working Group did not fulfill the requirements outlined in the preamble (see p.19).

Mutagenicity assays in which *in vitro* mammalian metabolism was taken into account have been performed with only three azo compounds: *para*-dimethylaminoazobenzene, *ortho*-aminoazotoluene and *para*-aminoazobenzene (Ames, 1974; Ames *et al.*, 1973; Commoner *et al.*, 1974). However, some other results, such as those obtained by direct mutagenicity tests that do not involve mammalian metabolism, tests on *Drosophila* and dominant lethal tests, which give valid information on the genetic activity of the compounds, are also included.

Dominant lethality is characterized by pre-implantation loss of non-viable blastocytes and early embryonic death. It is the expression of a heterozygous condition caused by deletion of a whole or part of a chromosome, and it is therefore not possible to confirm its genetic nature, although cytological examination of early cleavages in matings with a high dominant lethal incidence indicates a high rate of chromosomal aberrations. Nevertheless, results from dominant lethal tests were also included, assuming that a chemical agent that causes dominant lethality could do this by inducing a true mutation. For similar reasons, data on chromosomal aberrations are not considered to be useful for the evaluation of mutagenicity of chemicals unless they are accompanied by evidence of genotypic expression. The Working Group emphasized that more data are needed before the validity of dominant lethal tests for predicting the carcinogenicity of chemicals can be evaluated.

Epidemiological considerations

There is no published evidence to show whether the aromatic azo compounds considered, either singly or in combination, have caused cancer in man. Extensive independent searches by the Working Group and by the Information and Library Unit of the Central Toxicology Laboratory of Imperial Chemical Industries failed to reveal a single study in which the possible carcinogenic effect of these substances in man had been examined. One paper (Lipkin, 1972) made reference to the high levels of exposure to which workers in the azo-colour industry were subjected: concentrations of *ortho*-aminoazotoluene up to 8.3 mg/m^3 were reported to occur in air. However, there was no reference to observed effects in the exposed workers.

There is well-documented evidence of an increased risk of bladder cancer in workers engaged in the manufacture and use of dyestuff intermediates. The risk has been attributed to certain aromatic amines (Case & Pearson, 1954; Case *et al.*, 1954). The bladder cancer risk in the dyestuffs manufacturing industry was confirmed by Anthony & Thomas (1970); however, except for inconclusive data on certain occupational groups (tailors, hairdressers), bladder cancer rates were not shown to be increased in workers using, as opposed to manufacturing, dyestuffs. No specific reference to azo compounds was made in these studies, but the possibility of their presence and the possibility of a contributing effect cannot be excluded.

References

Ames, B.N. (1974) Carcinogens are mutagens: a simple method for detection. In: Program for XIth International Cancer Congress, Florence, 1974, Vol. 1, Geneva, UICC, pp. 15-16

Ames, B.N., Durston, W.E., Yamasaki, E. & Lee, F.D. (1973) Carcinogens are mutagens: a simple test system combining liver homogenates for activation and bacteria for detection. Proc. nat. Acad. Sci., 70, 2281-2285

Anthony, H.M. & Thomas, G.M. (1970) Tumors of the urinary bladder: an analysis of the occupations of 1,030 patients in Leeds, England. J. nat. Cancer Inst., 45, 879-895

Association of Public Analysts (1957) Separation and identification of food colours permitted by the colouring matters in food regulations, London

Bastianutti, J. (1963) Paper chromatographic method for the detection of artificial fat-soluble dyes in oils and fats of animal and plant origin. Boll. Lab. chim. provinciali, 14, 16-22

British Food Manufacturing Industries Research Association. Trace Material Committee (1963) The extraction and identification of permitted food colouring matters with special reference to the changes undergone during processing and storage. Analyst, 88, 864-871

British Standards Institution (1960) Methods for the analysis of water-soluble coal-tar dyes permitted for use in foods. BS3210:1960, London

Case, R.A.M. & Pearson, J.T. (1954) Tumours of the urinary bladder in workmen engaged in the manufacture and use of certain dyestuff intermediates in the British chemical industry. II. Further consideration of the role of aniline and of the manufacture of auramine and magenta (fuchsine) as possible causative agents. Brit. J. industr. Med., 11, 213-216

Case, R.A.M., Hosker, M.E., McDonald, D.B. & Pearson, J.T. (1954) Tumours of the urinary bladder in workmen engaged in the manufacture and use of certain dyestuff intermediates in the British chemical industry. I. The role of aniline, benzidine, *alpha*-naphthylamine and *beta*-naphthylamine. Brit. J. industr. Med., 11, 75-104

Cerma, E. (1960) The polarographic determination of food dyes. Rass. chim., 12, 13-20

Ciglar, J., Kolsek, J. & Perpar, M. (1962) Zur Papierchromatographie der basischer Farbstoffe. Chem. Ztg, 86, 41-43

Commoner, B., Vithayathil, A.J. & Henry, J.I. (1974) Detection of metabolic carcinogen intermediates in urine of carcinogen-fed rats by means of bacterial mutagenesis. Nature (Lond.), 249, 850-852

DFG (Deutsche Forschungsgemeinschaft) (1955) Kommission zur Bearbeitung des Lebensmittelfarbstoffproblems, *Toxikologische Daten von Farbstoffen und ihre Zulassung für Lebensmittel in verschiedenen Ländern*, Mitt. 6(1), Wiesbaden, Steiner Verlag

DFG (Deutsche Forschungsgemeinschaft) (1956) Farbstoff-Kommission, *Vergleichsmuster der vorgeschlagenen synthetischen Lebensmittelfarbstoffe mit Papierchromatogrammen und Spektren in UV, Sichtbaren und IR-Bereich*, Wiesbaden, Steiner Verlag

DFG (Deutsche Forschungsgemeinschaft) (1957) Farbstoff-Kommission, *Toxikologische Daten von Farbstoffen und ihre Zulassung für Lebensmittel in verschiedenen Ländern*, Mitt. 6(2), Wiesbaden, Steiner Verlag

DFG (Deutsche Forschungsgemeinschaft) (1962) Farbstoff-Kommission, Mitt. 11, Neuauflage der Mitt. vom 20. Dez. 56 (gleichzeitig Zus. fass. der "Resolution" v. April 1950 und der Mitt. 1, 2, 4, 5, 7, 9, 10, March 5), Wiesbaden, Steiner Verlag

DFG (Deutsche Forschungsgemeinschaft) (1964) Farbstoff-Kommission, *Untersuchungsmethoden zur Prüfung der Reinheit von Lebensmittelfarbstoffen*, Mitt. 12, Wiesbaden, Steiner Verlag

Dolinsky, M. & Stein, Ch. (1962) Application of a liquid anion exchange resin to the separation of FD & C colors from foods. *J. Ass. off. analyt. Chem.*, 45, 767-769

FAO (1963) *Specifications for identity and purity of food additives*, Vol. II, *Food Colors*, Rome

Fujii, S., Kamikura, M. & Oka, N. (1965) Dye standards of National Institute of Hygienic Sciences. *Bull. Nat. Inst. Hyg. Sci. (Tokyo)*, 83, 72-74

Hoodless, R.A., Thomson, J. & Arnold, J.E. (1971) Separation and identification of food colours. II. Identification of synthetic oil-soluble food colours using thin-layer chromatography. *J. Chromat.*, 56, 332-337

Horwitz, W., ed. (1970) *Official Methods of Analysis of the Association of Official Analytical Chemists*, 11th ed., Washington DC, Association of Official Analytical Chemists

Illi, J. (1963) Zur Isolierung von künstlichen Farbstoffen aus Lebensmitteln mit Hilfe von saurem (anionotropem) aktivem Aluminiumoxyd. *Mitt. Lebensmitt. Hyg.*, 54, 434-437

Inoue, T., Kamikura, M. & Murakami, N. (1967) Dye standards of National Institute of Hygienic Sciences. *Bull. Nat. Inst. Hyg. Sci. (Tokyo)*, 85, 150-152

Inoue, T., Kamikura, M. & Murakami, N. (1968) Dye standards of National Institute of Hygienic Sciences. Bull. Nat. Inst. Hyg. Sci. (Tokyo), 86, 136-139

Japan Food Hygiene Association (1974) Japanese Standards of Food Additives, 3rd ed., Tokyo, Ministry of Health and Welfare

Koether, B. (1960) Über die quantitative Bestimmung von 15 zum Färben von Lebensmitteln verwendeten Farbstoffen. Dtsch. Lebensmitt.-Rdsch., 56, 7-13

Lehmann, G., Collet, P., Malin, H.G. & Ashworth, M.R.F. (1970) Rapid method for detection and identification of synthetic water-soluble coloring matters in foods and drugs. J. Ass. off. analyt. Chem., 53, 1182-1188

Lehmann, G., Arackal, T. & Morán, M. (1973) Beiträge zur Analytik von Farbstoffen. XIV. Bestimmung fettlöslicher, synthetischer Farbstoffe in Fetten und Schokolade. Z. Lebensmitt. Untersuch., 153, 155-157

Lipkin, I.L. (1972) Occupational hygiene in the production of o-aminoazo-toluene. Gig. Tr. Prof. Zabol., 16, 13-16

Marmion, D.M. (1974) Applications of nuclear magnetic resonance spectroscopy to certifiable food colors. J. Ass. off. analyt. Chem., 57, 495-507

Matrka, M., Kroupa, J. & Spevak, A. (1971) Analysis of dyes and dye intermediates. XIII. Determination of some dyes containing amino- or imino-groups by titration with a nitrite-containing solution. Coll. Cs. chem. Commun., 36, 1379-1387

Miller, J.A. & Miller, E.C. (1953) The carcinogenic aminoazo dyes. Advanc. Cancer Res., 1, 339-396

Mottier, M. (1956) Remarques sur l'extraction et la chromatographie sur alumine de diverses colorants. Mitt. Lebensmitt. Hyg., 47, 372-386

Nagy, F. & Sohár, J. (1962a) Contributions to the oscillopolarographic examination of food colours. Elelmiszervizsgalati Közlemények, 8, 106-114

Nagy, F. & Sohár, J. (1962b) Beitrag zum oszillopolarographischen Analytik der Lebensmittelfarbstoffe. Chem. Zvesti, 16, 389-394

Oi, N. & Inaba, E. (1967) Analyses of drugs and chemicals by infrared absorption spectroscopy. XII. Analyses of water-soluble azo food dyes by use of high molecular weight amines. Yakugaku Zasshi, 87, 741-743

Pla Delfina, J.M. (1962) A systematic method for identification of food, drug and cosmetic azo dyes. J. Soc. Cosmet. Chem., 13, 214-244

Przybylski, W. & McKeown, G.G. (1960a) Absorption spectra of 1-arylazo-2-naphthol food colors. J. Ass. off. analyt. Chem., 43, 800-804

Przybylski, W. & McKeown, G.G. (1960b) Determination of coal-tar colors on oranges. J. Ass. off. analyt. Chem., 43, 274-278

Radomski, J.L. (1974) Toxicology of food colors. Ann. Rev. Pharmacol., 14, 127-137

Sasaki, H. & Iwata, T. (1972) Analytical studies of food dyes. IV. Direct densitometry of paper chromatograms of food and other dyes by transparent methods. Shokuhin Eiseigaku Zasshi, 13, 120-126

Singh, M. (1974) Determination of uncombined intermediates in FD & C Yellow No. 6 by high-pressure liquid chromatography. J. Ass. off. analyt. Chem., 57, 358-364

Sohár, J. & Sohár, P. (1963) Extraction of colors from foods with quarternary ammonium compounds. Structure of the formed compounds. Magyar Kém. Folyoirat, 69, 402-406

Stahl, E. (1967) Dünnschicht-Chromatographie, 2 Aufl., Berlin, Heidelberg, New York, Springer Verlag

Szokolay, A. (1963) Beitrag zum papierchromatographischen und spektrophotometrischen Nachweis fettlöslicher synthetischer Farbstoffe in Lebensmitteln und Cosmetica. Z. Lebensmitt. Forsch., 120, 295-299

Terayama, H. (1967) Aminoazo carcinogenesis - methods and biochemical problems. Meth. Cancer Res., 1, 399-449

Thaler, M. & Sommer, G. (1953a) Studien zur Farbstoffanalytik. IV. Die papierchromatographische Trennung wasserlöslicher Teerfarbstoffe. Z. Lebensmitt. Forsch., 97, 345-365

Thaler, M. & Sommer, G. (1953b) Studien zur Farbstoffanalytik. V. Nachweis und Identifizierung wasserlöslicher Teerfarbstoffe in Lebensmitteln. Z. Lebensmitt. Forsch., 97, 441-446

Truhaut, R. (1955) Sur l'action cancérigène de certaines matières colorantes. Importance en hygiène alimentaire, en thérapeutique et en hygiène générale. Ann. pharm. fr., 13, 36-51

US Code of Federal Regulations (1974) Food and Drugs, Title 21, part 8.510, Washington DC, US Government Printing Office

Woidich, H. (1967) Fremde Stoffe-Farbstoffe. In: Handbuch für Lebensmittelchemie, II/2, Berlin, Springer Verlag, pp. 1247-1355

Wollenweber, P. (1962) Dunnschicht-chromatographische Trennungen von Farbstoffen an Cellulose-Schichten. J. Chromat., 7, 557-560

Zollinger, H. (1958) *Die Chemie der Azofarbstoffe*, Basel, Birkhäuserverlag

Zollinger, H. (1961) *Azo and Diazo Chemistry of Aliphatic and Aromatic Compounds*, New York, Interscience

THE MONOGRAPHS

AMARANTH

1. Chemical and Physical Data

1.1 Synonyms and trade names

Colour Index No.: 16185

Colour Index Name: C.I. Food Red 9

Chem. Abstr. Reg. Serial No.: 915-67-3

Chem. Abstr. Name: 3-Hydroxy-4-[(4-sulpho-1-naphthalenyl)azo]-2,7-naphthalenedisulphonic acid, trisodium salt

For other names of which the Working Group was aware see index, p. 297.

1.2 Chemical formula and molecular weight

$C_{20}H_{11}N_2Na_3O_{10}S_3$ Mol. wt: 604.5

1.3 Chemical and physical properties of the pure substance

(a) Description: Dark red-brown crystals

(b) Absorption spectroscopy: λ_{max} 522.5 nm in water, 520 nm in 0.02N ammonium acetate solution

(c) Solubility: Slightly soluble in water (7.2 g/100 ml at 26°C); very slightly soluble in ethanol and cellosolve

(d) Stability: Stable to light in aqueous solution

1.4 Technical products and impurities

Specifications for amaranth are given by the British Standards Institution (1960) together with appropriate analytical methods; to comply with this standard the product must contain a minimum of 85% amaranth. Food, drug and cosmetic specifications in the US (US Code of Federal Regulations, 1974), and the standard set by FAO/WHO (1966) also require a minimum of 85% amaranth. Specifications for a colour reference standard given by Inoue *et al.* (1967) require a minimum of 99% pure colour.

2. Production, Use, Occurrence and Analysis

For important background information on this section, see preamble, p. 17.

2.1 Production and use

Amaranth was first synthesized by H. Baum in 1878 (Society of Dyers and Colourists, 1971). It can be made by coupling diazotized naphthionic acid (1-naphthylamine-4-sulphonic acid) with 2-naphthol-3,6-disulphonic acid (Richter, 1958), and Zuckerman (1964) reported that this is the process used for commercial production.

Large-scale production of amaranth in the US was first reported in 1914, and in 1921, 14,500 kg of this colour were produced (US Tariff Commission, 1922). In 1972, six US companies manufactured about 440,000 kg of amaranth (US Tariff Commission, 1974). Separate data on US imports and exports were not available.

There are probably 18 producers of amaranth in Western Europe, with a combined total annual production of approximately 300,000 kg.

In Japan, in 1973, five manufacturers produced about 97,000 kg of this colour. Exports in 1972 were 6,500 kg, and 16,000 kg in 1973; separate data on imports were not available.

Amaranth is used for dyeing textiles, paper, phenol-formaldehyde resins, wood and leather (Society of Dyers and Colourists, 1971); and Merck & Co. (1968) report its use as an indicator in hydrazine titrations and in colour photography.

The Deutsche Forschungsgemeinschaft (DFG, 1955) reported that amaranth was approved for food use in many countries throughout the world; known exceptions at that time were Finland, Yugoslavia and the USSR. A more recent edition (DFG, 1957) reported India as an additional exception, but indicated that the material had been approved in Finland and Yugoslavia. At present, many Western European countries permit its use in foodstuffs (DeGiacomi, 1974). Approval for its use in food in Japan was withdrawn prior to 1966, although it was allowed for certain non-food usages (Japan Food Hygiene Association, 1974).

Zuckerman (1964) reported that in the US amaranth is used in the colouring of gelatin, maraschino cherries, sausage casings, frozen desserts, carbonated beverages, dry drink powders, sweets and confectionary products not containing oils and fats, bakery products and cereals, puddings, aqueous drug solutions, tablets, capsules, mouthwashes, bath salts and hair rinses. That this colour is widely used in drugs in the US was shown by a Pharmaceutical Manufacturers Association survey, which reported that it is used in at least 1370 drug products (Anon., 1972).

In the US, during the first nine months of 1967, the following consumption pattern for amaranth in foods, drugs and cosmetics has been reported (Anon., 1968): sweets and confections (30,700 kg); beverages (128,500 kg); dessert powders (28,350 kg); cereals (7,100 kg); maraschino cherries (3,700 kg); pet foods (30,500 kg); bakery goods (19,800 kg); ice cream, sherbet and dairy products (13,500 kg); sausages (16,400 kg); snack foods (1,700 kg); meat inks (6 kg); miscellaneous (21,000 kg). Total food consumption was thus about 300,000 kg, consumption in pharmaceuticals was about 9,600 kg, and consumption in cosmetics 1,500 kg. The same source also estimated the maximum quantity of this colour ingested per person in the US per day, per food category: sweets and confections (2.3 mg); beverages (6.4 mg); dessert powders (2.2 mg); cereals (0.2 mg); maraschino cherries (0.1 mg); bakery goods (3.7 mg); ice cream, sherbet and dairy products (1.6 mg); sausages (0.7 mg); snack foods (0.1 mg); and miscellaneous (0.4 mg). These individual consumptions totalled a maximum intake of 17.7 mg per person per day.

The Joint FAO/WHO Expert Committee on Food Additives, which provides information to those concerned with regulating the use of chemical substances in food, recommends an acceptable daily intake (ADI) for man of 0-0.75 mg/kg bw, 50% less than the previous ADI quoted by that committee (FAO/WHO, 1972).

2.2 Occurrence

Amaranth is not known to occur in nature.

2.3 Analysis

See section, "General Remarks on the Substances Considered", p. 28.

3. Biological Data Relevant to the Evaluation of Carcinogenic Risk to Man

Two reviews on azo compounds, including amaranth, and their carcinogenic activity have been published (Radomski, 1974; Truhaut, 1955).

3.1 Carcinogenicity and related studies in animals

(a) Oral administration

Mouse: No tumours attributed to the treatment were observed in a group of 20 mice (sex and strain unspecified) following administration of weekly doses of 15-20 mg amaranth given over 5 days a week for life. The colour was fed as an aqueous solution added to brown bread. The last surviving mouse died 477 days (about 15 months) after the start of treatment, but survival rates were not reported. Autopsies were carried out on 18 mice, and sections were examined for 7. No mention was made of controls (Cook et al., 1940). [The limited number of animals used was noted by the Working Group.]

Feeding studies with C3Hf and C57Bl mice have been reported briefly (US Food and Drug Administration, unpublished study quoted in FAO/WHO, 1966). Diets containing 10,000 and 20,000 mg/kg amaranth, respectively, were fed to 100 animals of each strain; 200 of each strain served as controls. No tumours were observed. [No further details were available.]

Rat: A group of 5 male and 5 female Wistar rats was fed a diet containing 40,000 mg amaranth per kg of diet for up to 18 months. In 1/7 rats living to a tumour-bearing age, a mesenteric lymphosarcoma was observed. No tumours occurred in 50 controls surviving for 20 months or more (Willheim & Ivy, 1953). [The limited number of animals used was noted by the Working Group.]

Groups of 15 male and 15 female rats (strain unspecified) were fed diets containing 0, 300, 3000 or 15,000 mg amaranth per kg of diet for 64 weeks, after which all survivors were killed; no increase in the incidence of tumours was seen in test as compared to control animals (Mannel et al., 1958). [The short duration of the experiment was noted by the Working Group.]

Two-year feeding studies were carried out with Osborne-Mendel and Sprague-Dawley rats given concentrations of 10,000 and 20,000 mg amaranth per kg of diet. One hundred animals were used in each group and in a control group. There was no statistically significant increase in the incidence of tumours (US Food and Drug Administration, unpublished study quoted in FAO/WHO, 1966). [No further details were available.]

A group of 10 rats received a diet containing 2000 mg amaranth per kg of diet for 417 days (total dose, 11 g/animal). During an observation period of 830 days, 1 intestinal carcinoma was reported in 1 animal (Hecht, unpublished study quoted in DFG, 1957). [No further details were available.]

A group of 50 non-inbred rats received amaranth paste (containing 65-75% pure chemical in dry paste) in the diet at a concentration of 20,000-40,000 mg/kg of diet for 25 months; each rat thus received about 1 g/kg bw/day and a total dose of 245 g/animal. Sarcomas of the peritoneum and intestine were observed in 11/18 rats surviving 19-25 months, compared with 0/35 in controls (Baigusheva, 1968).

A group of 50 non-inbred rats was fed a diet containing chemically pure amaranth at a concentration of 20,000 mg/kg of diet for up to 33 months (total intake, 43-196 g/animal). In 13/48 rats surviving at the appearance of the first tumour, 15 tumours were observed, including 3 lymphomas, 3 subcutaneous sarcomas, 1 mammary adenofibroma, 3 adenocarcinomas of the intestine, 1 hepatoma, 1 rabdomyosarcoma, 1 skin epithelioma, 1 Zymbal gland carcinoma and 1 sebaceous gland carcinoma. No tumours were reported in 50 controls surviving up to 33 months (Andrianova, 1970).

Dog: A seven-year toxicity study was carried out on female beagle dogs. Five dogs were fed 20,000 mg amaranth in the diet, and three animals were used as controls. No histopathological or other abnormalities were reported (US Food and Drug Administration, unpublished study quoted in FAO/WHO, 1966). [No further details were available.]

(b) Subcutaneous and/or intramuscular injection

Rat: A group of 11 rats received s.c. injections of 0.5 ml of a 1% solution of amaranth twice a week for one year (total dose, 500 mg/animal). No tumours were seen after 879 days (Hecht, unpublished study quoted in DFG, 1957). [No further experimental data were available to the Working Group.]

A group of 9 male and 9 female Osborne-Mendel rats was given weekly s.c. injections of 1 ml of a 2-3% aqueous solution of amaranth (20-30 mg/dose) for 94-99 weeks. No local or distant tumours were reported (Nelson & Hagan, 1953). [No further experimental data were available to the Working Group.]

3.2 Other relevant biological data

(a) Animals

According to Hecht (unpublished study quoted in DFG, 1957), the LD_{50} of amaranth in rats both by i.p. and i.v. administration is above 1000 mg/kg bw. Rats fed 20 mg/animal/day for 78 weeks show 68% mortality, compared to 13% in controls; vacuolar dystrophy with eventual fatty degeneration of the liver cells was observed (Gales *et al.*, 1972). Amaranth has no cathartic action under conditions in which yellow AB and yellow OB do (Radomski & Deichmann, 1956).

In rats given a single oral dose of 100 mg amaranth, 0.45% was found in the faeces after 48 hours. Absorption from the intestinal tract after oral administration of 50 mg/kg bw was 2.8% of the dose. 1-Amino-4-

naphthalene sulphonic acid, one of the metabolites of amaranth, is absorbed to the extent of 18% after its oral administration (Radomski & Mellinger, 1962).

When given by intrasplenic infusion to rats with cannulated bile ducts, amaranth was entirely excreted in bile (93.5%) (Radomski & Mellinger, 1962); 53% (43-79%) was excreted in bile in the experiments of Ryan & Wright (1961).

Amaranth is rapidly reduced by a suspension of bacteria obtained from the large intestine and caecum of rats (Roxon et al., 1967); Ryan et al. (1968) found that it is reduced by rat liver homogenates as well as by rat intestinal contents. Products of reductive cleavage of amaranth, namely, 1-amino-4-naphthalene sulphonic acid and 1-amino-2-hydroxy-3,6-naphthalene disulphonic acid (R-amino salt), are found in the urine of rats fed the colour (Radomski & Mellinger, 1962). It is clear from these findings, however, that reduction products appearing in urine and bile are absorbed from the intestine after the colour has been reduced by bacterial flora.

Dose-related foetotoxic effects of amaranth (Collins & McLaughlin, 1972) and of sodium naphthionate and the R-amino salt, known metabolites of amaranth (Collins & McLaughlin, 1973), have been described. In a three-generation study with four different dose levels, Collins et al. (1975a,b) found no indication of adverse effects of amaranth on the reproductive system or of teratogenicity. The only effect observed was a decrease in the weaning index in one of the four F_1 generations. Tests in which a composite sample of amaranth from different manufacturers was given at dose levels of 15, 50 and 150 mg/kg bw to pregnant rats and at doses of 1.5, 5 and 15 mg/kg bw to pregnant rabbits showed no evidence of adverse effects (Keplinger et al., 1974).

3.3 Observations in man

No data were available to the Working Group.

4. Comments on Data Reported and Evaluation

4.1 Animal data

Amaranth has been tested by the oral route in mice, rats and dogs and by the subcutaneous route in rats. Two oral studies in rats indicating a carcinogenic effect do not allow a definite evaluation: in one study the compound used contained 25-35% of unspecified impurities; in the other, the absence of spontaneous tumours in controls after 33 months is considered to be very unusual.

Other oral studies in mice, rats and dogs gave negative results but were inadequately reported. Subcutaneous experiments in rats could not be evaluated because of the small numbers of animals used or insufficient reporting.

The carcinogenicity of this compound could not be evaluated.

4.2 Human data

No case reports or epidemiological studies were available to the Working Group.

5. References

Andrianova, M.M. (1970) Carcinogenous properties of red food pigments - amaranth, SX purple and 4R purple. Vop. Pitan., 29, 61-65

Anon. (1968) Guidelines for good manufacturing practice: use of certified FD & C colors in food. Food Technology, 22, 946-949

Anon. (1972) FDA's Red No. 2 restrictions are protested by PMA group in view of NAS/NRC's data. Chemical Marketing Reporter, 11 September, pp. 7, 23

Baigusheva, M.M. (1968) Carcinogenic properties of the amaranth paste. Vop. Pitan., 27, 46-50

British Standards Institution (1960) Methods for the analysis of water-soluble coal-tar dyes permitted for use in foods. BS3210:1960, London

Collins, T.F.X. & McLaughlin, J. (1972) Teratology studies on food colourings. I. Embryotoxicity of amaranth (FD & C Red No. 2) in rats. Fd Cosmet. Toxicol., 10, 619-624

Collins, T.F.X. & McLaughlin, J. (1973) Teratology studies on food colourings. II. Embryotoxicity of R-salt and metabolites of amaranth (FD & C Red No. 2) in rats. Fd Cosmet. Toxicol., 11, 355-365

Collins, T.F.X., Keller, H.V., Black, T.N. & Ruggles, D.I. (1975a) Long-term effects of dietary amaranth in rats. I. Effects on reproduction. Toxicology, 3, 115-128

Collins, T.F.X., Black, T.N. & Ruggles, D.I. (1975b) Long-term effects of dietary amaranth in rats. II. Effects on fetal development. Toxicology, 3, 129-140

Cook, J.W., Hewett, C.L., Kennaway, E.L. & Kennaway, N.M. (1940) Effects produced in the livers of mice by azonaphthalenes and related compounds. Amer. J. Cancer, 40, 62-77

DeGiacomi, R., ed. (1974) Food Processing and Packaging Directory 1974, 13th ed., London, IPC Consumer Industries Press Ltd, pp. 797-802

DFG (Deutsche Forschungsgemeinschaft) (1955) Kommission zur Bearbeitung des Lebensmittelfarbstoffproblems, Toxikologische Daten von Farbstoffen und ihre Zulassung für Lebensmittel in verschiedenen Ländern, Mitt. 6(1), Wiesbaden, Steiner Verlag

DFG (Deutsche Forschungsgemeinschaft) (1957) Farbstoff-Kommission, Toxikologische Daten von Farbstoffen und ihre Zulassung für Lebensmittel in verschiedenen Ländern, Mitt. 6(2), Wiesbaden, Steiner Verlag, p. 40

FAO/WHO (1966) Joint Expert Committee on Food Additives. Specifications for identity and purity and toxicological evaluation of food colours, FAO Nutr. Mtgs Rep. Ser. No. 38B, WHO/Food Add./66.25, p. 23

FAO/WHO (1972) 16th Report of the Joint FAO/WHO Expert Committee on Food Additives. Evaluation of mercury, lead, cadmium and the food additives amaranth, diethylpyrocarbonate and octyl gallate. WHO Food Additive Series No. 4, Wld Hlth Org. techn. Rep. Ser., No. 505, p. 65

Gales, V., Preda, N., Popa, L., Sendrea, D. & Simu, G. (1972) Recherches toxicologiques sur le colorant amaranthe. J. europ. Toxicol., 5, 167-173

Inoue, T., Kamikura, M. & Murakami, N. (1967) Dye standards of National Institute of Hygienic Sciences. Bull. Nat. Inst. Hyg. Sci. (Tokyo), 85, 150-152

Japan Food Hygiene Association (1974) Japanese Standards of Food Additives, 3rd ed., Tokyo, Ministry of Health and Welfare

Keplinger, M.L., Wright, P.L., Plank, J.B. & Calandra, J.C. (1974) Teratologic studies with FD & C Red No. 2 in rats and rabbits. Toxicol. appl. Pharmacol., 28, 209-215

Mannell, W.A., Grice, H.C., Lu, F.C. & Allmark, M.G. (1958) Chronic toxicity studies on food colours. IV. Observations on the toxicity of tartrazine, amaranth and sunset yellow in rats. J. Pharm. Pharmacol., 10, 625-634

Merck & Co. (1968) The Merck Index, 8th ed., Rahway, N.J., p. 48

Nelson, A.A. & Hagan, E.C. (1953) Production of fibrosarcomas in rats at site of subcutaneous injection of various food dyes. Fed. Proc., 12, 397-398

Radomski, J.L. (1974) Toxicology of food colors. Ann. Rev. Pharmacol., 14, 127-137

Radomski, J.L. & Deichmann, W.B. (1956) Cathartic action and metabolism of certain coal-tar food dyes. J. Pharmacol. exp. Ther., 118, 322-327

Radomski, J.L. & Mellinger, T.J. (1962) The absorption, fate and excretion in rats of the water-soluble azo dyes, FD & C red No. 2, FD & C red No. 4 and FD & C Yellow No. 6. J. Pharmacol. exp. Ther., 136, 259-266

Richter, F. (1958) Beilstein's Handbuch der Organischen Chemie, Vol. 16, p. I-305

Roxon, J.J., Ryan, A.J. & Wright, S.E. (1967) Reduction of water-soluble azo dyes by intestinal bacteria. Fd Cosmet. Toxicol., 5, 367-369

Ryan, A.J. & Wright, S.E. (1961) The excretion of some azo dyes in rat bile. J. Pharm. Pharmacol., *13*, 492-495

Ryan, A.J., Roxon, J.J. & Sivayavirojana, A. (1968) Bacterial azo reduction: a metabolic reaction in mammals. Nature (Lond.). *219*, 854-855

Society of Dyers and Colourists (1971) Colour Index, 3rd ed., Vol. I, Bradford, Yorkshire, Deanhouse Piccadilly, p. 1132

Truhaut, R. (1955) Sur l'action cancérigène de certaines matières colorantes. Importance en hygiène alimentaire, en thérapeutique et en hygiène générale. Ann. pharm. fr., *13*, 36-51

US Code of Federal Regulations (1974) Food and Drugs, Title 21, Part 9.61, Washington DC, US Government Printing Office, p. 195

US Tariff Commission (1922) Census of Dyes and Other Synthetic Organic Chemicals, 1921, Tariff Information Series No. 26, Washington DC, US Government Printing Office, pp. 47, 63

US Tariff Commission (1974) Synthetic Organic Chemicals, US Production and Sales, 1972, TC Publication 681, Washington DC, US Government Printing Office, p. 63

Willheim, R. & Ivy, A.C. (1953) A preliminary study concerning the possibility of dietary carcinogenesis. Gastroenterology, *23*, 1-19

Zuckerman, S. (1964) Colors for Food, Drugs and Cosmetics. In: Kirk, R.E. & Othmer, D.F., eds, Encyclopedia of Chemical Technology, 2nd ed., Vol. 5, New York, John Wiley & Sons, p. 866

para-AMINOAZOBENZENE

1. Chemical and Physical Data

1.1 Synonyms and trade names

Colour Index No.: 11000

Colour Index Name: C.I. Solvent Yellow 1

Chem. Abstr. Reg. Serial No.: 60-09-3

Chem. Abstr. Name: 4-(Phenylazo) benzenamine
For other names of which the Working Group was aware, see index, p. 297.

1.2 Chemical formula and molecular weight

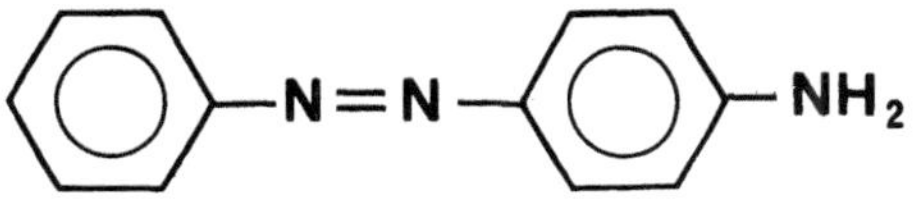

$C_{12}H_{11}N_3$ Mol. wt: 197.2

1.3 Chemical and physical properties of the pure substance

(a) Description: Brownish-yellow needles with a bluish coat
(b) Melting-point: 124-126°C
(c) Boiling-point: >360°C
(d) Solubility: Soluble in ethanol, benzene, chloroform and ether; slightly soluble in water

1.4 Technical products and impurities

According to US industrial sources, *para*-aminoazobenzene is not used in foods, drugs or cosmetics; thus its manufacture and testing do not conform to rigid chemical specifications, and it s composition varies in order to meet customer shade and intensity requirements.

2. Production, Use, Occurrence and Analysis

For important background information on this section, see preamble, p. 17.

2.1 Production and use

para-Aminoazobenzene was first prepared by Ch. Mène in 1861 (Society of Dyers and Colourists, 1971). It can be synthesized by diazotizing aniline and coupling the resulting diazoaminobenzene with a mixture of aniline and aniline hydrochloride (Vogel, 1956), but it is not known whether this method is used for commercial production.

Large-scale production of *para*-aminoazobenzene in the US was first reported in 1924 (US Tariff Commission, 1925). In 1972, only one US manufacturer reported production of this colour, so separate production data were not published; it was included in a miscellaneous category with at least 20 other colours, with a total combined production of about 465,000 kg (US Tariff Commission, 1974). Separate data on US imports and exports were not available.

In Western Europe, there may be about seven producers of *para*-aminoazobenzene, but current production is believed to be small. It is probably not produced in Japan, although it has been imported on an irregular basis.

para-Aminoazobenzene is reportedly used as a dye for lacquers, varnishes, wax products, oil stains and styrene resins (Society of Dyers and Colourists, 1971) and as an intermediate in the manufacture of acid yellow, diazo dyes and indulines (Merck & Co., 1968).

2.2 Occurrence

para-Aminoazobenzene is not known to occur in nature.

2.3 Analysis

See section, "General Remarks on the Substances Considered", p. 28.

3. Biological Data Relevant to the Evaluation of Carcinogenic Risk to Man

Three reviews on azo compounds, including *para*-aminoazobenzene, and their carcinogenic activity have been published (Miller & Miller, 1953; Terayama, 1967; Truhaut, 1955).

3.1 Carcinogenicity and related studies in animals

(a) Oral administration

Rat: A group of 16 male Wistar rats was fed a restricted diet (the glucose of the low protein diet was replaced by boiled potatoes) containing 12% casein plus a concentration of 2000-10,000 mg *para*-aminoazobenzene (AAB) per kg of diet for up to 104 weeks. Liver tumours developed in 7/16 rats. Two of the tumours, liver-cell carcinomas with metastases, were malignant, the first one developing at 525 days; no adenocarcinomas were observed. No liver tumours occurred in 8 male and 8 female controls (average life-span, 77 weeks). N,N-Dimethyl-4-aminoazobenzene, tested in a similar diet, produced liver-cell carcinomas in 5/8 males and 3/7 females (1 with metastases) and malignant bile duct tumours in 4/8 males and 2/8 females (Kirby & Peacock, 1947).

A group of 8 male and 7 female Wistar rats was fed a restricted diet (the boiled potatoes of the above diet were replaced by rice starch) containing 2500 mg AAB per kg of diet for 5 months, followed by 1500 mg/kg for 2 months and 1000 mg/kg for a further 11 months, at which time the concentration was reduced to 800 mg/kg of diet. Six rats survived 2 years of treatment No liver tumours were observed (Kirby, 1947).

A group of 32 male Donryu rats (11 weeks old at the start of treatment) was fed a diet containing 800 mg AAB per kg of diet for up to 60 weeks. Eighteen rats survived for 60 weeks and were killed at the end of treatment; only 1 fibrosarcoma was observed in the peritoneal cavity of 1 rat (Odashima & Hashimoto, 1968). [The Working Group noted the short duration of the experiment.]

(b) Skin application

Rat: A group of 6 male stock albino rats was painted twice weekly on the dorsal skin with 1 ml of a 0.2% solution of AAB in acetone for life (mean length of treatment, 123 weeks). Skin tumours occurred in all rats, including 4 squamous-cell carcinomas, 8 basal-cell carcinomas, 2 anaplastic carcinomas, 1 squamous papilloma and 3 miscellaenous tumours. No skin tumours occurred in 6 controls painted with acetone for life. No liver tumours were found in either control or treated animals (Fare, 1966).

(c) Subcutaneous and/or intramuscular injection

Mouse: Kirby (1945) found no local or liver tumours in 29 stock mice fed a restricted diet or in 7 stock mice fed a normal diet and given s.c. injections of 0.25 ml of a 2-3% solution of AAB in arachis oil every two weeks. Seven mice survived between 300 and 626 days, thus receiving total doses of 98-192 mg AAB.

Rat: A group of 20 male Charles River CD rats was given s.c. injections of 2.3 mg AAB in 0.2 ml tricaprylin twice weekly for 12 weeks. No local or other tumours occurred in 19 rats surviving at 14 months when the experiment was terminated. No local tumours, but one papilloma of the skin, occurred in 20 control rats injected with the vehicle only (Poirier et al., 1967).

(d) Intraperitoneal injection

Rat: A group of 20 female Charles River rats was given i.p. injections of 100 mg/kg bw AAB in 0.6 ml of an aqueous solution containing 1.7% gum acacia and 0.9% sodium chloride thrice weekly for 2 weeks, followed by similar injections of 75 mg/kg bw thrice weekly for 3 weeks. Of 16 rats surviving at 1 year, 1 developed a benign mammary tumour; 2/17 controls had 1 benign and 1 malignant mammary tumour. No other tumours were observed. However, 6 i.p. injections of 40 mg/kg bw N-hydroxy-2-acetylaminofluorene followed by another 6 i.p. injections of 30 mg/kg bw produced a high incidence of malignant mammary tumours and 1 cholangioma, 1 fibroma of the skin and 2 Zymbal gland carcinomas in a similar group of rats (Sato et al., 1966). [The Working Group noted the short duration of the study.]

(e) Other experimental systems

Of 39 frogs (Rana pipiens) given single injections of 0.3-0.5 mg AAB in 0.1 ml olive oil directly beneath the kidney capsule, 30 developed 'kidney nodules' between 3 weeks and 6 months after the injection; 9/23 of these, when examined histologically, were shown to be renal adenocarcinomas. Of 192 untreated frogs, 10 (5%) developed kidney nodules, 6 of which included renal adenocarcinomas (Strauss & Mateyko, 1964).

3.2 Other relevant biological data

(a) Animals

Metabolism of AAB involves N-hydroxylation, hydroxylation of the aromatic rings, N-acetylation and O-conjugation with sulphuric or glucuronic acids. The urine of rats, mice or hamsters injected with AAB contains N-hydroxy-N-acetyl-AAB in conjugated form (Sato et al., 1966). Metabolites in the urine of rats administered the colour by stomach tube include 4'-hydroxy-AAB sulphate, 3-hydroxy-AAB sulphate, 3,4'-dihydroxy-AAB sulphate, N-acetyl-4'-hydroxy-AAB sulphate, para-acetamidoacetanilide and conjugated forms of ortho- and para-aminophenol (Ishidate & Hashimoto, 1962).

AAB administered intraperitoneally to rats at a level of 60 mg/kg bw causes cyanosis and occasional exertional dyspnoea, due to the induction of methaemoglobinaemia (Lin et al., 1972).

This compound has been reported to be non-mutagenic when tested in Drosophila for the production of X-linked recessive lethals (the purity of the compound was not defined) (Demerec et al., 1949). AAB of undefined purity (Schuchardt, Munich) dissolved in dimethyl sulphoxide was found to induce reverse mutations in Salmonella TA1538 in the presence of a rat-liver microsomal system (Ames et al., 1973).

3.3 Observations in man

No data were available to the Working Group.

4. Comments on Data Reported and Evaluation[1]

4.1 Animal data

para-Aminoazobenzene is carcinogenic in rats following its oral

---

[1] See also the section, "Animal Data in Relation to the Evaluation of Risk to Man" in the introduction to this volume, p. 15.

administration, producing liver tumours, and by application to the skin, producing epidermal tumours. Experiments involving its subcutaneous injection in mice and rats or its intraperitoneal injection in rats could not be evaluated because of the limited numbers of animals used or the inadequate duration of the studies.

4.2 Human data

No case reports or epidemiological studies were available to the Working Group.

5. References

Ames, B.N., Durston, W.E., Yamasaki, E. & Lee, F.D. (1973) Carcinogens are mutagens: a simple test system combining liver homogenates for activation and bacteria for detection. Proc. nat. Acad. Sci., 70, 2281-2285

Demerec, M., Wallace, B., Witkin, E.M. & Bertani, G. (1949) The Gene. In: Carnegie Institution of Washington Yearbook, 1948-1949, No. 48, Washington DC, pp. 154-166

Fare, G. (1966) Rat skin carcinogenesis by topical application of some azo dyes. Cancer Res., 26, 2406-2408

Ishidate, M. & Hashimoto, Y. (1962) Metabolism of 4-dimethylaminoazobenzene and related compounds. II. Metabolites of 4-dimethylamincazobenzene and 4-aminoazobenzene in rat urine. Chem. Pharm. Bull., 10, 125-133

Kirby, A.H.M. (1945) Studies in carcinogenesis with azo compounds. I. The action of four azo dyes in mixed and pure strain mice. Cancer Res., 5, 673-682

Kirby, A.H.M. (1947) Studies in carcinogenesis with azo compounds. III. The action of (A) four azo compounds in Wistar rats fed restricted diets; (B) N,N-diethyl-p-aminoazobenzene in mice. Cancer Res., 7, 333-341

Kirby, A.H.M. & Peacock, P.R. (1947) The induction of liver tumours by 4-aminoazobenzene and its N:N-dimethyl derivative in rats on a restricted diet. J. Path. Bact., 59, 1-7

Lin, J.-K., Hsu, S.-M. & Wu, Y.-H. (1972) Methemoglobin - induced by carcinogenic aminoazo dyes in rats. Biochem. Pharmacol., 21, 2147-2150

Merck & Co. (1968) The Merck Index, 8th ed., Rahway, N.J., p. 53

Miller, J.A. & Miller, E.C. (1953) The carcinogenic aminoazo dyes. Advanc. Cancer Res., 1, 339-396

Odashima, S. & Hashimoto, Y. (1968) Carcinogenicity and target organs of methoxyl derivatives of 4-aminoazobenzene in rats. I. 3-Methoxy- and 3,4'-dimethoxy-4-aminoazobenzene. Gann, 59, 131-143

Poirier, L.A., Miller, J.A., Miller, E.C. & Sato, K. (1967) N-Benzoyloxy-N-methyl-4-aminoazobenzene: its carcinogenic activity in the rat and its reactions with proteins and nucleic acids and their constituents *in vitro*. Cancer Res., 27, 1600-1613

Sato, K., Poirier, L.A., Miller, J.A. & Miller, E.C. (1966) Studies on the N-hydroxylation and carcinogenicity of 4-aminoazobenzene and related compounds. Cancer Res., 26, 1678-1687

Society of Dyers and Colourists (1971) *Colour Index*, 3rd ed., Vol. III, Bradford, Yorkshire, Deanhouse Piccadilly, p. 3566

Strauss, E. & Mateyko, G.M. (1964) Chemical induction of neoplasms in the kidney of *Rana pipiens*. *Cancer Res.*, 24, 1969-1977

Terayama, H. (1967) Aminoazo carcinogenesis - methods and biochemical problems. *Methods Cancer Res.*, 1, 399-449

Truhaut, R. (1955) Sur l'action cancérigène de certaines matières colorantes. Importance en hygiène alimentaire, en thérapeutique et en hygiène générale. *Ann. pharm. fr.*, 13, 36-51

US Tariff Commission (1925) *Census of Dyes and Other Synthetic Organic Chemicals, 1924*, Tariff Information Series No. 33, Washington DC, US Government Printing Office, p. 66

US Tariff Commission (1974) *Synthetic Organic Chemicals, US Production and Sales, 1972*, TC Publication 681, Washington DC, US Government Printing Office, p. 64

Vogel, A.I. (1956) *Practical Organic Chemistry*, 3rd ed., London, Longmans, p. 627

ortho-AMINOAZOTOLUENE

1. Chemical and Physical Data

1.1 Synonyms and trade names

Colour Index No.: 11160

Colour Index Name: C.I. Solvent Yellow 3

Chem. Abstr. Reg. Serial No.: 97-56-3

Chem. Abstr. Name: 2-Methyl-4-[(2-methylphenyl)azo]-benzenamine

For other names of which the Working Group was aware see index, p. 297.

1.2 Chemical formula and molecular weight

$C_{14}H_{15}N_3$ Mol. wt: 225.3

1.3 Chemical and physical properties of the pure substance

(a) Description: Golden crystals

(b) Melting-point: 101-102°C

(c) Absorption spectroscopy: λ_{max} 326 and 490 nm (in 50% alcoholic 1N HCl)

(d) Solubility: Practically insoluble in water; soluble in ethanol, ether, chloroform, acetone, cellosolve and toluene

1.4 Technical products and impurities

According to US industrial sources, *ortho*-aminoazotoluene is not used in foods, drugs or cosmetics; thus its manufacture and testing do not conform to rigid chemical specifications and its composition varies in order to meet customer shade and intensity requirements.

2. Production, Use, Occurrence and Analysis

For important background information on this section, see preamble, p. 17.

2.1 Production and use

ortho-Aminoazotoluene was first prepared by R. Nietski in 1877. It can be synthesized by diazotizing *ortho*-toluidine (Society of Dyers and Colourists, 1971a), but it is not known whether this method is used for commercial production.

Large-scale production of *ortho*-aminoazotoluene in the US was first reported in 1914 (US Tariff Commission, 1922). In 1972, only two US manufacturers reported production of this colour, so separate production data were not reported; it was included in a miscellaneous category with at least 20 other colours, with a total production of about 465,000 kg (US Tariff Commission, 1974).

In Western Europe, there may be about five producers of *ortho*-aminoazotoluene, but production is believed to be small. Japan has neither produced nor imported *ortho*-aminoazotoluene during the past five years.

ortho-Aminoazotoluene is used to colour oils, fats and waxes (Society of Dyers and Colourists, 1971b). The Deutsche Forschungsgemeinschaft (DFG, 1957) reported that it was not approved for general food use in any of the countries surveyed.

2.2 Occurrence

ortho-Aminoazotoluene is not known to occur in nature.

2.3 Analysis

See section, "General Remarks on the Substances Considered", p. 28.

3. Biological Data Relevant to the Evaluation of Carcinogenic Risk to Man

Three reviews on azo compounds, including *ortho*-aminoazotoluene, and their carcinogenic properties have been published (Miller & Miller, 1953; Terayama, 1967; Truhaut, 1955).

3.1 Carcinogenicity and related studies in animals

(a) Oral administration

Mouse: The oldest report on the induction of tumours in mice given *ortho*-aminoazotoluene (AAT) orally is that of Nishiyama (1935). Of 40 mice given 300 mg AAT per kg of diet, 7 survived for 11 months and 6 developed liver tumours. Morosenskaya (1938) reported liver tumours in 14 mice given total doses of 0.5 g AAT in olive oil over a period of 4 months. Of the original 108 mice, 30 survived at 7 months. The production of liver tumours (diagnosed as hepatomas) in mice administered AAT in the diet was confirmed in several subsequent experiments (Baumann et al., 1939; Morosenskaya, 1939; Shelton, 1954; Silverstone, 1948; Vylegjanin, 1945).

Lung tumours and lung haemangioendotheliomas have also been reported in mice fed AAT. A group of 17 male and 19 female C mice, without contemporary controls, was fed a diet containing 300 mg AAT per kg of diet (total dose, 100-130 mg) for up to 223 days. Pulmonary tumours occurred in 10 males and 16 females and haemangioendotheliomas in 2 males and 6 females. These findings confirmed those of an earlier experiment in mice fed AAT at a concentration of 600 mg/kg of diet; however, in that study the dose reduced survival (Andervont et al., 1944). The incidence of haemangioendotheliomas in untreated C strain females was known to be less than 5% (Andervont, 1950).

No dose-response studies are available, although dietary concentrations greater than 300 mg/kg of diet have been found to be effective. In an investigation lasting 115 days, female A mice of the Heston subline were fed a diet containing 500 mg AAT per kg of diet for 88 days, followed by control diet or the AAT test diet for 115 days. The numbers of mice developing liver tumours were 7/24 (29%) and 18/22 (82%), respectively. No tumours occurred in 20 controls, 74% of which survived 120 days. A high riboflavin diet did not protect mice from developing liver tumours. When pellets of diethylstilboestrol were implanted also, ingestion of the colour for only 60 days was sufficient to produce the maximum percentage of liver tumours (82%) (Shelton, 1955).

Rat: Yoshida (1932) fed 26 male albino rats a diet containing 1000 mg AAT per kg of diet for up to 344 days. Of 6 rats surviving longer than 186 days, 4 developed liver tumours described as hepatomas (total dose, 1.9-3.4 g). Three rats dying before 186 days developed adenomatous changes of the liver. This observation was confirmed in several other reports (Sasaki, 1935; Sasaki & Yoshida, 1935; Sumita, 1935; Yoshida, 1933). Liver lesions diagnosed as hepatomas*, liver adenomas, liver carcinomas and cholangiomas were reported. No dose-response study has been reported, although the lowest effective dietary concentration given was 200 mg/kg of diet.

Some studies reported the occasional occurrence of peritoneal fibrosarcomas in addition to liver tumours (Isibasi, 1935) and of bladder papillomas (Maruya, 1938; Yoshida, 1935).

Hamster: In a study lasting 110 weeks, 25 male and 15 female Syrian golden hamsters were fed a diet containing 1000 mg AAT per kg of diet for 49 weeks. Nine males and only 1 female survived 70 or more weeks. Nineteen liver tumours (9 liver-cell carcinomas and 10 hepatomas) occurred in 17/21 males surviving at 43 weeks, the time of appearance of the first tumour; hepatomas were observed in 3/3 females surviving at 59 weeks, the time of appearance of the first tumour. Tumours of the urinary bladder, including papillomas and papillary and transitional-cell carcinomas, occurred in 15/16 males surviving at the time of appearance of the first tumour (55 weeks) and in 5/9 females surviving at the time of appearance of the first tumour (45 weeks). Also, 1 carcinoma and 1 papilloma of the gall bladder were observed in 2 females dying at the 59th and 65th weeks; 3 females had mammary adenocarcinomas believed to be related to the treatment. Of 33 male and 38 female controls, of which 26 males and 14 females survived 70 or more weeks, 7 males and 6 females developed tumours: 3 animals had cholangiomas, 1 developed a myxoma, 1 a sarcoma of the pleura, 2 angiomas, 2 adrenal cortical adenomas, 2 lymphomas, 1 a papilloma of the forestomach and 1 a liver-cell carcinoma (Tomatis *et al.*, 1961).

---

* This term was used by the Japanese workers to describe hepatocellular carcinoma.

Dog: Ten Irish terriers or mongrel dogs were administered 5 or 20 mg/kg bw/day AAT. All animals fed 20 mg/kg bw/day died within 8 weeks. Of the 4 which survived 30-62 months 2 developed carcinomas of the urinary bladder, 1 an adenocarcinoma of the liver and gall bladder and 1 an adenocarcinoma of the gall bladder with a cholangioma and a hepatoma in the liver. Among 40 dogs administered other compounds during 33-74 months, no such tumours were observed (Nelson & Woodard, 1953).

(b) Skin application

Mouse: Morosenskaya (1938) reported that of 40 mice painted with a 1% solution of AAT in benzene every other day for 6 months and surviving 7 months, 22 developed liver tumours. Similar results were obtained with a concentration of 0.5% in benzene (Morosenskaya, 1939), and with 1% 3 times per week for 8 months (Khramkova & Guelstein, 1965). Several other studies have demonstrated that repeated skin painting with AAT induced liver tumours in mice.

(c) Subcutaneous and/or intramuscular administration

Mouse: Shear (1937) reported that 6 s.c. administrations of 10 mg AAT as crystals given over 12 months induced liver carcinomas in 13/16 male and female A or M mice dying between 11-14 months. Andervont (1939), Andervont & Edwards (1943), Andervont & Shimkin (1940) and Andervont et al. (1942) reported the induction of lung tumours in A and C mice given repeated s.c. injections of AAT. Incidences were about 82% and 54%, respectively (Andervont et al., 1942). Law (1941) also reported the occurrence of local fibrosarcomas in 13/30 C57Bl mice given a total of 5 mg AAT in three s.c. injections during the first 2 months of the experiment, followed by implantation of a pellet of 5 mg AAT. No controls were used.

The occurrence of sarcomas in 8/10 C mice injected subcutaneously with AAT in oil was reported by Turner & Mulliken (1942). Andervont (1950) reported the occurrence of haemangioendotheliomas at various sites (fat pads and lungs) in mice of different strains.

C3H mice were injected subcutaneously with 10 mg AAT moistened with glycerol at monthly intervals for 7 months. Only hepatomas were reported to have occurred in 30/53 males and 24/34 females, compared with 22/45 male and 1/30 female controls, at the age of 15 months (Andervont, 1958).

Newborn mouse: Single s.c. injections of 0.4 or 0.7 mg AAT in gelatin were given to A/Jax mice aged less than 1 day and kept for 15 months. Incidences of hepatomas were 12/26 in males and 5/27 in females; no hepatomas were found in controls. A total of 43/53 mice also had lung adenomas, compared with 21/94 in controls (Nishizuka et al., 1965).

Rat: Furuwaka (1939) observed liver tumours in 12/21 albino rats surviving 230-410 days after the beginning of a treatment of weekly s.c. injections of 5-50 mg AAT. The first hepatoma appeared at 280 days.

Other species: Aoji (1936) described the occurrence of liver adenocarcinomas in 3/15 fowl following repeated s.c. injections into the chest region of 0.4-0.8 ml of a 10% solution at 1-2 day intervals. The experiment lasted for 265 days. Yamasaki & Sato (1937) found papillomas of the bladder in 3/14 rabbits after daily s.c. injections of 1 ml of a 1% solution of AAT in olive oil for 216 days.

(d) Intraperitoneal administration

Mouse: Akamatsu et al. (1967) gave single i.p. injections of 20 mg AAT to male early adult C3H/HeOs mice and kept them for 92 weeks. Of the treated mice, 28/56 developed hepatocarcinomas, compared with 102/323 controls (50% and 31.6%, respectively). The same treatment in C57Bl mice induced hepatomas in 6/24 males, compared with 1/143 controls, and in 8/30 treated females, compared with 1/171 controls.

(e) Other experimental systems

Bladder implantation and/or instillation: Clayson et al. (1968) implanted paraffin wax pellets containing 12.5% AAT into the bladders of 60 (C57xIF)F_1 mice. Of 52 survivors at 40 weeks (when the experiment was terminated), 9 had bladder carcinomas (17%), compared with 6 bladder carcinomas in 142 controls receiving paraffin wax pellets alone and surviving at 40 weeks (4%) ($P<0.01$). Of 9 rabbits given daily instillations into the bladder of 5 ml of a 1% solution of AAT in olive oil, 1 developed a papilloma of the bladder after 119 days and 1 a papillary carcinoma after

208 days. Papillomas of the bladder developed in 3/6 rabbits given 10 ml of a saturated solution of AAT in water daily for 16-357 days (Yamasaki & Sato, 1937).

Perinatal exposure: Of 71 C3H/A mice born to females that had been painted repeatedly with AAT during pregnancy and lactation, 21 developed lung adenomas (30%) and 46 had liver tumours (65%). Incidences were slightly lower in mice born to females treated during pregnancy only. Of 21 mice whose mothers received AAT before delivery only, 19% had lung adenomas and 43% liver tumours. Of 56 mice born after the end of the treatment, 7% had lung adenomas and 16% had liver tumours. In the F_2 generation, with no further treatment, 12/195 (6%) developed liver tumours and 20/195 (10%) had lung adenomas. In 302 control mice, the incidence of liver tumours was 2% and that of lung adenomas, 5% (Gelstein, 1961).

3.2 Other relevant biological data

(a) Animals

Using autoradiography with ^{3}H-AAT and immunofluorescence, the compound was shown to be taken up by periportal areas of liver lobules. The radioactivity was distributed in all parts of the cells; however, by fluorescence microscopy the AAT-specific antigen was detected in cytoplasmic granules and around the membranes of the nucleus and nucleolus (Müller, 1967).

AAT caused disorganization of rough-surfaced endoplasmic reticulum, hypertrophy of smooth-surfaced endoplasmic reticulum, depletion of glycogen, formation of autophagic vacuoles and induction of mitochondrial abnormalities (Liu et al., 1969). The compound induced cell proliferation and mitotic irregularities in the liver (Maini & Stich, 1961).

The azo linkage of AAT is easily reduced by yeast to give ortho-toluidine and 2-methyl-1,4-phenylenediamine; azobenzene or derivatives of azobenzene without an amino or a hydroxyl group are not reduced under the same conditions (Mecke & Schmähl, 1957).

The bile of rats dosed with AAT contains the N-glucuronide of AAT, the N-glucuronide of the corresponding 2-hydroxymethyl derivative (i.e., 4-

amino-2-hydroxymethyl-3'-methylazobenzene), the sulphate and glucuronides of 4-amino-4'-hydroxyazotoluene and the N-glucuronide-O-sulphate of 4'-hydroxyazotoluene (Samejima et al., 1967). In rabbits, para-toluene-diamine is formed and is excreted mainly as the diacetyl derivative (Hashimoto, 1935).

The livers of mice and rats dosed with AAT contain four previously unidentified compounds, one of which was found later to be 4,4'-bis(ortho-tolylazo)-2,2'-dimethylazobenzene (Matsumoto & Terayama, 1965).

After oral dosing with ^{3}H-AAT for 2-8 weeks, radioactivity was found in nucleic acids and protein. Radioactivity could no longer be detected bound to protein after 28 days, but was present in both RNA and DNA 84 days after a single dose of ^{3}H-AAT (Lawson, 1970).

AAT of undefined purity (Schuchardt, Munich) dissolved in dimethyl sulphoxide was found to induce reverse mutations in Salmonella TA1538 in the presence of a rat-liver microsomal system (Ames et al., 1973). Another batch of AAT of undefined purity (Eastman Kodak) was shown to produce mutants resistant to T1 bacteriophage in Escherichia coli B/r (Scherr et al., 1954) and auxotrophic mutants in the fungus Neurospora (Barratt & Tatum, 1951, 1958).

(b) Man

Allergic reactions to AAT include eczema of the hands and arms (Castelain, 1967; Meara & Martin-Scott, 1953; Zina & Bonu, 1965).

3.3 Observations in man

No data were available to the Working Group.

4. Comments on Data Reported and Evaluation

4.1 Animal data

ortho-Aminoazotoluene is carcinogenic in mice, rats, hamsters and dogs following its oral administration, producing mainly tumours of the liver, gall-bladder, lung and urinary bladder. It also produced a carcinogenic effect following its administration by other routes in mice and rats. There is some evidence that it produces papillomas of the bladder in rabbits following its administration by direct bladder instillation and in mice after bladder implantation. It is effective in single doses in newborn mice.

4.2 Human data

No case reports or epidemiological studies were available to the Working Group.

5. References

Akamatsu, Y., Takemura, T., Ikegami, R., Takahashi, A. & Miyajima, H. (1967) Growth behavior of hepatomas in o-aminoazotoluene-treated mice in comparison with spontaneous hepatomas. Gann, 58, 323-330

Ames, B.N., Durston, W.E., Yamasaki, E. & Lee, F.D. (1973) Carcinogens are mutagens: a simple test system combining liver homogenates for activation and bacteria for detection. Proc. nat. Acad. Sci., 70, 2281-2285

Andervont, H.B. (1939) The induction of pulmonary tumors in strain A mice by injection of 2-amino-5-azotoluene or 3:4:5:6-dibenzcarbazole. Publ. Hlth Rep., 54, 1529-1533

Andervont, H.B. (1950) Induction of hemangio-endotheliomas and sarcomas in mice with o-aminoazotoluene. J. nat. Cancer Inst., 10, 927-941

Andervont, H.B. (1958) Induction of hepatomas in strain C3H mice with 4-o-tolylazo-o-toluidine and carbon tetrachloride. J. nat. Cancer Inst., 20, 431-438

Andervont, H.B. & Edwards, J.E. (1943) Response of strain A female mice to small amounts of o-aminoazotoluene. J. nat. Cancer Inst., 3, 355-358

Andervont, H.B. & Shimkin, M.B. (1940) Biologic testing of carcinogens. II. Pulmonary tumor-induction technique. J. nat. Cancer Inst., 1, 225-239

Andervont, H.B., Grady, H.G. & Edwards, J.E. (1942) Induction of hepatic lesions, hepatomas, pulmonary tumors and hemangio-endotheliomas in mice with o-aminoazotoluene. J. nat. Cancer Inst., 3, 131-153

Andervont, H.B., White, J.W. & Edwards, J.E. (1944) Effect of two azo compounds when added to the diet of mice. J. nat. Cancer Inst., 4, 583-586

Aoji, Sh. (1936) An experimental study on the changes of fowl organs by o-amido-azo-toluol. III. Changes of the mature fowl's liver by o-amido-azo-toluol. Jap. J. Obstet. Gynec., 19, 457-466

Barratt, R.W. & Tatum, E.L. (1951) An evaluation of some carcinogens as mutagens. Cancer Res., 11, 234

Barratt, R.W. & Tatum, E.L. (1958) Carcinogenic mutagens. Ann. N.Y. Acad. Sci., 71, 1072-1084

Baumann, C.A., Jacobi, H.P. & Rusch, H.P. (1939) The effect of diet on experimental tumor production. Amer. J. Hyg., 30, 1-6

Castelain, M.P.Y. (1967) Eczéma des mains à épisodes multiples par sensibilisation à l'amino-azotoluene. Bull. Soc. fr. derm. Syph., 74, 561

Clayson, D.B., Pringle, J.A.S., Bonser, G.M. & Wood, M. (1968) The technique of bladder implantation: further results and an assessment. Brit. J. Cancer, 22, 825-832

DFG (Deutsche Forschungsgemeinschaft) (1957) Farbstoff-Kommission, Toxikologische Daten von Farbstoffen und ihre Zulassung für Lebensmittel in verschiedenen Ländern, Mitt. 6(2), Wiesbaden, Steiner Verlag, p. 146

Furukawa, R. (1939) Experimentelle Entstehung des Leberkrebses durch subkutane Injektion von Olivenöllösung des o-Amidoazotoluols. Nagasaki Igaku Zasshi, 17, 2370-2387

Gelstein, V.I. (1961) Incidence of tumours in descendants of mice treated with orthoaminoazotoluene. Vop. Onkol., 7, 58-64

Hashimoto, T. (1935) Über den Abbau von o-Amidoazotoluol im Tierkörper. Gann, 29, 306-309

Isibasi, M. (1935) Ein Fütterungsversuch mit o-Amidoazotoluol. Tr. Jap. Path. Soc., 25, 690-693

Khramkova, N.I. & Guelstein, V.I. (1965) Antigenic structure of mouse hepatomas. V. Organospecific liver antigens and embryonic α-globulin in hepatomas of mice induced with orthoaminoazotoluene (AAT). Neoplasma, 12, 239-250

Law, L.W. (1941) The cancer-producing properties of azo compounds in mice. Cancer Res., 1, 397-401

Lawson, T.A. (1970) The effect of prolonged feeding of ortho-aminoazotoluene on binding to cellular constituents in mouse liver. Chem.-biol. Interact., 2, 9-16

Liu, L.B., Domingo, E.O., Stenger, R.J., Warren, K.S., Confer, D.B. & Johnson, E.A. (1969) An ultrastructural study of the toxic and carcinogenic effects of 2-amino-5-azotoluene on the livers of Schistosome-infected and -uninfected mice. Cancer Res., 29, 837-847

Maini, M.M. & Stich, H.F. (1961) Chromosomes of tumor cells. II. Effect of various liver carcinogens on mitosis of hepatic cells. J. nat. Cancer Inst., 26, 1413-1427

Maruya, H. (1938) On the renal changes of albino rats induced by the oral administration of 14 azo compounds and 5 aromatic amino compounds. Tr. Jap. Path. Soc., 28, 541-547

Matsumoto, M. & Terayama, H. (1965) Mechanism of liver carcinogenesis by certain aminoazo dyes. VIII. Characterization of some unknown dyes found in liver of mice given o-aminoazotoluene. Gann, 56, 339-351

Meara, R.H. & Martin-Scott, I. (1953) Contact dermatitis due to aminoazotoluene. Brit. med. J., ii, 1142-1143

Mecke, R. & Schmähl, D. (1957) Die Spaltbarkeit der Azo-Brücke durch Hefe. Arzneimittel.-Forsch., 7, 335-340

Miller, J.A. & Miller, E.C. (1953) The carcinogenic aminoazo dyes. Advanc. Cancer Res., 1, 339-396

Morosenskaya, L.S. (1938) *ortho*-Aminoazotoluene. Arch. Sci. biol. Moscow, 56, 189-200

Morosenskaya, L.S. (1939) On the local effect of *ortho* aminoazotoluene and the distant tumours elicited by it outside the liver. Arch. Sci. biol. Moscow, 56, 53-58

Müller, M. (1967) Autoradiographische, fluoreszenzimmunologische und morphologische Untersuchungen zur Verteilung und Wirkung von o-Aminoazotoluol in der Mäuseleber. Arch. Geschwülstforsch., 30, 97-108

Nelson, A.A. & Woodard, G. (1953) Tumors of the urinary bladder, gall bladder and liver in dogs fed o-aminoazotoluene or p-dimethylaminoazobenzene. J. nat. Cancer Inst., 13, 1497-1509

Nishiyama, Y. (1935) Experimentelle Hepatombildung durch Fütterung mit o-Amidoazotoluol bei der Maus. Gann, 29, 285-294

Nishizuka, Y., Ito, K. & Nakakuki, K. (1965) Liver tumor induction by a single injection of o-aminoazotoluene to newborn mice. Gann, 56, 135-142

Samejima, K., Tamura, Z. & Ishidate, M. (1967) Metabolism of 4-dimethylaminoazobenzene and related compounds. IV. Metabolites of o-aminoazotoluene in rat bile. Chem. pharm. Bull., 15, 964-975

Sasaki, T. (1935) *ortho*-Aminoazotoluene. Gann, 29, 52-64

Sasaki, T. & Yoshida, T. (1935) Experimentelle Erzeugung des Leberkarzinoms durch Fütterung mit o-Amidoazotoluol. Virchows Arch. Path. Anat., 295, 175-200

Scherr, G.H., Fishman, M. & Weaver, R.H. (1954) The mutagenicity of some carcinogenic compounds for *Escherichia coli*. Genetics, 39, 141-149

Shear, M.J. (1937) Studies in carcinogenesis. IV. Development of liver tumors in pure strain mice following the injection of 2-amino-5-azotoluene. Amer. J. Cancer, 29, 269-284

Shelton, E. (1954) Production of liver tumors in mice with 2-amino-5-azo-toluene. Proc. Amer. Ass. Cancer Res., 1, 44

Shelton, E. (1955) Hepatomas in mice. I. Factors affecting the rapid induction of a high incidence of hepatomas by o-aminoazotoluene. J. nat. Cancer Inst., 16, 107-128

Silverstone, H. (1948) The effect of rice diets on the formation of induced and spontaneous hepatomas in mice. Cancer Res., 8, 309-317

Society of Dyers and Colourists (1971a) Colour Index, 3rd ed., Vol. III, Bradford, Yorkshire, Deanhouse Piccadilly, p. 3566

Society of Dyers and Colourists (1971b) Colour Index, 3rd ed., Vol. IV, Bradford, Yorkshire, Deanhouse Piccadilly, p. 4017

Sumita, S. (1935) Studien über die Umstimmung des Gewebsstoffwechsels. Mitt. med. ges. Tokyo, 49, 875-891

Terayama, H. (1967) Aminoazo carcinogenesis - methods and biochemical problems. Methods Cancer Res., 1, 399-449

Tomatis, L., Della Porta, G. & Shubik, P. (1961) Urinary bladder and liver cell tumors induced in hamsters with o-aminoazotoluene. Cancer Res., 21, 1513-1517

Truhaut, R. (1955) Sur l'action cancérigène de certaines matières colorantes. Importance en hygiène alimentaire, en thérapeutique et en hygiène générale. Ann. pharm. fr., 13, 36-51

Turner, J.C. & Mulliken, B. (1942) Production of subcutaneous sarcoma by azo dyes and the influence thereon of liver feeding. Proc. Soc. exp. Biol. (N.Y.)., 49, 317-319

US Tariff Commission (1922) Census of Dyes and Other Synthetic Organic Chemicals, 1921, Tariff Information Series No. 26, Washington DC, US Government Printing Office, p. 47

US Tariff Commission (1974) Synthetic Organic Chemicals, US Production and Sales, 1972, TC Publication 681, Washington DC, US Government Printing Office, p. 64

Vylegjanin, N.I. (1945) Some particularities of the carcinogenicity of o-aminoazotoluene. Byull. eksp. Biol. Med., 20, 3-6

Yamasaki, J. & Sato, S. (1937) Experimentelle Erzeugung von Blasengeschwülste durch Anilin und o-Aminoazotoluol. Jap. J. Dermatol. Urol., 42, 332-342

Yoshida, T. (1932) Über die experimentelle Erzeugung von Hepatom durch die Fütterung mit o-Amido-azotoluol. Proc. imp. Acad. Jap., 8, 464-467

Yoshida, T. (1933) Über die serienweise Verfolgung der Veränderungen der Leber bei der experimentellen Hepatomerzeugung durch o-Aminoazotoluol. Tr. Jap. Path. Soc., 23, 636-638

Yoshida, T. (1935) Über die nebensächlich beobachteten Harnblasenepitheliome der mit o-Amidoazotoluol gefütterten Hepatomratten. Gann, 29, 295-300

Zina, G. & Bonu, G. (1965) Il ruolo dei coloranti azoici come allergeni primari da contatto. Minerv. Dermatol., 40, 307-314

AZOBENZENE

1. Chemical and Physical Data

1.1 Synonyms and trade names

Chem. Abstr. Reg. Serial No.: 103-33-3

Chem. Abstr. Name: Diphenyldiazene

For other names of which the Working Group was aware see index, p. 297.

1.2 Chemical formula and molecular weight

$C_{12}H_{10}N_2$ Mol. wt: 182.2

1.3 Chemical and physical properties of the pure substance

(a) Description: Orange-red leaflets or crystals

(b) Melting-point: 68°C

(c) Boiling-point: 293°C

(d) Refractive index: n_D^{78} 1.6266

(e) Density: d_4^{20} 1.203

(f) Solubility: Insoluble in water; soluble in ethanol, ether and glacial acetic acid

(g) Volatility: The vapour pressure is 1 mm Hg at 103°C.

1.4 Technical products and impurities

No data were available to the Working Group.

2. Production, Use, Occurrence and Analysis

For important background information on this section, see preamble, p. 17.

2.1 Production and use

Azobenzene can be synthesized by reduction of nitrobenzene under suitable conditions.

US production of azobenzene was first reported in 1921; it was included in a group of chemicals which were identified as having been produced for research and experimental purposes and no production figure was reported (US Tariff Commission, 1922). Commercial production of a number of cyclic intermediates, including this colour, was reported to the US Tariff Commission up to the end of 1953, but production figures for azobenzene were never reported separately (US Tariff Commission, 1954). It is now supplied only in small quantities for research purposes. Separate data on US imports and exports were not available.

The two major commercial producers of azobenzene in Western Europe are in the Federal Republic of Germany (Firmenhandbuch Chemische Industrie, 1973), although it is probably also produced in other European countries, for laboratory purposes only. It is believed that azobenzene was at one time manufactured by about eight Japanese companies, apparently as an intermediate in the manufacture of benzidine; however, it it no longer manufactured on a commercial basis in that country.

Azobenzene may have been used in the US as an unisolated intermediate for the production of benzidine and its salts, and in 1972 about 700,000 kg of benzidine were produced. The sole major US producer of benzidine for commercial sale voluntarily stopped production in 1973, but it may still be manufactured for sale by small regional producers. At least one large US manufacturer reportedly has used, and may still use, benzidine as a dye intermediate; however, it is not known whether azobenzene has been used in its preparation (Bell, 1973).

Martin (1971) reported that azobenzene is an acaricide and can be used as a fumigant or smoke in greenhouses for control of mites; however, it is not believed to be made commercially for this purpose. Other sources have reported its use as an intermediate in the manufacture of insecticides (Römpp, 1966) and in the manufacture of dyes and rubber accelerators (Condensed Chemical Dictionary, 1971). It may be used in Western Europe as an intermediate in the manufacture of pyrazolone derivatives.

2.2 Occurrence

Azobenzene is not known to occur in nature.

2.3 Analysis

See section, "General Remarks on the Substances Considered", p. 28.

3. Biological Data Relevant to the Evaluation of Carcinogenic Risk to Man

3.1 Carcinogenicity and related studies in animals

(a) Oral administration

Mouse: In a study reported as a preliminary note, groups of 18 male and 18 female (C57BL/6xC3H/Anf)F_1 mice and the same numbers of (C57BL/6xAKR)F_1 mice received 21.5 mg/kg bw azobenzene in 0.5% gelatin by stomach tube when the animals were 7 days of age. The same absolute amount was then given daily until the animals were 28 days of age, when they were transferred to a diet containing azobenzene at a concentration of 56 mg/kg of diet; treatment was continued for up to 80 weeks. An excess of hepatomas, as compared to controls, was found in male (C57BL/6xC3H/Anf)F_1 mice, i.e., 8/18 *versus* 8/73. Hepatomas and tumours at other sites occurred sporadically in female mice of the same strain and in both sexes of (C57BL/6xAKR)F_1 mice, to the same extent as in the controls. The results were considered by the authors as "requiring additional evaluation" (Innes, 1968; Innes *et al.*, 1969).

(b) Subcutaneous and/or intramuscular administration

Mouse: Groups of 18 male and 18 female (C57BL/6xC3H/Anf)F_1 mice and the same numbers of (C57BL/6xAKR)F_1 mice received single s.c. injections of 1000 mg/kg bw azobenzene in dimethylsulphoxide at the age of 28 days. Groups of 24 mice of each sex of each strain received the solvent only.

Animals were observed until 80 weeks of age, and survival rates were equally good in treated and control animals. The following tumours were observed: 2 reticulum-cell sarcomas, 2 hepatomas and 1 lung adenoma in treated (C57BL/6xC3H/Anf)F_1 mice; 1 hepatoma, 1 angioma of the spleen and 1 lung adenoma in control mice of the same strain; 1 malignant lymphoma, 1 leiomyosarcoma and 1 hepatoma in treated (C57BL/6xAKR)F_1 mice; and 1 reticulum-cell sarcoma and 3 lung adenomas in control mice of that strain (Innes, 1968).

Rat: A group of 50 female Sherman rats received weekly s.c. injections of 30 mg azobenzene in olive oil (total dose, 3.1 g). Thirty-seven rats survived for 300 or more days. No liver or local tumours were observed, but one rat developed a carcinoma of the Zymbal gland after 796 days. Benzidine tested in the same system (15 mg/injection; total dose, 0.95 g; 152 animals at start, 24 surviving 300 or more days) produced a high incidence of liver-cell, Zymbal gland and intestinal tumours; however, liver-cell tumours were observed in males only (Spitz et al., 1950).

3.2 Other relevant biological data

(a) Animals

The oral LD_{50} of azobenzene in rats is 1000 mg/kg bw (Christensen, 1973); intraperitoneal injection of 100 mg azobenzene into rats causes some deaths (Elson & Warren, 1944).

Following the administration of azobenzene by i.p. injection to rats, aniline and a water-soluble compound that gives benzidine on acidification were found in the urine (Elson & Warren, 1944).

Of 500 mg/kg bw azobenzene given to rabbits, 30% appears in the faeces; of the absorbed azobenzene, 60% is excreted in the urine as the glucuronide, 20% as the sulphate and 23% unchanged (Bray et al., 1951).

The azo linkage of absorbed colour is reduced in the liver by microsomal NADPH-dependent reductase (Fouts et al., 1957). It induces microsomal enzymes in rat liver. Sudan III and scarlet red increase oxidative metabolism of methyl groups of 7,12-dimethylbenzanthracene, but azobenzene increases ring oxidation (Levin & Conney, 1967). It causes mitochondrial swelling in the liver, but to a lesser extent than do carcinogenic derivatives of aminoazobenzene (Arcos *et al.*, 1960).

Azobenzene binds to bovine serum albumin (Helmer *et al.*, 1968). The interaction of azobenzene and other azo compounds with proteins involves secondary valences (Watters & Cantero, 1967).

Azobenzene and some other azo compounds cause methaemoglobinaemia, but there is no correlation between carcinogenic activity and formation of methaemoglobin (Neish, 1959).

This compound has been reported to be non-mutagenic when tested in *Drosophila* for the production of X-linked recessive lethals (the purity of the compound was not defined) (Demerec *et al.*, 1949).

3.3 Observations in man

No data were available to the Working Group.

4. Comments on Data Reported and Evaluation[1]

4.1 Animal data

Azobenzene was tested by the oral route in mice and by the subcutaneous route in mice and rats. In the oral study in mice it produced an excess of liver-cell tumours over the controls in males but not in females in one of the two strains used. Subcutaneous studies in mice and rats were negative, but they cannot be evaluated because the adequacy of the dose used could not be assessed.

4.2 Human data

No case reports or epidemiological studies were available to the Working Group.

---

[1] See also the section, "Animal Data in Relation to the Evaluation of Risk to Man" in the introduction to this volume, p. 15.

5. References

Arcos, J.C., Gosch, H.H. & Zickafoose, D. (1960) Fine structural alterations in cell particles during chemical carcinogenesis. III. Selective action of hepatic carcinogens on different types of mitochondrial swelling. J. Biophys. biochem. Cytol., 10, 23-36

Bell, D.R. (1973) Final Environmental Impact Statement, Proposed Regulation (Administrative Action), Handling of Certain Carcinogens, Washington DC, US Occupational Safety and Health Administration, p. 5

Bray, H.G., Clowes, R.C. & Thorpe, W.V. (1951) The metabolism of azobenzene and p-hydroxyazobenzene in the rabbit. Biochem. J., 49, 115

Christensen, H.E., ed. (1973) The Toxic Substances List, 1973 Edition, Rockville, Maryland, US Department of Health, Education and Welfare

Condensed Chemical Dictionary (1971) 8th ed., New York, Van Nostrand Reinhold, p. 87

Demerec, M., Wallace, B., Witkin, E.M. & Bertani, G. (1949) The Gene. In: Carnegie Institution of Washington Yearbook, 1948-1949, No. 48, Washington DC, pp. 154-166

Elson, L.A. & Warren, F.L. (1944) The metabolsim of azo compounds. I. Azobenzene. Biochem. J., 38, 217-220

Firmenhandbuch Chemische Industrie (1973) Frankfurt/Main, Verband des Chemischen Industries e.V.

Fouts, J.R., Kamm, J.J. & Brodie, B.B. (1957) Enzymatic reduction of prontosil and other azo dyes. J. Pharmacol. exp. Ther., 120, 291-300

Helmer, F., Kiehs, K. & Hansch, C. (1968) The linear free-energy relationship between partition coefficients and the binding and conformational perturbation of macromolecules by small organic compounds. Biochemistry, 7, 2858-2863

Innes, J.R.M. (1968) Evaluation of carcinogenic, teratogenic and mutagenic activities of selected pesticides and industrial chemicals, Vol. 1, Carcinogenic study. Bionetics Research Labs, Inc., Bethesda National Technical Information Service, US Department of Commerce

Innes, J.R.M., Ulland, B.M., Valerio, M.G., Petrucelli, L., Fishbein, L., Hart, E.R., Pallotta, A.J., Bates, R.R., Falk, H.L., Gart, J.J., Klein, M., Mitchell, I. & Peters, J. (1969) Bioassay of pesticides and industrial chemicals for tumorigenicity in mice. A preliminary note. J. nat. Cancer Inst., 42, 1101-1114

Levin, W. & Conney, A.H. (1967) Stimulatory effect of polycyclic hydrocarbons and aromatic azo derivatives on the metabolism of 7,12-dimethylbenz(a)anthracene. Cancer Res., 27, 1931-1938

Martin, H., ed. (1971) Pesticide Manual, 2nd ed., Ombersley, British Crop Protection Council, p. 29

Neish, W.J.P. (1959) Lack of correlation between the methaemoglobinogenic activity of azo dyes and their carcinogenicity. Naturwissenschaften, 46, 535

Römpp, H. (1966) Chemie-Lexicon, 6th ed., Stuttgart, Frank'sche Verlagbuchshandlung, pp. 290-291

Spitz, S., Maguigan, W.H. & Dobriner, K. (1950) The carcinogenic action of benzidine. Cancer, 3, 789-804

US Tariff Commission (1922) Census of Dyes and Other Synthetic Organic Chemicals, 1921, Tariff Information Series No. 26, Washington DC, US Government Printing Office, p. 27

US Tariff Commission (1954) Synthetic Organic Chemicals, US Production and Sales, 1953, Report No. 194, Second Series, Washington DC, US Government Printing Office, p. 63

Watters, C. & Cantero, A. (1967) Protein azo dyes interaction in vitro; possible role of secondary valences in carcinogenesis. Brit. J. Cancer, 21, 393-400

CARMOISINE

1. Chemical and Physical Data

1.1 Synonyms and trade names

Colour Index No.: 14720

Colour Index Name: C.I. Food Red 3

Chem. Abstr. Reg. Serial No.: 3567-69-9

Chem Abstr. Name: 4-Hydroxy-3-[(4-sulpho-1-naphthalenyl)azo]-1-naphthalenesulphonic acid, disodium salt

For other names of which the Working Group was aware see index, p. 297.

1.2 Chemical formula and molecular weight

$C_{20}H_{12}N_2Na_2O_7S_2$ Mol. wt: 502.5

1.3 Chemical and physical properties of the pure substance

(a) Description: Reddish-brown crystals

(b) Absorption spectroscopy: λ_{max} 516 nm (in 0.02N ammonium acetate solution)

(c) Solubility: Soluble in water; slightly soluble in ethanol; insoluble in vegetable oils

1.4 Technical products and impurities

Specifications for carmoisine are given by the British Standards Institution (1960) together with appropriate analytical methods: the product must contain a minimum of 85% carmoisine. The FAO/WHO (1966)

standard also requires a minimum of 85% pure colour.

According to US industrial sources, when carmoisine is not used in foods, drugs or cosmetics, its manufacture and testing do not conform to rigid chemical specifications and its composition may vary in order to meet customer shade and intensity requirements.

2. Production, Use, Occurrence and Analysis

For important background information on this section, see preamble, p. 17.

2.1 Production and use

Carmoisine was first synthesized by O.N. Witt in 1883 (Society of Dyers and Colourists, 1971). It can be made by coupling diazotized 4-aminonaphthalene sulphonic acid with 4-hydroxynaphthalene sulphonic acid (Richter, 1951), but it is not known whether this method is used for commercial production.

Large-scale production of carmoisine in the US was first reported in 1914; in 1921, ten US manufacturers reported a total production of 106,000 kg (US Tariff Commission, 1922). In 1972, it was manufactured by five companies; however, separate production data were not reported and it was included in a group of at least 33 other acid red colours, with a total production of 642,000 kg (US Tariff Commission, 1974). Separate data on US imports and exports were not available.

In Western Europe, there are probably 15 manufacturers who produce this colour, and it is believed that current production is more than 100,000 kg per year. In Japan, one manufacturer reported production of 4000 kg in 1973 and 2700 kg in 1972. Exports in 1972 were 60 kg; there were no reported imports.

Carmoisine is reportedly used for dyeing wool and leather and to stain wood. In the US, it was used to colour cosmetics until October 4, 1966, when it was removed from the approved list for this usage (US Code of Federal Regulations, 1974). It is believed to have been used in face lotions and soaps in Japan from 1956-1966 (Pharmacopoeia of Japan, 1971).

According to one source, carmoisine has been used in EEC countries for colouring food, cosmetics and drugs (Society of Dyers and Colourists, 1971). The Deutsche Forschungsgemeinschaft (DFG, 1955) indicated that this substance was approved for use in foods in Australia, Austria, Belgium, the Federal Republic of Germany, The Netherlands, New Zealand, Norway, South Africa, Spain, Sweden, Switzerland, Yugoslavia and the United Kingdom. A more recent edition (DFG, 1957) reported approvals also in Denmark, Egypt, Finland and India, but indicated that approval had been withdrawn in Switzerland. Approval for its use in food was withdrawn in Japan prior to 1966 (Japan Food Hygiene Association, 1974), and DeGiacomi (1974) has reported that Finland, Norway and Sweden also no longer permit use of this colour in foodstuffs.

2.2 Occurrence

Carmoisine is not known to occur in nature.

2.3 Analysis

See section, "General Remarks on the Substances Considered", p. 28.

3. Biological Data Relevant to the Evaluation of Carcinogenic Risk to Man

3.1 Carcinogenicity and related studies in animals

(a) Oral administration

Mouse: Groups of 30 male and 30 female ASH/CS1 mice were fed a diet containing 100, 500, 2500 or 12,500 mg carmoisine per kg of diet for 80 weeks. A group of 60 males and 60 females was used as controls. About 50-70% of the mice survived for 80 weeks. The incidences of lung tumours, kidney tumours and lymphoblastomas were similar in treated animals and in controls. Tumours occurring in control mice but not in treated mice included 1 liver adenoma, 2 fibrosarcomas, 1 tumour of the ovary and 2 lymphomas; tumours occurring in treated mice but not in controls included 1 mammary adenocarcinoma in 1 female given the highest dose and a lymphosarcoma in a male given 2500 mg carmoisine per kg of diet (Mason *et al.*, 1974).

Rat: In a group of 10 rats fed a diet containing 2000 mg carmoisine per kg of diet for 417 days (equivalent to an approximate daily intake of 100 mg/kg bw, and a total intake of 11 g/animal), no tumours were reported to have occurred in animals observed up to 838 days. In two further groups of 10 rats given drinking-water containing 1% of the colour for 209 or 250 days (equivalent to a daily intake of 1.2 or 0.94 g/kg bw, and a total intake of 51 or 52 g/animal), no tumours were reported to have occurred in animals observed for 919 or 545 days, respectively (Hecht, unpublished study quoted in DFG, 1957). [No further details were reported.]

(b) Subcutaneous and/or intramuscular administration

Mouse: A group of 15 male and 15 female mice (strain unspecified) was given twice weekly s.c. injections of 0.1 ml of a 3% suspension of carmoisine in arachis oil (equivalent to 6 mg/week) for 6 months. At this time the dose was increased to 6% (12 mg/week), and administration was continued for a further 6 months (total dose, 468 mg). Thereafter the mice were allowed to survive as long as possible. A group of 60 controls of both sexes was injected twice weekly with 0.1 ml arachis oil. Mortality was high in the early part of the experiment. No subcutaneous tumours or hepatomas occurred in 12 treated mice dying between 20-90 weeks; lymphomas occurred in 0/1 males and 7/11 females compared with 1/9 and 4/9 controls. An intestinal tumour occurring in 1 male was not considered to be related to the treatment (Bonser *et al.*, 1956).

Rat: A group of 10 rats received twice weekly s.c. injections of 0.5 ml of a 1% aqueous solution of carmoisine for 1 year (total dose, 500 mg). Of rats observed up to 938 days, 1 developed an axillary tumour diagnosed as a spindle-cell sarcoma. In a further experiment involving the same treatment, no tumours were reported to have occurred in rats observed up to 521 days (Hecht, unpublished study quoted in DFG, 1957). [No further details were reported.]

3.2 Other relevant biological data

(a) Animals

The acute i.p. LD_{50} of carmoisine in rats and mice is about 1 g/kg bw; that by i.v. injection in mice is 0.8 g/kg bw (DFG, 1957; Gaunt *et al.*, 1967);

orally administered doses of up to 8 g/kg bw in mice and 10 g/kg bw in rats were not lethal. In groups of 16 male and 16 female rats fed diets containing 0 (control), 500, 1000, 5000 and 10,000 mg carmoisine per kg of diet for 3 months, the only adverse effect seen was kidney enlargement in females fed a diet containing the highest level (Gaunt *et al.*, 1967). The sample tested confirmed to the specifications drawn up by the British Standards Institution.

Following i.v. administration of 1 mg carmoisine to rats, 30-40% of the colour was excreted unchanged in the bile (Ryan & Wright, 1961). It is reduced by lactic acid bacteria (Eisenbrand & Pfeil, 1955).

3.3 Observations in man

No data were available to the Working Group.

4. Comments on Data Reported and Evaluation

4.1 Animal data

Carmoisine was tested in mice and rats by the oral and subcutaneous routes. The test by the oral route in mice was negative. The other studies could not be evaluated because of the small numbers of animals used.

4.2 Human data

No case reports or epidemiological studies were available to the Working Group.

5. References

Bonser, G.M., Clayson, D.B. & Jull, J.W. (1956) The induction of tumours of the subcutaneous tissues, liver and intestine in the mouse by certain dyestuffs and their intermediates. *Brit. J. Cancer*, 10, 653-667

British Standards Institution (1960) Methods for the analysis of water-soluble coal-tar dyes permitted for use in foods. *BS3210:1960*, London

DeGiacomi, R., ed. (1974) *Food Processing and Packaging Directory 1974*, 13th ed., London, IPC Consumer Industries Press Ltd, pp. 797-802

DFG (Deutsche Forschungsgemeinschaft) (1955) Kommission zur Bearbeitung des Lebensmittelfarbstoffproblems, *Toxikologische Daten von Farbstoffen und ihre Zulassung für Lebensmittel in verschiedenen Ländern*, Mitt. 6(1), Wiesbaden, Steiner Verlag

DFG (Deutsche Forschungsgemeinschaft) (1957) Farbstoff-Kommission, *Toxikologische Daten von Farbstoffen und ihre Zulassung für Lebensmittel in verschiedenen Ländern*, Mitt. 6(2), Wiesbaden, Steiner Verlag, p. 38

Eisenbrand, J. & Pfeil, D. (1955) Über die Reduktion von Azofarbstoffen, insbesondere von Azorubin durch Milchsäurebakterien. *Naturwissenschaften*, 42, 97-98

FAO/WHO (1966) Joint Expert Committee on Food Additives. Specifications for identity and purity and toxicological evaluation of food colours, *FAO Nutr. Mtgs Rep. Ser. No. 38B, WHO/Food Add./66.25*, p. 106

Gaunt, I.F., Farmer, M., Grasso, P. & Gangolli, S.D. (1967) Acute (mouse and rat) and short-term (rat) toxicity studies on carmoisine. *Fd Cosmet. Toxicol.*, 5, 179-185

Japan Food Hygiene Association (1974) *Japanese Standards of Food Additives*, 3rd ed., Tokyo, Ministry of Health and Welfare

Mason, P.L., Gaunt, I.F., Butterworth, K.R., Hardy, J., Kiss, I.S. & Grasso, P. (1974) Long-term toxicity studies of carmoisine in mice. *Fd Cosmet. Toxicol.*, 12, 601-607

Pharmacopoeia of Japan (1971) 8th ed., Tokyo, Ministry of Health and Welfare

Richter, F. (1951) *Beilsteins Handbuch der Organischen Chemie*, Berlin, Springer Verlag, Vol. 16, II, p. 129

Ryan, A.J. & Wright, S.E. (1961) The excretion of some azo dyes in rat bile. *J. Pharm. Pharmacol.*, 13, 492-495

Society of Dyers and Colourists (1971) *Colour Index*, 3rd ed., Vol. III, Bradford, Yorkshire, Deanhouse Piccadilly, pp. 2781-2788

US Code of Federal Regulations (1974) *Food and Drugs*, Title 21, part 8.510, Washington DC, US Government Printing Office, p. 181

US Tariff Commission (1922) *Census of Dyes and Other Synthetic Chemicals, 1921*, Tariff Information Series No. 26, Washington DC, US Government Printing Office, p. 63

US Tariff Commission (1974) *Synthetic Organic Chemicals, US Production and Sales, 1972*, TC Publication 681, Washington DC, US Government Printing Office, pp. 57, 68

CHRYSOIDINE

1. Chemical and Physical Data

1.1 Synonyms and trade names

Colour Index No.: 11270

Colour Index Name: C.I. Basic Orange 2

Chem. Abstr. Reg. Serial No.: 532-82-1

Chem. Abstr. Name: 4-(Phenylazo)-1,3-benzenediamine, monohydrochloride

For other names of which the Working Group was aware see index, p. 297.

1.2 Chemical formula and molecular weight

$$\left[\text{C}_6\text{H}_5-\text{N}=\text{N}-\text{C}_6\text{H}_3(\text{NH}_2)-\text{NH}_2 \right] \text{HCl}$$

$C_{12}H_{13}ClN_4$ Mol. wt: 248.7

1.3 Chemical and physical properties of the pure substance

(a) Description: Reddish-brown crystals

(b) Melting-point: 118-118.5°C

(c) Solubility: At 15°C: in water, 5.5%; in ethanol, 4.75%; in cellosolve, 6.0%; in ethylene glycol, 9.5%; in xylene, 0.005%; slightly soluble in acetone; practically insoluble in benzene

1.4 Technical products and impurities

According to US industrial sources, since chrysoidine is not used in foods, drugs or cosmetics, its manufacture and testing do not conform to rigid chemical specifications and its composition varies in order to meet customer shade and intensity requirements.

2. Production, Use, Occurrence and Analysis

For important background information on this section, see preamble, p. 17.

2.1 Production and use

Chrysoidine was first prepared by H. Caro in 1875 (Society of Dyers and Colourists, 1971). It can be synthesized by coupling diazotized aniline with *meta*-phenylenediamine (Vogel, 1956), but it is not known whether this is the method used for commercial production.

Large-scale production of chrysoidine in the US was first reported in 1914, and in 1921 a total of 115,000 kg were manufactured (US Tariff Commission, 1922). Seven US manufacturers reported a total production of about 203,000 kg in 1972 (US Tariff Commission, 1974), and imports through the principal US custom districts in that year were less than 300 kg (US Tariff Commission, 1973). Separate data on exports were not available.

Chrysoidine may be produced by as many as 12 manufacturers in Western Europe, and it has been estimated that a few hundred thousand kg per year are produced presently. One Japanese manufacturer produced 70,000 kg of the colour in 1972 and 67,000 kg in 1973. Exports from that country were 10,000 kg in 1972 and 4,000 kg in 1973.

It has been reported that chrysoidine is used as a colourant in textiles, paper, leather, inks, and wood and biological stains (Society of Dyers and Colourists, 1971); it is also used as an antiseptic in the form of either the thiocyanate or hydrochloride citrate salt (Merck & Co., 1968). Truhaut (1967) reports the use of chrysoidine as a disinfectant in the treatment of throat infections; however, the particular salt employed is not identified. The Deutsche Forschungsgemeinschaft (DFG, 1955, 1957) reported that it was approved for food use in Egypt, Italy, Poland, Rumania and Switzerland.

A Joint FAO/WHO Expert Committee of Food Additives, which provides information to those concerned with regulating the use of chemical substances in food, considers chrysoidine, on the basis of toxicological evidence, to be unsafe for use in food (FAO/WHO, 1973).

2.2 Occurrence

Chrysoidine is not known to occur in nature.

2.3 Analysis

See section, "General Remarks on the Substances Considered", p. 28.

3. Biological Data Relevant to the Evaluation of Carcinogenic Risk to Man

A review on azo compounds, including chrysoidine, and their carcinogenic properties has been published (Truhaut, 1955).

3.1 Carcinogenicity and related studies in animals

(a) Oral administration

Mouse: A group of 60 male and 60 female C57BL mice was fed a low vitamin diet containing 2000 mg chrysoidine per kg of diet for 13 months, after which a control diet was given for the remainder of their life-span. Two other groups of 100 (50 males and 50 females) and 130 (60 males and 70 females) mice served as controls. In the chrysoidine-treated animals liver tumours (25 adenomas and 50 adenocarcinomas) were observed in 75/104 mice, the first tumour being observed after 10-11 months. Metastases to the lungs occurred in 3 animals. In the control groups 1/89 and 2/117 animals developed liver tumours without metastases to the lungs. In addition, 28/104 treated mice developed leukaemias and reticulum-cell sarcomas, compared with 9/89 and 12/117 in the control groups (Albert, 1956).

Rat: Maruya (1938) reported that no tumours occurred in a group of 10 rats fed a diet containing 1000 mg chrysoidine per kg of diet for 51-366 days.

3.2 Other relevant biological data

(a) Animals

When chrysoidine was fed to mice, only very small amounts (23.8 mμmoles/kg protein after 7 days) were found bound to liver proteins (Piekarski & Marciszewski, 1966).

It has an antifungal activity, and at a concentration of 100 mg/l it inhibited the *in vitro* growth of six species of fungi (Zsolnai, 1962).

(b) Man

A derivate of chrysoidine, sulphamidochrysoidine, which is used in man for the treatment and prevention of streptococcal infection, especially of erysipelas, can provoke allergic reactions in certain cases (Nitti & Bovet, 1936).

3.3 Observations in man

No data were available to the Working Group.

4. Comments on Data Reported and Evaluation[1]

4.1 Animal data

Chrysoidine is carcinogenic in mice following its oral administration, producing liver-cell tumours, leukaemia and reticulum-cell sarcomas. Tests in rats were too briefly reported to be evaluated.

4.2 Human data

No case reports or epidemiological studies were available to the Working Group.

---

[1] See also the section, "Animal Data in Relation to the Evaluation of Risk to Man" in the introduction to this volume, p. 15.

5. References

Albert, Z. (1956) Effect of prolonged feeding with chrysoidin on the formation of adenoma and cancer of the liver in mice. Arch. Immunol. Ter. dosw., 4, 189-242

DFG (Deutsche Forschungsgemeinschaft) (1955) Kommission zur Bearbeitung des Lebensmittelfarbstoffproblems, Toxikologische Daten von Farbstoffen und ihre Zulassung für Lebensmittel in verschiedenen Ländern, Mitt. 6(1), Wiesbaden, Steiner Verlag

DFG (Deutsche Forschungsgemeinschaft) (1957) Farbstoff-Kommission, Toxikologische Daten von Farbstoffen und ihre Zulassung für Lebensmittel in verschiedenen Ländern, Mitt. 6(2), Wiesbaden, Steiner Verlag, p. 3

FAO/WHO (1973) List of Additives Evaluated for their Safety-In-Use in Food. First Series, CAC/FAL 1-1973, p. 45

Maruya, M. (1938) On the renal changes of albino rats induced by the oral administration of 14 azo-compounds and 5 aromatic amino-compounds. Tr. Jap. Path. Soc., 28, 541-547

Merck & Co. (1968) The Merck Index, 8th ed., Rahway, N.J., p. 261

Nitti, F. & Bovet, D. (1936) Recherches expérimentales sur les phénomènes allergiques provoqués par la sulfamidochrysoidine. Rev. Immunol., 2, 460-464

Piekarski, L. & Marciszewski, H. (1966) Affinity of carcinogenic chrysoidine for proteins of mice liver. Rocz. Panstw. Zakl. Hig., 17, 485-489

Society of Dyers and Colourists (1971) Colour Index, 3rd ed., Vol. I, Bradford, Yorkshire, Deanhouse Piccadilly, p. 1623

Truhaut, R. (1955) Sur l'action cancérigène de certaines matières colorantes. Importance en hygiène alimentaire, en thérapeutique et en hygiène générale. Ann. pharm. fr., 13, 36-51

Truhaut, R., ed. (1967) Considérations générales sur les risques de cancérisation pouvant résulter de l'emploi de certains agents chimiques en thérapeutique. In: UICC Monograph Series, Vol. 7, Potential Carcinogenic Hazard from Drugs, Heidelberg, Springer Verlag, p. 16

US Tariff Commission (1922) Census of Dyes and Other Synthetic Organic Chemicals, 1921, Tariff Information Series No. 26, Washington DC, US Government Printing Office, p. 63

US Tariff Commission (1973) Imports of Benzenoid Chemicals and Products, 1972, TC Publication 601, Washington DC, US Government Printing Office, p. 48

US Tariff Commission (1974) Synthetic Organic Chemicals, US Production and Sales, 1972, TC Publication 681, Washington DC, US Government Printing Office, p. 60

Vogel, A.I. (1956) Practical Organic Chemistry, 3rd ed., London, Longmans, p. 623

Zsolnai, T. (1962) Versuch zur Entdeckung neuer Fungistatika. VI. Hydrazin-Derivate und organische Basen bzw. ihre Salze. Biochem. Pharmacol., 11, 995-1016

C.I. DISPERSE YELLOW 3

1. Chemical and Physical Data

1.1 Synonyms and trade names

Colour Index No.: 11855

Colour Index Name: C.I. Disperse Yellow 3

Chem. Abstr. Reg. Serial No.: 2832-40-8

Chem. Abstr. Name: N-{4-[(2-Hydroxy-5-methylphenyl)azo]phenyl}-acetamide

For other names of which the Working Group was aware see index, p. 297.

1.2 Chemical formula and molecular weight

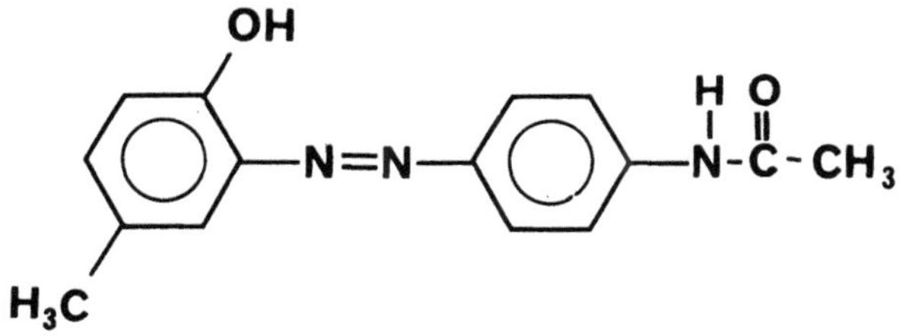

$C_{15}H_{15}N_3O_2$ Mol. wt: 269.3

1.3 Chemical and physical properties of the pure substance

(a) Solubility: Soluble in acetone, ethanol and benzene

1.4 Technical products and impurities

According to US industrial sources, C.I. Disperse Yellow 3 is not used in foods, drugs and cosmetics; thus, its manufacture and testing do not conform to rigid chemical specifications, and its composition varies in order to meet customer shade and intensity requirements.

2. Production, Use, Occurrence and Analysis

For important background information on this section, see preamble, p. 17.

2.1 Production and use

C.I. Disperse Yellow 3 was first prepared by Fischer & Müller (1926) by coupling diazotized 4-acetamidoaniline with *para*-cresol, but it is not known whether this method is used for commercial production.

Large-scale production of C.I. Disperse Yellow 3 in the US was first reported in 1941 (US Tariff Commission, 1945). In 1972, a total of 1,277,000 kg was produced by seven manufacturers (US Tariff Commission, 1974); US imports in that year were 125 kg (US Tariff Commission, 1973). Separate data on US exports were not available.

There may be as many as 11 manufacturers of this colour in Western Europe, with an estimated annual total production of 1 million kg. Production of C.I. Disperse Yellow 3 by three Japanese manufacturers was 82,000 kg in 1972 and 44,000 kg in 1973. No exports were reported in 1972, but in 1973 a total of 18,000 kg was exported. Separate data on imports were not available.

C.I. Disperse Yellow 3 is reportedly used for dyeing textiles, sheepskins and furs, for colouring polymethyl methacrylate and nylon and in the surface-dyeing of cellulose acetate (Society of Dyers and Colourists, 1971).

2.2 Occurrence

C.I. Disperse Yellow 3 is not known to occur in nature.

2.3 Analysis

See section, "General Remarks on the Substances Considered", p. 28.

3. Biological Data Relevant to the Evaluation of Carcinogenic Risk to Man

3.1 Carcinogenicity and related studies in animals

(a) Other experimental systems

<u>Bladder implantation and/or instillation</u>: One adenoma and 6 carcinomas of the bladder were observed in 7/23 stock <u>mice</u> surviving 25 weeks after the implantation of pellets of C.I. Disperse Yellow 3 in cholesterol (amount not stated). A total of 4 papillomas and 5 carcinomas of the bladder occurred in 77 mice given implants of cholesterol alone and surviving at 25 weeks. The results were of borderline significance (Boyland et al., 1964).

3.2 Other relevant biological data

No information was available on the absorption, metabolism or excretion of C.I. Disperse Yellow 3. It appears to be responsible for allergic, contact-type dermatitis induced by nylon stockings tinted by this colour (Foussereau et al., 1972). Cross-hypersensitivity was found with para-phenylenediamine amongst 13 reported cases of sensitivity to C.I. Disperse Yellow 3 (Dobkevitch & Baer, 1947).

3.3 Observations in man

No data were available to the Working Group.

4. Comments on Data Reported and Evaluation

4.1 Animal data

C.I. Disperse Yellow 3 was tested in mice by bladder implantation in cholesterol. The results were of borderline significance. An evaluation of the carcinogenicity of this compound could not be made in the absence of other information.

4.2 Human data

No case reports or epidemiological studies were available to the Working Group.

5. References

Boyland, E., Busby, E.R., Dukes, C.E., Grover, P.L. & Manson, D. (1964) Further experiments on implantation of materials into the urinary bladder of mice. Brit. J. Cancer, 18, 575-581

Dobkevitch, S. & Baer, R.L. (1947) Eczematous cross-hypersensitivity to azodyes in nylon stockings and to *para*phenylenediamine. J. invest. Derm., 9, 203-211

Fischer, E. & Müller, E. (1926) German Patent 469,514, April 24

Foussereau, J., Tanahaski, Y., Grosshans, E., Liman-Mestiri, S. & Khochnevis, A. (1972) Allergic eczema from Disperse Yellow 3 in nylon stockings and socks. Trans. St. Johns Hosp. Derm. Soc., 58, 75-80

Society of Dyers and Colourists (1971) Colour Index, 3rd ed., Vol. II, Bradford, Yorkshire, Deanhouse Piccadilly, p. 2484

US Tariff Commission (1945) Synthetic Organic Chemicals, US Production and Sales, 1941-43, Report No. 153, Washington DC, US Government Printing Office, p. 81

US Tariff Commission (1973) Imports of Benzenoid Chemicals and Products, 1972, TC Publication 601, Washington DC, US Government Printing Office, p. 54

US Tariff Commission (1974) Synthetic Organic Chemicals, US Production and Sales, 1972, TC Publication 681, Washington DC, US Government Printing Office, p. 62

CITRUS RED NO. 2

1. Chemical and Physical Data

1.1 Synonyms and trade names

Colour Index No.: 12156

Colour Index Name: C.I. Solvent Red 80

Chem. Abstr. Reg. Serial No.: 6358-53-8

Chem. Abstr. Name: 1-[(2,5-Dimethoxyphenyl)azo]-2-naphthalenol

For other names of which the Working Group was aware see index, p. 297.

1.2 Chemical formula and molecular weight

$C_{18}H_{16}N_2O_3$ Mol. wt: 308.3

1.3 Chemical and physical properties of the pure substance

(a) Melting-point: 155-157°C

(b) Solubility: Slightly soluble in water; partially soluble in ethanol and vegetable oils

1.4 Technical products and impurities

Citrus red No. 2 used in food must contain a minimum of 98% pure chemical (FAO/WHO, 1966; US Code of Federal Regulations, 1974).

2. Production, Use, Occurrence and Analysis

For important background information on this section, see preamble, p. 17.

2.1 Production and use

Citrus red No. 2 was first prepared by H.W. Elley & H.W. Daudt in 1940 (Society of Dyers and Colourists, 1971). It is synthesized commercially by coupling diazotized 2,5-dimethoxyaniline with 2-naphthol (Elley & Daudt, 1941; Zuckerman, 1964).

Large-scale production of this colour in the US was first reported in 1960 (US Tariff Commission, 1961); it has not been reported to the US Tariff Commission in recent years but is probably still being manufactured by two US companies. Separate data on US imports and exports were not available.

Citrus red No. 2 is not believed to be produced commercially in Western Europe or Japan, although 1000 kg were produced in Japan in 1972.

In the US, this colour is permitted only for colouring the skins of oranges that are not intended or used for processing, at a level not exceeding 2 ppm on the basis of the weight of the whole fruit (US Code of Federal Regulations, 1974).

The Joint FAO/WHO Expert Committee on Food Additives, which provides information to those concerned with regulating the use of chemical substances in food, considers citrus red No. 2, on the basis of toxicological evidence, to be unsafe for use in food (FAO/WHO, 1973).

2.2 Occurrence

Citrus red No. 2 is not known to occur in nature.

2.3 Analysis

See section, "General Remarks on the Substances Considered", p. 28.

3. Biological Data Relevant to the Evaluation of Carcinogenic Risk to Man

A review on azo compounds, including citrus red No. 2, and their carcinogenicity has been published (Radomski, 1974).

3.1 Carcinogenicity and related studies in animals

(a) Oral administration

Mouse: Groups of 20 male and 20 female stock mice were fed a diet containing 0, 500 or 2500 mg citrus red No. 2 per kg of diet for up to 2 years. None of the control males survived longer than 22 months after the start of treatment, but, in other groups, about 50% of animals survived for 2 years. Of 20 treated mice examined, hyperplasia of the bladder wall was seen in 6, 2 had bladder papillomas and 1 male receiving the highest dose level had a papillary carcinoma of the bladder. No changes were reported to have occurred in the bladders of control animals (Dacre, 1965).

Groups of 50 male and 50 female stock mice were fed a diet containing 0, 100, 300 or 1000 mg citrus red No. 2 per kg of diet for 80 weeks. The total numbers of survivors for each group of 100 mice after 80 weeks were 37, 38, 45 and 38, respectively; the total numbers of benign and malignant tumours found were 16 in controls, compared with 22, 15 and 9 in the three treated groups. The tumours were mainly adenocarcinomas of the lung and lymphosarcomas; they occurred in both treated and control animals. A small number of malignant tumours in various organs (ureter, kidney, thyroid, colon) were found in treated and not in control animals, but the increase was not significant (Sharratt et al., 1966).

Rat: Groups of 20 male and 20 female albino rats were fed a diet containing 0, 500 or 2500 mg citrus red No. 2 per kg of diet for 2 years. About 50% of the animals survived the 2 years of treatment, except for males fed the highest dietary level, in which case only 20% survived. Papillomas of the urinary bladder were observed in 4/28 rats examined, and hyperplasia of the bladder in 10/28 rats. No such changes were reported to have occurred in controls (Dacre, 1965).

(b) Subcutaneous and/or intramuscular injection

Mouse: Two groups of 50 male and 50 female stock mice received weekly s.c. injections of a 10% suspension of citrus red No. 2 in 0.1 ml trioctanoin or 0.1 ml trioctanoin alone for 35 weeks, followed by a further 15 injections given every three weeks. All surviving animals (42 control and 44 treated animals) were killed 80 weeks after the start of treatment. The total number of benign and malignant tumours occurring in the controls examined was 24, compared with 37 in treated mice. In treated females, the incidence of malignant tumours (mainly adenocarcinomas of the lung and lymphosarcomas) in autopsied animals was significantly greater (11/50 *versus* 25/48; P<0.01) and more tumours occurred earlier (between weeks 60-70) (Sharratt *et al.*, 1966).

Rat: Two groups of 50 male and 50 female rats were given once-weekly s.c. injections of 0.2 ml tricaprylin containing 20 mg citrus red No. 2 or 0.2 ml tricaprylin alone for 2 years, alternately into the axillary and inguinal regions. Persistent nodular encapsulations of the injected material within a thin fibrous wall were noted, but no tumours were found at the injection sites (Painter & Scala, unpublished study quoted in FAO/WHO, 1966). [No further details were available.]

(c) Other experimental systems

Bladder implantation and/or instillation: A group of 53 (C57xIF)F_1 mice, 10-12 weeks of age at the start of the experiment, was used for the implantation of pellets weighing 15-17 mg and containing a 12.5% suspension of citrus red No. 2 in crushed paraffin wax. A total of 7/50 mice (14%) developed bladder carcinomas within 40 weeks, compared with 6/142 mice (4.2%) given implants of paraffin wax alone. The difference was statistically significant (P<0.01) (Clayson *et al.*, 1968).

3.2 Other relevant biological data

(a) Animals

Citrus red No. 2 is easily reduced by the intestinal contents of rats, rabbits or dogs. After its oral administration to rats, small amounts of the colour are seen in fat but not in other tissues. When it was given in corn oil only small amounts of the colour were found in faeces; however, when it was administered in a dry diet 26% was found in the faeces (Radomski, 1961).

When citrus red No. 2 was administered to rats with cannulated bile ducts, six red-coloured, water-soluble metabolites were detected in bile, and traces of 1-amino-2-naphthol glucuronide and 1-amino-2-naphthol sulphate were present in urine. The urine of normal rats dosed with the colour contained six metabolites: one of the two red-coloured metabolites was the O-glucuronide of citrus red No. 2 (2,5-dimethoxyphenylazo-2-naphthyl glucuronide); two of the products were unidentified; two others were 1-amino-2-naphthol glucuronide and 1-amino-2-naphthol sulphate. The urine of dogs given the colour contained 12 metabolites, one of which, 1-amino-2-naphthol sulphate, was present in high concentrations; however, 1-amino-2-naphthyl glucuronide was not detected (Radomski, 1962).

(b) Man

1-Amino-2-naphthyl glucuronide is a metabolite of citrus red No. 2 in humans (Radomski, 1962).

3.3 Observations in man

No data were available to the Working Group.

4. Comments on Data Reported and Evaluation[1]

4.1 Animal data

Citrus red No. 2 is carcinogenic in mice and rats. Following its oral administration it produced hyperplasia and tumours of the bladder. Given subcutaneously, it produced adenocarcinomas of the lung and lymphosarcomas in female mice. Its administration in mice by bladder implantation produced carcinomas of that organ.

4.2 Human data

No case reports or epidemiological studies were available to the Working Group.

---

[1]See also the section, "Animal Data in Relation to the Evaluation of Risk to Man" in the introduction to this volume, p. 15.

5. References

Clayson, D.B., Pringle, J.A.S., Bonser, G.M. & Wood, M. (1968) The technique of bladder implantation: further results and an assessment. Brit. J. Cancer, 22, 825-832

Dacre, J.C. (1965) Chronic toxicity and carcinogenicity studies on citrus red No. 2. Proc. Univ. Otago med. Sch., 43, 31-33

Elley, H.W. & Daudt, H.W. (1941) US Patent 2,224,904 (to E.I. DuPont de Nemours & Co.)

FAO/WHO (1966) Toxicological evaluation of some food colours, emulsifiers, stabilizers, anticaking agents and certain other substances. FAO Nutr. Rep. Mtgs Ser. No. 46A; WHO/Food Add./70.36

FAO/WHO (1973) List of Additives Evaluated for their Safety-in-Use in Food, First Series, CAC/FAL 1-1973, p. 45

Radomski, J.L. (1961) The absorption, fate and excretion of citrus red No. 2 (2,5-dimethoxyphenyl-azo-2-naphthol) and Ext. D & C Red No. 14 (1-xylylazo-2-naphthol). J. Pharmacol. exp. Ther., 134, 100-109

Radomski, J.L. (1962) 1-Amino-2-naphthyl glucuronide, a metabolite of 2,5-dimethoxy-2-naphthol and 1-xylylazo-2-naphthol. J. Pharmacol. exp. Ther., 136, 378-385

Radomski, J.L. (1974) Toxicology of food colors. Ann. Rev. Pharmacol., 14, 127-137

Sharratt, M., Frazer, A.C. & Paranjoti, I.S. (1966) Biological effects of citrus red No. 2 in the mouse. Fd Cosmet. Toxicol., 4, 493-502

Society of Dyers and Colourists (1971) Colour Index, 3rd ed., Bradford, Yorkshire, Deanhouse Piccadilly

US Code of Federal Regulations (1974) Food and Drugs, Title 21, part 8.201, Washington DC, US Government Printing Office, p. 159

US Tariff Commission (1961) Synthetic Organic Chemicals, US Production and Sales, 1960, TC Publication 681, Washington DC, US Government Printing Office, p. 105

Zuckerman, S. (1964) Colors for Foods, Drugs and Cosmetics. In: Kirk, R.E. & Othmer, D.F., eds, Encyclopedia of Chemical Technology, 2nd ed., Vol. 5, New York, John Wiley & Sons, p. 867

D & C RED NO. 9

1. Chemical and Physical Data

1.1 Synonyms and trade names

Colour Index No.: 15585:1

Colour Index Name: C.I. Pigment Red 53, Ba salt

Chem. Abstr. Reg. Serial No.: 5160-02-1

Chem. Abstr. Name: 5-Chloro-2-[(2-hydroxy-1-naphthalenyl)azo]-4-methylbenzenesulphonic acid, barium salt

For other names of which the Working Group was aware see index, p. 297.

1.2 Chemical formula and molecular weight

$C_{17}H_{13}ClN_2O_4S \cdot \frac{1}{2} Ba$ Mol. wt: 445.5

1.3 Chemical and physical properties of the pure substance

(a) Description: Orange-red crystals

(b) Absorption spectroscopy: λ_{max} 487 nm (in acidified, dilute ethanol)

(c) Solubility: Slightly soluble in water and ethanol; insoluble in acetone and benzene

1.4 Technical products and impurities

D & C Red No. 9 used in drugs and cosmetics must contain a minimum of 87% pure compound (US Code of Federal Regulations, 1974a). Specifications for a colour reference standard given by Inoue et al. (1968) require a minimum of 96.5% pure colour.

2. Production, Use, Occurrence and Analysis

For important background information on this section, see preamble, p. 17.

2.1 Production and use

D & C Red No. 9 was first prepared by K. Schirmacher in 1902 (Society of Dyers and Colourists, 1971). It can be synthesized by coupling diazotized 2-amino-5-chloro-*para*-toluenesulphonic acid with 2-naphthol and boiling with barium chloride (Lang, 1941), and it is believed that this is the method used for its commercial production (Zuckerman, 1964).

Production of D & C Red No. 9 was first reported in the US in 1940 (US Tariff Commission, 1941). In 1972, 13 manufacturers reported production of 1,272,000 kg (US Tariff Commission, 1974), and imports in that year were 26,600 kg (US Tariff Commission, 1973). Separate data on exports were not available.

In Western Europe, there may be as many as seven producers of this colour, but production data were not available. In Japan, 11 companies reported a total production of 1,310,000 kg in 1972 and of 1,500,000 kg in 1973; small quantities of the colour are exported.

D & C Red No. 9 is reportedly used in the manufacture of its alkaline earth metal salts, which are used in the manufacture of pigments for colouring printing inks, plastics and rubber (Society of Dyers and Colourists, 1971).

In the US D & C Red No. 9 is provisionally approved for use in cosmetics (generally lipstick) and in drugs, provided that ingestion will correspond to no more than approximately 0.1 ppm in the daily diet. If the level of pure colour in lipstick is expressed as percent weight no more than 6% is permitted; there are no restrictions for levels in externally applied drugs and cosmetics (US Code of Federal Regulations, 1974b). It may still be used in cosmetics in EEC countries, and has so been used in Japan.

2.2 Occurrence

D & C Red No. 9 is not known to occur in nature.

2.3 Analysis

See section, "General Remarks on the Substances Considered", p. 28.

3. Biological Data Relevant to the Evaluation of Carcinogenic Risk to Man

A review on azo compounds, including D & C Red No. 9, and their carcinogenicity has been published (Radomski, 1974).

3.1 Carcinogenicity and related studies in animals

(a) Oral administration

Rat: Groups of 25 male and 25 female Osborne-Mendel rats were fed 0 (control), 100, 500, 2500 or 10,000 mg D & C Red No. 9 per kg of diet. About 80% of rats in all groups survived 18 months or longer, and all surviving rats were killed at 103-108 weeks. The total numbers of rats developing tumours in the respective groups were: 22/50 (controls), 19/50, 23/50, 27/50 and 21/50. Tumours included pituitary adenomas and adenocarcinomas, mammary fibroadenomas and adenocarcinomas, fibromas and fibrosarcomas (localization not specified), lymphosarcomas, epidermoid carcinomas, adenomas and adenocarcinomas of the thyroid, adrenal adenomas, interstitial-cell adenomas of the testis, liposarcomas of the kidney, kidney pelvic carcinomas, malignant, mixed mesodermal tumours and uterine polyp and pulmonary adenocarcinomas. Tumours not occurring in control animals included fibrosarcomas (localization not specified) in 5 treated rats of the various treatment groups; 3 epidermoid carcinomas and 1 interstitial-cell adenoma of the testis in rats fed the lowest level; 1 thyroid adenocarcinoma, 1 adrenal adenoma, 2 interstitial-cell adenomas of the testis, 1 kidney pelvic carcinoma, 1 malignant, mixed mesodermal tumour, 1 pulmonary adenocarcinoma and 1 uterine polyp in rats fed the highest dose level; 1 thyroid adenoma in rats fed the 500 mg/kg level; and 1 thyroid adenocarcinoma in rats fed the 2500 mg/kg level (Davis & Fitzhugh, 1962). [The difference was not significant for each tumour type.]

3.2 Other relevant biological data

(a) Animals

Groups of 5 male and 5 female Osborne-Mendel rats were fed 2500, 5000,

10,000 or 20,000 mg D & C Red No. 9 per kg of diet for 20 weeks. Splenomegaly occurred in all treated rats (Davis & Fitzhugh, 1962).

No data on the metabolism of this colour were available to the Working Group.

3.3 **Observations in man**

No data were available to the Working Group.

4. Comments on Data Reported and Evaluation

4.1 **Animal data**

D & C Red No. 9 was only tested in rats by the oral route. No evidence of carcinogenicity was observed in this test.

4.2 **Human data**

No case reports or epidemiological studies were available to the Working Group.

5. References

Davis, K.J. & Fitzhugh, O.G. (1962) Pathological changes noted in rats fed D&C Red No. 9 for two years. Toxicol. appl. Pharmacol., 4, 200-205

Inoue, T., Kamikura, M. & Murakami, N. (1968) Dye standards of National Institute of Hygiene Sciences. Lithol rubine BCA standard, lake red C standard and lake red CBA standard. Bull. nat. Inst. Hyg. Sci. (Tokyo), 86, 136-139

Lang, J.W. (1941) US Patent 2,249,314 (assigned to E.I. DuPont de Nemours & Co. Inc.)

Radomski, J.L. (1974) Toxicology of food colors. Ann. Rev. Pharmacol., 14, 127-137

Society of Dyers and Colourists (1971) Colour Index, 3rd ed., Vol. IV, Bradford, Yorkshire, Deanhouse Piccadilly, p. 3309

US Code of Federal Regulations (1974a) Food and Drugs, Title 21, part 9.154, Washington DC, US Government Printing Office, p. 198

US Code of Federal Regulations (1974b) Food and Drugs, Title 21, part 8.503, Washington DC, US Government Printing Office, p. 179

US Tariff Commission (1941) Synthetic Organic Chemicals, US Production and Sales, 1940, Report No. 148, Second Series, Washington DC, US Government Printing Office, p. 35

US Tariff Commission (1973) Imports of Benzenoid Chemicals and Products, 1972, TC Publication 601, Washington DC, US Government Printing Office, p. 75

US Tariff Commission (1974) Synthetic Organic Chemicals, US Production and Sales, 1972, TC Publication 681, Washington DC, US Government Printing Office, p. 94

Zuckerman, S. (1964) Colors for Foods, Drugs and Cosmetics. In: Kirk, R.E. & Othmer, D.F., eds, Encyclopedia of Chemical Technology, 2nd ed., Vol. 5, New York, John Wiley & Sons, p. 869

DIACETYLAMINOAZOTOLUENE

1. Chemical and Physical Data

1.1 Synonyms and trade names

Chem. Abstr. Reg. Serial No.: 83-63-6

Chem Abstr. Name: N-Acetyl-N-{2-methyl-4-[(2-methylphenyl)azo]-phenyl}acetamide

For other names of which the Working Group was aware, see index, p. 297.

1.2 Chemical formula and molecular weight

$C_{18}H_{19}N_3O_2$ Mol. wt: 309.4

1.3 Chemical and physical properties of the pure substance

(a) **Description**: Exists in two crystalline forms: (i) brick-red needles; (ii) red prisms

(b) **Melting-point**: (i) 65°C; (ii) 75°C

(c) **Solubility**: Insoluble in water; soluble in acetone, ethanol, benzene, chloroform and ether

1.4 Technical products and impurities

No data were available to the Working Group.

2. Production, Use, Occurrence and Analysis

For important background information on this section, see preamble, p. 17.

2.1 Production and use

Diacetylaminoazotoluene can be synthesized by treating aminoazotoluene with acetic anhydride (or acetyl chloride) in the presence of sodium acetate

(Merck & Co., 1968). It is not known whether this method is used for commercial production of the chemical.

Diacetylaminoazotoluene is not produced commercially in the US or Japan, but it is believed that two companies in the Federal Republic of Germany produce several hundred kg per year.

The Merck Index reports that this chemical is used in human and veterinary medicine, in a 2% ointment or 5% dusting powder to stimulate wound epithelization (Merck & Co., 1968). Another source has reported that it is used in veterinary medicine for the treatment of oedema of the lung, udder and cerebrum (Römpp, 1966).

2.2 Occurrence

Diacetylaminoazotoluene is not known to occur in nature.

2.3 Analysis

See section, "General Remarks on the Substances Considered", p. 28.

3. Biological Data Relevant to the Evaluation of Carcinogenic Risk to Man

3.1 Carcinogenicity and related studies in animals

(a) Oral administration

Rat: A group of 39 albino rats was fed a polished-rice diet containing 1000 mg diacetylaminoazotoluene per kg of diet for up to 412 days; 34 died from the toxic effects produced by the colour before 322 days. Two rats dying on day 322 and day 360 had developed liver cancers, and 4 rats dying between day 360 and day 412 had multiple papillomas of the bladder with an invasive pattern. The rat which died on day 360 had both lesions (Harada, 1936). [No data were available concerning controls.]

Kinosita (1936) reported that hepatomas occurred within 300 days in rats given diacetylaminoazotoluene in olive oil. [No further details were reported.]

3.2 Other relevant biological data

No data were available to the Working Group.

3.3 Observations in man

No data were available to the Working Group.

4. Comments on Data Reported and Evaluation

4.1 Animal data

Diacetylaminoazotoluene was only tested by the oral route in rats. Although the authors claimed hepatocarcinogenicity, the studies could not be evaluated due to inadequate reporting.

4.2 Human data

No case reports or epidemiological studies were available to the Working Group.

5. References

Harada, M. (1936) Diacetylaminoazotoluol. Osaka Igaku Zasshi, 35, 2295-2299

Kinosita, R. (1936) Diacetylaminoazotoluene. Osaka Igaku Zasshi, 35, 403-404

Merck & Co. (1968) The Merck Index, 8th ed., Rahway, N.J., p. 1060

Römpp, H. (1966) Chemie-Lexikon, 6th ed., Stuttgart, Frank'sche Verlagsbuchhandlung, p. 852

2,6-DIAMINO-3-(PHENYLAZO) PYRIDINE (HYDROCHLORIDE)

1. Chemical and Physical Data

1.1 Synonyms and trade names

Chem. Abstr. Reg. Serial Nos:

(i) Free base: 94-78-0
(ii) Hydrochloride: 136-40-3

Chem. Abstr. Names:

(i) 3-(Phenylazo)-2,6-pyridinediamine
(ii) 3-(Phenylazo)-2,6-pyridinediamine hydrochloride

For other names of which the Working Group was aware see index, p. 297.

1.2 Chemical formulae and molecular weights

(i)

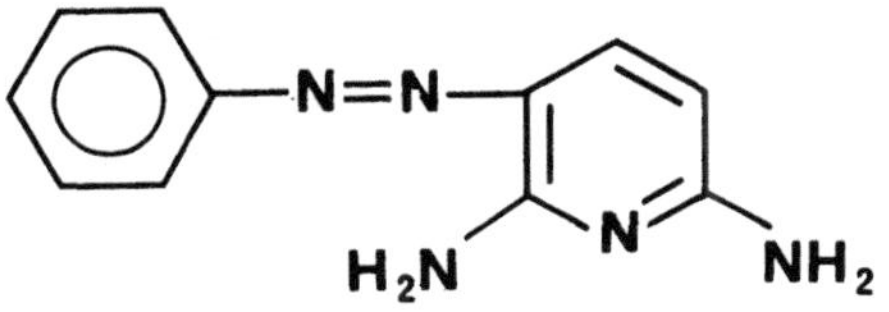

$C_{11}H_{11}N_5$ Mol. wt: 213.2

(ii)

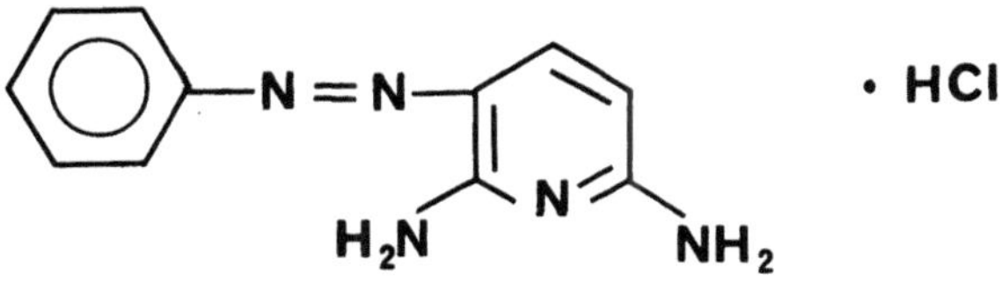

$C_{11}H_{12}ClN_5$ Mol. wt: 249.7

1.3 Chemical and physical properties of the pure substance

(i) Free base

(a) Description: Brownish-yellow crystals

(b) Melting-point: 139°C

(c) Absorption spectroscopy: λ_{max} 238 nm (in ethanol)

(ii) Hydrochloride

(a) Description: Brick-red micro-crystals; slight violet lustre

(b) Melting-point: 235°C

(c) Solubility: Slightly soluble in cold water (1 part in 300); soluble in boiling water (1 part in 20); slightly soluble in ethanol and lanolin; soluble in glacial acetic acid, glycerol, ethylene and propylene glycols; insoluble in acetone, benzene, chloroform, ether and toluene

1.4 Technical products and impurities

2,6-Diamino-3-(phenylazo)pyridine hydrochloride is available in the US in a purified grade in the form of 100 mg tablets or in various solutions (American Society of Hospital Pharmacists, 1972).

2. Production, Use, Occurrence and Analysis

For important background information on this section, see preamble, p. 17.

2.1 Production and use

The first published report of the synthesis of 2,6-diamino-3-(phenylazo)pyridine hydrochloride appears to have been in 1914 (Tchichibabin & Zeide, 1914). The free base can be synthesized by diazotizing aniline and reacting the product with 2,6-diaminopyridine (Shreve et al., 1943), but it is not known whether this is the method used for commercial production.

Although commercial production of the free base has not been reported in the US, it is undoubtedly made as an unisolated intermediate in the production of the hydrochloride. Large-scale production of the hydrochloride in the US was first reported in 1944; in 1972, only two US companies reported production, so separate production data were not published. No data on US imports and exports were available.

There are only two major producers of the hydrochloride in Western Europe, in Italy and Switzerland, and their estimated total annual production is 10-25 thousand kg. The hydrochloride is not currently produced commercially in Japan.

One US producer has reported that 2,6-diamino-3-(phenylazo) pyridine hydrochloride may frequently be used in combination with sulphonamides to treat cystitis, prostatitis, urethritis and pyelonephritis, as a local anesthetic prior to urethral medication and to treat infections of the mouth and conjunctiva (American Society of Hospital Pharmacists, 1972).

2.2 Occurrence

Neither 2,6-diamino-3-(phenylazo) pyridine nor its hydrochloride are known to occur in nature.

2.3 Analysis

See section, "General Remarks on the Substances Considered", p. 28.

3. Biological Data Relevant to the Evaluation of Carcinogenic Risk to Man

3.1 Carcinogenicity and related studies in animals

(a) Other experimental systems

Bladder implantation and/or instillation: A group of 20 stock mice was given single bladder implantations of 9-11 mg pellets containing 1 part 2,6-diamino-3-(phenylazo) pyridine in 4 parts of cholesterol. Of 14 mice surviving 30-52 weeks, at which time all remaining animals were killed, 2 developed papillomas or adenomas and 2 developed carcinomas of the bladder. Of 24 mice surviving 30 weeks and given pellets of cholesterol alone, 1 mouse developed a carcinoma of the bladder after 52 weeks (Allen et al., 1957). [The statistical significance of these results is borderline.]

3.2 Other relevant biological data

(a) Animals

In rats the i.p. LD_{50} for the hydrochloride (pyridium) is about 270 mg/kg bw, while that for the neutralized compound is 520 mg/kg bw (Walton & Lawson, 1934). In mice, the maximum tolerated i.v. dose of pyridium is 125-165 mg/kg bw (Ostromislensky, 1926), and the i.p. LD_{50} has been reported to be >600 mg/kg bw (Burba, 1967). In rabbits, the maximum tolerated i.v. dose is 100 mg/kg bw, and the s.c. or i.m. dose is 150 mg/kg bw (Ostromislensky, 1926).

Following oral administration of 150 mg/kg bw 2,6-diamino-3-(phenylazo) pyridine to rabbits, aniline, *para*-aminophenol, N-acetyl-*para*-aminophenol, *ortho*-aminophenol, 2,3,6-triaminopyridine and unchanged drug appear in the urine. Free N-acetyl-*para*-aminophenol is also present in the plasma of treated rabbits (Johnson & Burba, 1965). When 75 mg/kg bw 2,3,6-triaminopyridine are administered orally or intraperitoneally to rabbits, 15% is excreted unchanged and 1-25% as metabolites; it is more acutely toxic than is the parent component (Burba, 1967).

(b) Man

In humans, orally administered doses of 200 mg pyridium are completely excreted within 14-48 hours, mainly in the urine but partly in the faeces (Riaboff, 1932): about 80% of an orally administered dose of 600 mg is eliminated in the urine within 24 hours. About 8% appears as aniline, 27% as *para*-aminophenol, 20% as N-acetyl-*para*-aminophenol, *ortho*-aminophenol and 2,3,6-triaminopyridine, and 45% appears as unchanged pyridium (Johnson & Burba, 1965). Given at a dose of 324 mg every 4 hours, pyridium shows no ill-effects, and no red-blood cells, albumin or casts appear in the urine (Riaboff, 1932). Daily doses of 600 mg 2,6-diamino-3-(phenylazo) pyridine for 2 weeks to 1 month cause no abnormal methaemoglobin levels (Walton & Lawson, 1934). Toxic symptoms which occur in humans overdosed with pyridium include methaemoglobinaemia, Heinz-body formation, haemolytic anaemia, renal failure, hepatic enlargement, jaundice and hypersensitivity hepatitis (Alano & Webster, 1970; Bloch & Porter, 1969; Cohen & Bovasso, 1971; Crawford *et al.*, 1951; Gabor *et al.*, 1964;

Goldfinger & Marx, 1972; Greenberg & Wong, 1964; Hood & Toth, 1966; Sand & Edelmann, 1961; Wander & Pascoe, 1965).

3.3 Observations in man

No data were available to the Working Group.

4. Comments on Data Reported and Evaluation

4.1 Animal data

2,6-Diamino-3-(phenylazo) pyridine was tested only in mice by implantation of cholesterol pellets containing this substance into the urinary bladders, in which it produced benign and malignant tumours. However, the statistical significance of this experiment is doubtful (see also preamble, p. 21). No evaluation can be made.

4.2 Human data

No case reports or epidemiological studies were available to the Working Group.

5. References

Alano, F.A. & Webster, G.D., Jr (1970) Acute renal failure and pigmentation due to phenazopyridine (pyridium). *Ann. int. Med.*, 72, 89-91

Allen, M.J., Boyland, E., Dukes, C.E., Horning, E.S. & Watson, J.G. (1957) Cancer of the urinary bladder induced in mice with metabolites of aromatic amines and tryptophan. *Brit. J. Cancer*, 11, 212-228

American Society of Hospital Pharmacists (1972) *American Hospital Formulary Service*, Washington DC, Section 8:36

Bloch, A. & Porter, B. (1969) Phenylazopyridine poisoning. *Amer. J. Dis. Child.*, 117, 369

Burba, J.V. (1967) The metabolism and toxicity of 2,3,6-triaminopyridine, a metabolite of pyridium. *Canad. J. Biochem.*, 45, 773-780

Cohen, B.L. & Bovasso, G.J., Jr (1971) Acquired methemoglobinemia and hemolytic anemia following excessive pyridium (phenazopyridine hydrochloride) ingestion. *Clin. Pediat.*, 10, 537-540

Crawford, S.E., Moon, A.E., Jr, Panos, T.C. & Hooks, C.A. (1951) Methemoglobinemia associated with pyridium administration. *J. Amer. med. Ass.*, 146, 24-25

Gabor, E.P., Lowenstein, L. & de Leeuw, N.K.M. (1964) Hemolytic anemia induced by phenylazo-diamino-pyridine (pyridium). *Canad. med. Ass. J.*, 91, 756-759

Goldfinger, S.E. & Marx, S. (1972) Hypersensitivity hepatitis due to phenazopyridine hydrochloride. *New Engl. J. Med.*, 286, 1090-1091

Greenberg, M.S. & Wong, H. (1964) Methemoglobinemia and Heinz body hemolytic anemia due to phenazopyridine hydrochloride. *New Engl. J. Med.*, 271, 431-435

Hood, J.W. & Toth, W.N. (1966) Jaundice caused by phenazopyridine hydrochloride. *J. Amer. med. Ass.*, 198, 1366-1367

Johnson, W.J. & Burba, J. (1965) Metabolic fate of diamino phenylazopyridine (DPP). *Fed. Proc.*, 25, 734

Ostromislensky, J. (1926) *The Scientific Basis of Chemotherapy*, New York, Inter-American Medical Publishing Company

Riaboff, P.J. (1932) A study of pyridium as an urinary antiseptic with special reference to its elimination by the kidneys. *J. Urol.*, 27, 329-342

Sand, R.E. & Edelmann, C.M., Jr (1961) Pyridium-induced methemoglobinemia. J. Pediat., 58, 845-848

Shreve, R.N., Swaney, M.W. & Riechers, E.H. (1943) Studies in azo dyes. I. Preparation and bacteriostatic properties of azo derivatives of 2,6-diaminopyridine. J. Amer. chem. Soc., 65, 2241-2243

Tchichibabin, A.F. & Zeide, O.A. (1914) 2,6-Diamino-3-(phenylazo)pyridine. J. Russ. phys.-chem. Soc., 46, 1216

Walton, R.P. & Lawson, E.H. (1934) Pharmacology and toxicology of the azo dye, phenyl-azo-*alpha-alpha*-diaminopyridine (pyridium). J. Pharmacol. exp. Ther., 51, 200-216

Wander, H.J. & Pascoe, D.J. (1965) Phenylazopyridine hydrochlcride poisoning. Report of case and review of literature. Amer. J. Dis. Child., 110, 105-107

para-DIMETHYLAMINOAZOBENZENE

1. Chemical and Physical Data

1.1 Synonyms and trade names

Colour Index No.: 11020

Colour Index Name: C.I. Solvent Yellow 2

Chem. Abstr. Reg. Serial No.: 60-11-7

Chem. Abstr. Name: N,N-Dimethyl-4-(phenylazo)-benzenamine

For other names of which the Working Group was aware see index, p. 297.

1.2 Chemical formula and molecular weight

$C_{14}H_{15}N_3$ Mol. wt: 225.3

1.3 Chemical and physical properties of the pure substance

(a) Description: Yellow leaflets

(b) Melting-point: 114-117°C

(c) Solubility: Insoluble in water; soluble in ethanol, benzene, chloroform, ether, petroleum ether, mineral acids and oils

1.4 Technical products and impurities

According to US industrial sources, *para*-dimethylaminoazobenzene is not used in foods, drugs or cosmetics; thus its manufacture and testing do not conform to rigid chemical specifications, and its composition varies in order to meet customer shade and intensity requirements.

2. Production, Use, Occurrence and Analysis

For important background information on this section, see preamble, p. 17.

2.1 Production and use

para-Dimethylaminoazobenzene was first prepared by O.N. Witt in 1876 (Society of Dyers and Colourists, 1971). It can be synthesized by reacting aniline with dimethylaniline, followed by the addition of sodium nitrite in a sodium hydroxide solution (Griess, 1877), but it is not known whether this is the method used for commercial production.

Large-scale production of *para*-dimethylaminoazobenzene in the US was first reported in 1914, and in 1921 five manufacturers reported a total production of 8500 kg (US Tariff Commission, 1922). In 1972, three US manufacturers reported production of this colour; however, separate production data were not reported and it was included in a miscellaneous category with at least 20 other colours, with a total production of 465,500 kg (US Tariff Commission, 1974). Separate data on US imports and exports were not available.

In Western Europe, there may be as many as 14 producers of this colour, but current production is believed to be small. In Japan in 1972, three manufacturers reported production of 5500 kg.

para-Dimethylaminoazobenzene is reportedly used for colouring polishes and other wax products, polystyrene, petrol, soap, as an indicator (Society of Dyers and Colourists, 1971), and for the determination of free hydrochloric acid in gastric juice (Merck & Co., 1968).

The Deutsche Forschungsgemeinschaft (DFG, 1957) reported that this colour was not approved for general food use in any of the countries surveyed. In the US, it was withdrawn from the approved list of food additives in 1918, 6 months after its addition to the list, because contact dermatitis was observed in up to 90% of factory workers handling it (National Research Council, 1971).

The Joint FAO/WHO Expert Committee on Food Additives, which provides information to those concerned with regulating the use of chemical substances in food, considers *para*-dimethylaminoazobenzene, on the basis of toxicological evidence, to be unsafe for use in food (FAO/WHO, 1973).

2.2 Occurrence

para-Dimethylaminoazobenzene is not known to occur in nature.

2.3 Analysis

See section, "General Remarks on the Substances Considered", p. 28.

3. Biological Data Relevant to the Evaluation of Carcinogenic Risk to Man

para-Dimethylaminoazobenzene (DAB) is one of the most extensively studied chemical carcinogens. Three reviews on azo compounds, including DAB, and their carcinogenic properties have been published (Miller & Miller, 1953; Terayama, 1967; Truhaut, 1955).

3.1 Carcinogenicity and related studies in animals

(a) Oral administration

Mouse: Lung tumours were observed in 6/22 stock albino mice fed a diet containing 150 mg DAB per kg of diet for 4 months, starting at 6-8 weeks of age. Such tumours were reported to occur in about 15% of untreated mice at the age of 6 months (Jaffé, 1947).

In C3H/HeOs male mice fed a diet containing 600 mg DAB per kg of diet for 1 week, 1 month or 5 months, hepatomas were found in 1/19, 1/9 and 3/5 mice observed up to 45-61 weeks, compared with 102/323 controls observed up to 51-80 weeks. In C57BL mice given the same treatments, only 2/15 mice treated for 5 months developed hepatomas after 56-62 weeks, compared with 1/143 controls observed for 51-86 weeks (Akamatsu & Ikegami, 1968).

Rat: The occurrence of liver tumours in rats following the oral administration of DAB in their diet was reported as early as 1935 by Kinosita (1936). Liver tumours (solid, alveolar, trabecular or adenomatous) were produced after 50 or more days of treatment (smallest total dose, 176 mg DAB); in many cases, the tumours gave metastases in other organs (Kinosita, 1937). The production of liver tumours in rats has been confirmed in a large number of subsequent experiments. Rats of the Sherman, Wistar and Evans strains were found to be equally susceptible to the carcinogenicity of DAB administered at a concentration of 600 mg/kg of diet (Sugiura & Rhoads, 1941).

Dose-response aspects of the carcinogenicity of DAB in rats following its oral administration were investigated by Druckrey (1943, 1951, 1967). Druckrey & Küpfmüller (1948) gave daily dosages of 1, 3, 10, 20 or 30 mg DAB/rat for lifespan. All doses produced liver tumours, the induction time being inversely proportional to the daily dose and ranging between 34 days in rats given 30 mg DAB/day and 700 days in rats given 1 mg DAB/day. For rats given from 3-30 mg/rat/day, the total carcinogenic dose was about 1000 mg. Daily intakes of 0.1 and 0.3 mg/rat did not produce tumours (see also Fig. 1). In another experiment, rats were given daily dosages of 5 mg DAB/rat for 40, 60, 100, 140 or 200 days and then kept for life-span on a normal diet. The incidences of liver carcinomas were 20, 26, 49, 80 and 81%, respectively (Druckrey, 1967).

Hamster: A group of 5 hamsters was given 30 mg/day DAB; the occurrence of 1 "abdominal carcinoma, probably of hepatocellular origin" was reported before the end of the study (Fischer, 1954). No excess of tumours over those found in controls was found in a study on 15 hamsters of each sex given 5-10 mg DAB in corn oil by stomach tube three times weekly for 42 weeks (total dose, 1155 mg) and observed for lifespan (Terracini & Della Porta, 1961). [Only one dose level was used in this experiment, and exposure time was much shorter than lifespan.]

Guinea-pig: In a study lasting 18 months, 60 guinea-pigs were fed a diet containing 600-8000 mg DAB per kg of diet. No tumours were observed (Orr, 1940). [Time of exposure in this experiment was shorter than lifespan.]

Dog: Of 10 dogs (Irish terriers or mongrels) given 20 mg/kg bw/day DAB, 8 died within 16 months. Two dogs surviving 38 months (continuous treatment) and 48 months (treated for 16 months only) developed bladder papillomas with invasion. Of 9 dogs given 5 mg/kg bw/day, none developed bladder tumours within 63 months. No tumours were observed in 40 dogs fed various aromatic amines and other food dyes for 33-74 months (Nelson & Woodard, 1953).

(b) Subcutaneous and/or intramuscular administration

Mouse: Groups of 29 C57BL and 30 Dba mice, 2 months of age, were given three s.c. injections of DAB in olive oil (total dose, 5 mg); a 5 mg pellet of DAB was administered when the mice were 4 months of age. In C57BL mice, 6/29 developed fibrosarcomas at the injection site, the first tumour appearing at 112 days of age; however, only one of the Dba mice developed a local tumour after 476 days, and a hepatoma occurred in one other Dba mouse killed at 581 days. No controls were used (Law, 1941).

Groups of 17 male and 17 female C, 14 male and 18 female C57BL and 9 male and 10 female A strain mice were given nine monthly s.c. injections of 5 mg DAB in 0.25 ml olive oil (total dose, 45 mg). Two C57BL females killed after 41 weeks had fibrosarcomas at the injection site; no tumours were found in C and C57BL controls killed at the same time. In a second experiment, 10 male and 10 female A mice and 16 male and 14 female C mice were given monthly s.c. injections of 10 mg DAB in glycerol (total dose, 100 mg), and were killed at 12 months. Neither local tumours nor hepatic changes occurred (Andervont & Edwards, 1943).

Of 9 male and 3 female mice of a mixed strain fed a complete diet and surviving 250 or more days after repeated fortnightly s.c. injections of 0.25 ml of a 3% solution of DAB in arachis oil, 2 males developed subcutaneous sarcomas after 344 and 379 days. Two other males and 1 female dying after 429-438 days developed hepatomas (total dose, 187 mg). No subcutaneous sarcomas occurred in 3 mice surviving 250 or more days after similar injections of DAB but fed on a restricted diet (with boiled potatoes); 1 female dying after 382 days developed a hepatoma. No local tumours were observed in 8 male Cba mice given similar injections of DAB and fed a full diet, but 3 hepatomas were found in mice dying after 515-556 days (total dose, 232-247 mg). No liver tumours occurred in 6 male Cba mice surviving 250-426 days that had been injected with DAB and fed a restricted diet. Of 5 male and 7 female C57BL mice injected with DAB and on a full diet, 8 survived 250 or more days and 1 female developed a subcutaneous sarcoma. Four other females developed liver tumours, including 1 liver-cell carcinoma, between 446-615 days (total doses, 172, 187, 210 and 210 mg). In 5 male and 5 female stock controls autopsied between 157-342 days, no liver tumours were observed, and no tumours were seen in 2 male Cba controls killed at 153 and 254 days. Of the C57BL controls, 7 which were autopsied between 84-523 days and 2 which died after 426 and 523 days had developed benign liver tumours which, according to the authors, differed from those seen in treated mice. All the controls were fed a restricted diet (Kirby, 1945).

Newborn mouse: A group of male and female Swiss mice received s.c. injections of 0.2 mg DAB in arachis oil on each of the first 5 days of life. Survivors at weaning were 29 males and 27 females, and at 1 year (end of experiment), 28 males and 25 females. Liver tumours were found in 26/28 males, compared with 3/31 in controls, and in 4/25 females, compared with 0/25 in controls. Lung adenomas were observed in 6/53 treated mice, compared with 4/56 controls (Roe et al., 1971).

Rat: Of a group of rats given weekly s.c. injections of 15 mg DAB, 16 survived 150 days and 5 developed metastasizing liver-cell tumours (Maruya & Tanaka, 1936). In a more recent study, 20 male Charles River CD rats were given 24 s.c. injections of 2.7 mg DAB in tricaprylin; no tumours were observed in 18 survivors after 14 months, at which time the experiment was terminated (Poirier et al., 1967). [The amount of DAB injected in this experiment was less than 1/5 of that given in the previous one.]

Newborn rat: In 12 male and female newborn Wistar rats given single s.c. injections of 1.2 mg DAB in 0.02 ml olive oil within the first 12 hours of life, no tumours were observed in animals surviving up to 380 days (Baba & Takayama, 1961). [The length of this experiment was shorter than the usual lifespan of rats.]

(c) Intraperitoneal injection

Rat: Of 50 rats given weekly i.p. injections of 12.5 mg DAB in olive oil, 2/8 rats surviving 200 days developed hepatomas (Mori & Nakahara,

1940). This result was confirmed in a later study on 9 animals, 3 of which developed hepatic cancer (Mori et al., 1956).

(d) Skin application

Mouse: A group of 40 mice was given twice-weekly applications of a 1 or 3% solution of DAB in benzene; 22 survived for more than 1 year. No skin or liver tumours were observed; however, 1 mouse developed a subcutaneous sarcoma in the region of the neck after 23 months (Roussy & Guérin, 1946).

Rat: All of 6 male rats painted twice weekly with 1 ml of a 2% solution of DAB in acetone for life (90 weeks) developed skin tumours, including 3 squamous-cell, 11 basal-cell and 4 anaplastic carcinomas and 3 miscellaneous tumours, compared with 0/6 controls given acetone alone. No liver tumours were found in treated or control animals (Fare, 1966).

3.2 Other relevant biological data

(a) Animals

(i) Histological changes

Large doses of DAB (50-250 mg/kg bw) in rats cause hepatic degeneration within 24 hours (Orr & Price, 1948), followed by focal degeneration of some parenchymal cells around the portal spaces (Opie, 1947). After feeding of DAB, examination of the nuclear and sub-nuclear fractions of liver cells showed intranuclear changes (Rees et al., 1965); prolonged feeding causes liver cirrhosis in rats (Miller & Miller, 1953).

(ii) Biochemical changes

Biochemical changes caused by aminoazo compounds have been reviewed by Miller & Miller (1953) and by Terayama (1967). I.p. injection of DAB in rats induced some methaemoglobinaemia, but less than was induced by N-methylaminoazobenzene or by aminoazobenzene (Lin et al., 1972). Changes in the structure and function of the rough-surfaced endoplasmic reticulum of the rat liver were observed after a single i.p. dose of this substance (Ketterer et al., 1967a). DAB (and ethionine, but not non-carcinogenic analogues) increased the RNA methylase activity of rat and hamster liver cells (Hancock & Forrester, 1973).

I.p. injections of 0.5-3.0 mg/100 g DAB to pregnant hamsters increased the transformation ability of embryonic cells grown *in vitro*; these cells induced tumours when they were reimplanted in hamsters (DiPaolo et al., 1973).

(iii) Metabolism

DAB is metabolized *via* the following pathways: (1) reduction and cleavage of the azo group; (2) demethylation; (3) ring hydroxylation; (4) N-hydroxylation; (5) N-acetylation and O-conjugation of metabolites.

(1) Reduction and cleavage of the azo group

Rat liver homogenates containing DAB formed N,N'-dimethyl-*para*-phenylenediamine and aniline by reductive cleavage. The azo reductase, a flavoprotein, was localized in the microsomal liver fraction and was found to require NADPH as electron donor (Mueller & Miller, 1949). The urine of rats fed DAB contained *para*-aminophenol, N-acetyl-*para*-aminophenol, *para*-phenylenediamine and N,N'-diacetyl-*para*-phenylenediamine, showing that the azo linkage is reduced *in vivo* (Stevenson et al., 1942). Urine of rats given i.p. injections of DAB labelled with ^{3}H in one ring and ^{14}C in the other contained some 70% of the expected amount of *para*-aminophenol, but only 10% of the expected *para*-phenylenediamine (Robinson et al., 1964). Studies on the rates of reductive cleavage of various aminoazo colours indicated that a single parameter, such as azo reduction rate, could not be correlated with the carcinogenic potency (Matsumoto & Terayama, 1965).

Administration of terephthalic acid, dimethyl terephthalate or β-hydroxyethyl terephthalate to rats increased the azo reductase activity of rat liver, terephthalic acid more than the others; terephthalic acid and β-hydroxyethyl terephthalate reduced the amount of protein-bound dimethyl-aminoazobenzene in the livers (Yanai & Kuretani, 1968).

The feeding of rats on a diet containing brown rice, which gave a high incidence of tumours with DAB, reduced the ability of the liver to destroy the azo compound. The addition of yeast, or of riboflavin and casein but not of biotin or adenine, restored the ability of the liver to destroy the azo compound (Kensler, 1948, 1949). The azo linkage of DAB is readily reduced by yeast (Mecke & Schmähl, 1957) and by many strains of bacteria (Walker, 1970).

Administration of DAB reduced the activity of microsomal azo reductase in rat liver (Decloitre et al., 1972; Ketterer et al., 1968); this activity is greatly enhanced, however, by 3-methylcholanthrene treatment *in vivo* (Conney et al., 1956).

(2) Demethylation

DAB and its metabolite, *para*-monomethylaminoazobenzene (MAB), are demethylated before reduction of the azo linkage (Miller et al., 1945a). The N-demethylase is also localized in rat and mouse microsomal liver fraction and requires oxygen and NADPH as electron donor (Mueller & Miller, 1951).

When [^{14}C-dimethyl]-aminoazobenzene was fed to rats, most of the radioactivity was found in expired carbon dioxide (Boissonnas et al., 1949). Pretreatment of rats with 3-methylcholanthrene increased the microsomal liver N-demethylase activity *in vitro* (Conney et al., 1956). It has been reported that azo compounds that are demethylated slowly are weak carcinogens (Matsumoto & Terayama, 1961); but MacDonald et al. (1952) found no clear-cut correlation between rate of demethylation and carcinogenic activity.

(3) Ring hydroxylation

Rat liver can hydroxylate DAB and its metabolites, MAB, aniline and *para*-phenylenediamine derivatives, in the rings *in vivo* or *in vitro* (for review, see Terayama, 1967). The hydroxylating enzymes, like the N-demethylase activity, are localized in the microsomes in rat liver and require oxygen and NADPH *in vitro* (Booth & Boyland, 1957); they are dependent on dietary factors and are induced by polycyclic hydrocarbons (Terayama, 1967).

(4) N-Hydroxylation

N-Hydroxylation has been demonstrated in rat liver for several carcinogenic aromatic amines; it also requires oxygen and NADPH (for review, see Miller, 1970). Indirect evidence of the N-hydroxylation of MAB *in vivo* (Lin et al., 1968) is the formation of 3-methylmercapto-N-methyl-4-aminoazobenzene(3-methylmercapto-4-MAB) by alkaline treatment of liver proteins from rats fed DAB (Scribner et al., 1965) and the fact that the identical product is obtained by reacting N-benzoyloxy-MAB (a synthetic carcinogenic N-hydroxy-ester of MAB) with methionine or proteins (Poirier et al., 1967).

(5) <u>N-Acetylation and O-conjugation of metabolites</u>

Urine of rats administered DAB contained 50-60% in the form of sulphates or glucuronides of N-acetylated metabolites (Terayama, 1967).

Data concerning N-hydroxylation and the type of interaction of N-benzoyloxy-MAB with proteins and nucleic acids have led to the suggestion that esterification of N-OH-MAB may give rise to reactive metabolites (Miller, 1970). This proposal was further supported by *in vitro* experiments in which N-OH-MAB was converted by soluble sulphotransferase of rat liver to a reactive metabolite which reacted with methionine to form 3-methylmercapto-4-MAB (Miller, 1974).

(iv) <u>Protein binding</u>

Because the binding products of proteins and azo dyes are coloured, their formation in the liver with DAB and its metabolite MAB was easily recognized. These coloured proteins contain nucleoprotein (Miller & Miller, 1947) and are found only in the liver of rats and mice, the species in which DAB and MAB have been found to produce hepatomas (Miller & Miller, 1953).

More than half of the bound dye in all liver-cell fractions is associated with soluble proteins; of this, 80% is bound to a fraction which accounts for only 15% of the soluble proteins. The chemistry of the binding is considered in two metabolic studies (Miller & Miller, 1953; Sorof & Cohen, 1951). Three soluble liver proteins which bind DAB have been identified (Ketterer, 1972; Ketterer et al., 1967b). However, in experiments with rats administered DAB or MAB (uniformly ^{14}C-labelled in the aniline ring) by i.v. injection, the binding took place primarily in the liver microsomal fraction and subsequently passed over to the cytosol fraction. The same was true for ^{14}C-MAB in NADPH-fortified microsomal fractions *in vitro* containing cytosol (Hultin, 1957).

Diets high in riboflavin or supplemented with polycyclic hydrocarbons, which reduced tumour induction by the azo dyes, also lowered the binding of the dyes to protein fractions (Decloitre et al., 1973; Miller & Miller, 1953).

(v) Binding to nucleic acids

When tritium-labelled DAB was injected intraperitoneally into rats, it was covalently bound to various nucleic acid fractions of the liver and spleen: less was bound to DNA in the spleen than to DNA in the liver, and in the liver DNA binding was less than protein binding. The azo colour was also bound to all fractions in the livers of guinea-pigs. A ^{3}H-label in DNA was not liberated by hydrolyzing enzymes; and some of the azo colour remained bound to DNA 12 weeks after its injection into rats (Roberts & Warwick, 1966a,b; Warwick & Roberts, 1967).

The levels of binding of tritiated DAB and of the non-carcinogenic 2-methyl-4-dimethylaminoazobenzene to different cell fractions of rat liver and spleen following a single oral administration were similar, except that more DNA was bound to the carcinogen between 4 and 8 hours after administration (Albert & Warwick, 1972).

Feeding rats a high riboflavin diet, which inhibits the carcinogenic action of DAB, reduced the binding to both protein and DNA of a single injected dose of DAB, but to a greater extent to DNA. The binding of the carcinogenic 3'-methyl-4-dimethylaminoazobenzene to DNA was six times greater than that of 2-methyl-4-dimethylaminoazobenzene (Dingman & Sporn, 1967).

When ^{14}C-labelled DAB or 2-methyl-4-dimethylaminoazobenzene were given continuously to rats in the diet, the binding of 2-methyl-4-dimethylamino-azobenzene to liver proteins was slightly higher than that of the carcinogenic compound. DAB was, however, bound much more to the DNA of the liver than was the non-carcinogenic analogue (Chauveau & Benoit, 1973).

Degradation of the RNA and DNA from livers of rats given injections of MAB-prime ring-^{3}H yields derivatives which are identical to the compounds prepared by reactions of N-benzoyloxy-MAB with guanosine or deoxyguanosine. They were identified as N-(guanosin-8-yl)-MAB and N-(deoxy-guanosin-8-yl)-MAB (Miller, 1970).

(vi) *Effect of diet and other modifying factors on tumour incidence*

The carcinogenic action of DAB and other aminoazo compounds is influenced by diet: the addition of dried milk or yeast to a diet of brown rice and carrots with DAB delayed and reduced the incidence of tumours; riboflavin and casein added to the diet also reduced tumour incidence (Kensler, 1947). The addition of pyridoxine (Miller *et al.*, 1945b), vitamin B_{12} (Day *et al.*, 1950) or biotin (duVigneaud *et al.*, 1942) increased its carcinogenic action.

Administration of sodium glucuronate or glucuronolactone inhibited the development of tumours in rats treated with DAB (Odashima & Ishizawa, 1957). With diets containing DAB and 6% casein, cysteine supplementation increased the incidence of tumours when feeding was *ad libitum*, but decreased the carcinogenic action with paired feeding (White & Edwards, 1942a,b).

Of a number of oestrogens which delayed the carcinogenic action of DAB in male rats, 17-α-ethinyloestradiol was the most effective (Lacassagne *et al.*, 1968).

The carcinogenic action of DAB is reduced by treating animals with substances that increase the metabolism of foreign compounds, such as 3-methylcholanthrene and barbiturates (Ishidate, 1964). However, Odashima (1959) observed an increased incidence of hepatomas in experiments in which 3-methylcholanthrene was given after the administration of a sub-carcinogenic total dose of DAB.

The carcinogenic activity of DAB was less in rats that were treated at 10-11 weeks than in rats treated when they were 4-6 weeks old (Decloitre *et al.*, 1973).

(vii) *Mutagenicity data*

DAB has been reported to be non-mutagenic when tested in *Drosophila* for the production of X-linked recessive lethals (the purity of the compound was not defined) (Demerec *et al.*, 1949). It produced mutations at specific DNA regions (r-RNA and t-RNA genes) in *Drosophila* (Fahmy & Fahmy, 1972a,b).

DAB did not induce reverse mutations in *Salmonella* TA1538 in the presence of rat liver microsomal systems (Ames *et al.*, 1973), but they were produced in this strain when a urinary metabolite from rats fed DAB (purity not specified), following treatment with β-glucuronidase, was dissolved in dimethyl sulphoxide and assayed in the presence of a rat-liver microsomal system (Commoner *et al.*, 1974).

N-Benzoyloxy-N-methyl-4-aminoazobenzene, a synthetic N-hydroxy-ester, produced forward mutations in *Bacillus subtilis*, transforming DNA; however, N-methyl-4-aminoazobenzene, a demethylated metabolite of DAB, was inactive (Maher *et al.*, 1968).

(b) Man

Contact dermatitis has been observed in factory workers handling DAB (National Research Council, 1971).

3.3 Observations in man

No data were available to the Working Group.

4. Comments on Data Reported and Evaluation[1]

4.1 Animal data

para-Dimethylaminoazobenzene (DAB) is carcinogenic in rats, producing liver tumours after its administration by several routes, and in dogs, producing bladder tumours following its administration by the oral route. Results of oral administration studies were doubtful in mice and negative in hamsters and guinea-pigs; but these studies were of short duration, and the adequacy of the dose levels used was not known.

DAB has also been tested by subcutaneous injection in mice, and the results are suggestive of local and hepatic carcinogenicity. Treatment of newborn animals produced systemic carcinogenic effects in mice; the negative results obtained in rats are doubtful, since the period of

---

[1]See also the section, "Animal Data in Relation to the Evaluation of Risk to Man" in the introduction to this volume, p. 15.

observation was too short. Skin-painting with DAB produced epidermal tumours in rats but not in mice.

An extensive dose-response study was carried out in rats: the lowest effective dose was 1 mg/rat/day and the highest non-effective dose, 0.3 mg/rat/day.

4.2 Human data

No case reports or epidemiological studies were available to the Working Group.

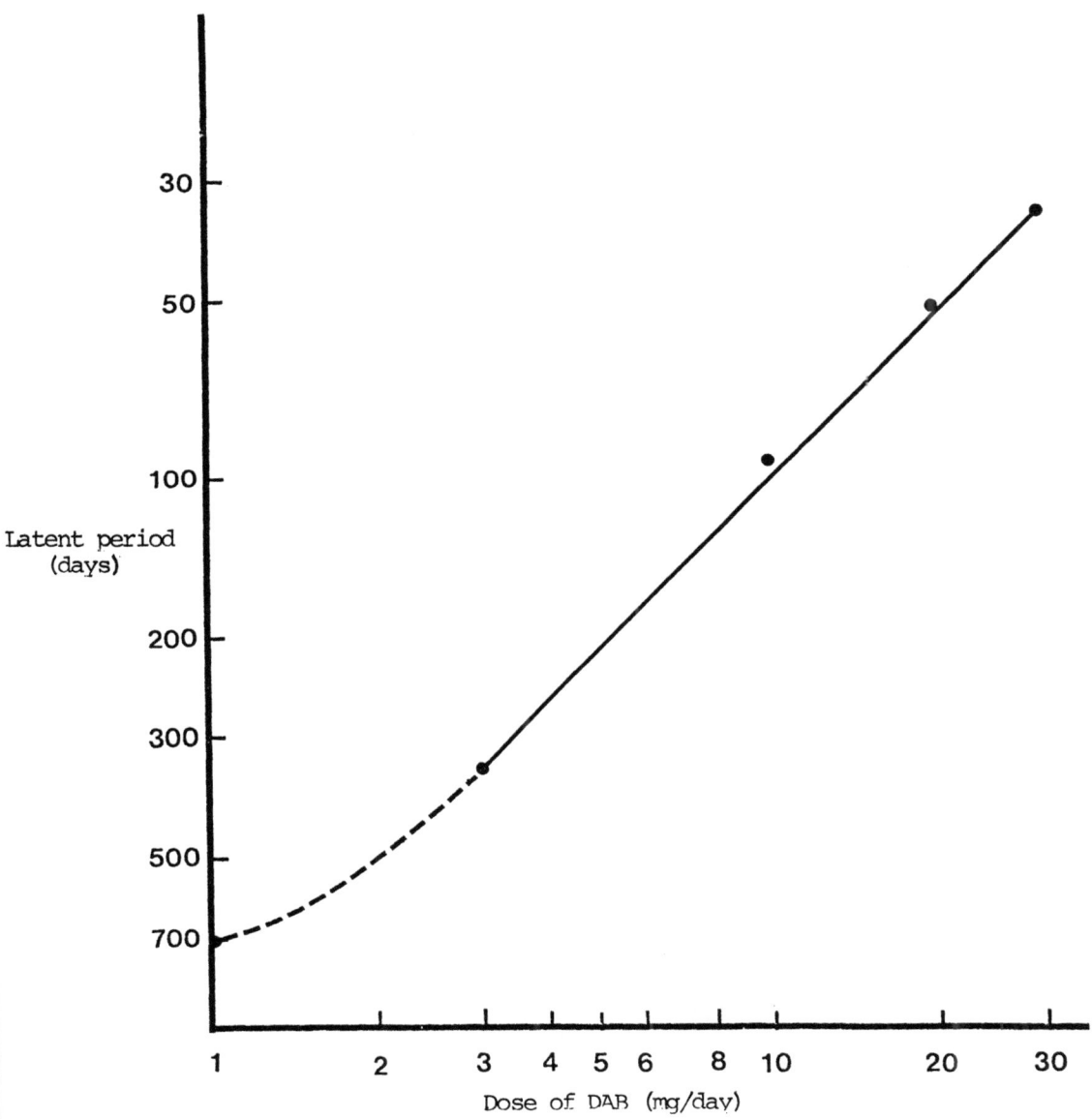

Figure 1*

Relationship between latent period for the appearance of liver cancer in rats fed DAB at different dose levels

* From Druckrey, 1951

5. References

Akamatsu, Y. & Ikegami, R. (1968) Induction of hepatoma and systemic amyloidosis in mice by 4-(dimethylamino)azobenzene feeding. Gann, 59, 201-206

Albert, A.E. & Warwick, G.P. (1972) The subcellular distribution of tritiated 4-dimethylaminoazobenzene and 2-methyl-4-dimethylaminoazobenzene in rat liver and spleen following a single oral administration. Chem.-biol. Interact., 5, 65-68

Ames, B.N., Durston, W.E., Yamasaki, E. & Lee, F.D. (1973) Carcinogens are mutagens: a simple test system combining liver homogenates for activation and bacteria for detection. Proc. nat. Acad. Sci., 70, 2281-2285

Andervont, H.B. & Edwards, J.E. (1943) Carcinogenic action of two azo compounds in mice. J. nat. Cancer Inst., 3, 349-354

Baba, T. & Takayama, S. (1961) Influence of p-dimethylaminoazobenzene (DAB) pretreatment in neonatal stage on the DAB hepato-carcinogenesis in the adult rats, with special reference to sex difference in the carcinogenesis. Gann, 52, 73-82

Boissonnas, R.A., Turner, R. & duVigneaud, V. (1949) Metabolic study of the methyl groups of butter yellow. J. biol. Chem., 180, 1053-1058

Booth, J. & Boyland, E. (1957) The biochemistry of aromatic amines. III. Enzymic hydroxylation by rat-liver microsomes. Biochem. J., 66, 73-78

Chauveau, J. & Benoit, A. (1973) Fixation au DNA et aux protéines hépatiques de deux composés azoïques de pouvoir cancérogène différent. C.R. Acad. Sci. (Paris), 276, 235-238

Commoner, B., Vithayathil, A.J. & Henry, J.I. (1974) Detection of metabolic carcinogen intermediates in urine of carcinogen-fed rats by means of bacterial mutagenesis. Nature (Lond.), 249, 850-852

Conney, A.H., Miller, E.C. & Miller, J.A. (1956) The metabolism of methylated aminoazo dyes. V. Evidence for induction of enzyme synthesis in the rat by 3-methylcholanthrene. Cancer Res., 16, 450-459

Day, P.L., Payne, L.D. & Dinning, J.S. (1950) Procarcinogenic effect of vitamin B_{12} on p-dimethylaminoazobenzene-fed rats. Proc. Soc. exp. Biol. (N.Y.), 74, 854-855

Decloitre, F., Meunier, M. & Auffret, M. (1972) Effet de l'ingestion du p-diméthylaminoazobenzène (DAB) et du 3'-méthyl-DAB sur les capacités d'activation du DAB et d'azoréduction des microsomes de foie de rat. C.R. Acad. Sci. (Paris), 274, 776-779

Decloitre, F., Chauveau, J. & Martin, M. (1973) Influence of age and 3-methylcholanthrene on azo-dye carcinogenesis and metabolism of *p*-dimethylaminoazobenzene in rat liver. Int. J. Cancer, 11, 676-680

Demerec, M., Wallace, B., Witkin, E.M. & Bertani, G. (1949) The Gene. In: Carnegie Institution of Washington Yearbook, 1948-1949, No. 48, Washington DC, pp. 154-166

DFG (Deutsche Forschungsgemeinschaft) (1957) Farbstoff-Kommission, Toxikologische Daten von Farbstoffen und ihre Zulassung für Lebensmittel in verschiedenen Ländern, Mitt. 6(2), Wiesbaden, Steiner Verlag, p. 145

Dingman, G.W. & Sporn, M.B. (1967) The binding of metabolites of aminoazo dyes to rat liver DNA *in vivo*. Cancer Res., 27, 938-944

DiPaolo, J.A., Nelson, R.L., Donovan, P.J. & Evans, C.H. (1973) Host-mediated *in vivo-in vitro* assay for chemical carcinogenesis. Arch. Path., 95, 380-385

Druckrey, H. (1943) Quantitative Grundlagen der Krebserzeugung. Klin. Wschr., 22, 532-534

Druckrey, H. (1951) Experimentelle Beiträge zum Mechanismus der cancerogenen Wirkung. Arzneimittel.-Forsch., 1, 383-394

Druckrey, H. (1967) Quantitative aspects in chemical carcinogenesis. In: Truhaut, R., ed., Potential Carcinogenic Hazards from Drugs, UICC Monogr. Series, 7, 60-78

Druckrey, H. & Küpfmüller, K. (1948) Quantitative Analyse der Krebsentstehung. Z. Naturforsch., 3b, 254-266

Fahmy, O.G. & Fahmy, M.J. (1972a) Mutagenic selectivity for the RNA-forming genes in relation to the carcinogenicity of alkylating agents and polycyclic aromatics. Cancer Res., 32, 550-557

Fahmy, O.G. & Fahmy, M.J. (1972b) Genetic properties of substituted derivatives of N-methyl-4-aminoazobenzene in relation to azo-dye carcinogenesis. Int. J. Cancer, 10, 194-206

FAO/WHO (1973) List of Additives Evaluated for their Safety-in-Use in Food, First Series, CAC/FAL 1-1973, p. 45

Fare, G. (1966) Rat skin carcinogenesis by topical applications of some azo dyes. Cancer Res., 26, 2405-2408

Fischer, W. (1954) Durch Buttergelb erzeugte Tumoren. Arch. Geschwülstforsch., 7, 301-320

Griess, P. (1877) *para*-Dimethylaminoazobenzene. Ber. dtsch. chem. Ges., 10, 525

Hancock, R.L. & Forrester, P.I. (1973) Increase in soluble RNA methylase activities by chemical carcinogens. Cancer Res., 33, 1747-1753

Hultin, T. (1957) Reactions of C^{14}-labeled carcinogenic azo dyes with rat liver proteins. Exp. Cell Res., 13, 47-59

Ishidate, M. (1964) Combined effect of carcinogens and co-carcinogens on metabolic process. Acta Un. int. Cancr, 20, 909-914

Jaffé, W.G. (1947) The response of mice to the simultaneous application of two different carcinogenic agents. Cancer Res., 7, 529-530

Kensler, C.J. (1947) Effect of diet on the production of liver tumors in the rat by N,N-dimethyl-p-aminoazobenzene. Ann. N.Y. Acad. Sci., 49, 29-40

Kensler, C.J. (1948) The influence of diet on the ability of rat-liver slices to destroy the carcinogen N,N-dimethyl-p-aminoazobenzene. Cancer, 1, 483-488

Kensler, C.J. (1949) The influence of diet on the riboflavin content and the ability of rat liver slices to destroy the carcinogen N,N-dimethyl-p-aminoazobenzene. J. biol. Chem., 179, 1079-1084

Ketterer, B. (1972) Proteins that bind carcinogen metabolites. Biochem. J., 126, 3P-4P

Ketterer, B., Holt, S.J. & Ross-Mansell, P. (1967a) The effect of a single intraperitoneal dose of the hepatocarcinogen 4-dimethylaminoazobenzene on the rough-surfaced endoplasmic reticulum of the liver of the rat. Biochem. J., 103, 692-698

Ketterer, B., Ross-Mansell, P. & Whitehead, J.K. (1967b) The isolation of carcinogen-binding protein from livers of rats given 4-dimethylaminoazobenzene. Biochem. J., 103, 316-324

Ketterer, B., Ross-Mansell, P. & Davidson, H. (1968) The effect of 4-dimethylaminoazobenzene and corn oil on azo-dye reductase in the rat liver. Biochem. J., 107, 15P-16P

Kinosita, R. (1936) Researches on the cancerogenesis of the various chemical substances. Gann, 30, 423-426

Kinosita, R. (1937) Special report. Studies on the cancerogenic chemical substances. Tr. Jap. Path. Soc., 27, 665-727

Kirby, A.H.M. (1945) Studies in carcinogenesis with azo compounds. I. The action of four azo dyes in mixed and pure strain mice. Cancer Res., 5, 673-682

Lacassagne, A., Jayle, M.F. & Hurst, L. (1968) Influence exercée par différents oestrogènes sur la cancérisation du foie du rat par le *para*-diméthyl-aminoazobenzène (DAB). C.R. Acad. Sci. (Paris), 267, 137-140

Law, L.W. (1941) The cancer producing properties of azo compounds in mice. Cancer Res., 1, 397-401

Lin, J-K., Miller, J.A. & Miller, E.C. (1968) Studies on structures of polar dyes derived from the liver proteins of rats fed N-methyl-4-aminoazobenzene. III. Tyrosine and homocysteine sulfoxide polar dyes. Biochemistry, 8, 1573-1583

Lin, J-K., Hsu, S-M. & Wu, Y-H. (1972) Methaemoglobin - induced by carcinogenic aminoazo dyes in rats. Biochem. Pharmacol., 21, 2147-2150

MacDonald, J.C., Plescia, A.M., Miller, E.C. & Miller, J.A. (1952) Studies on the metabolism of various N-methyl-C^{14}-subsituted aminoazo dyes. Cancer Res., 12, 280

Maher, V.M., Miller, E.C., Miller, J.A. & Szybalski, W. (1968) Mutations and decreases in density of transforming DNA produced by derivatives of the carcinogens 2-acetylaminofluorene and N-methyl-4-aminoazobenzene. Mol. Pharmacol., 4, 411-426

Maruya, H. & Tanaka, Y. (1936) Buttergelb. Osaka Igakkai Zasshi, 35, 2304

Matsumoto, M. & Terayama, H. (1961) Studies on the mechanism of liver carcinogenesis by certain aminoazo dyes. V. N-Demethylation of various aminoazobenzene derivatives by rat liver homogenate, with respect to the carcinogenic potency. Gann, 52, 239-245

Matsumoto, M. & Terayama, H. (1965) Studies on the mechanism of liver carcinogenesis by certain aminoazo dyes. VII. Reductive cleavage of various aminoazo dyes with rat-liver homogenate. Gann, 56, 169-175

Mecke, R. & Schmähl, D. (1957) Die Spaltbarkeit der Azo-Brücke durch Hefe. Arzneimittel.-Forsch., 7, 335-340

Merck & Co. (1968) The Merck Index, 8th ed., Rahway, N.J., p. 374

Miller, E.C. (1974) The metabolic activation of aromatic amines and amides. In: Program for XIth International Cancer Congress, Florence, 1974, Vol. I, Geneva, UICC, p. 11

Miller, E.C. & Miller, J.A. (1947) The presence and significance of bound aminoazo dyes in the livers of rats fed *p*-dimethylaminoazobenzene. Cancer Res., 7, 468-480

Miller, E.C., Baumann, C.A. & Rusch, H.P. (1945b) Certain effects of dietary pyridoxine and casein on the carcinogenicity of *p*-dimethyl-aminoazobenzene. Cancer Res., 5, 713-716

Miller, J.A. (1970) Carcinogenesis by chemicals: an overview. Cancer Res., 30, 559-576

Miller, J.A. & Miller, E.C. (1953) The carcinogenic aminoazo dyes. Advanc. Cancer Res., 1, 339-396

Miller, J.A., Miller, E.C. & Baumann, C.A. (1945a) On the methylation and demethylation of certain carcinogenic azo dyes in the rat. Cancer Res., 5, 162-168

Mori, K. & Nakahara, W. (1940) Effect of liver feeding on the production of malignant tumors, based on injections of carcinogenic substances. Gann, 34, 188-190

Mori, K., Ichii, S. & Sigeta, Y. (1956) Inhibition of experimental production of liver cancer by tobacco tar. Gann, 47, 97-103

Mueller, G.C. & Miller, J.A. (1949) The reductive cleavage of 4-dimethylaminoazobenzene by rat liver: the intracellular distribution of the enzyme system and its requirement for triphosphopyridine nucleotide. J. biol. Chem.., 180, 1125-1136

Mueller, G.C. & Miller, J.A. (1951) The oxidative demethylation of N-methylaminoazo dyes by rat liver homogenates. Cancer Res., 11, 271

National Research Council (1971) Food Colors, Washington DC, National Academy of Sciences, p. 7

Nelson, A.A. & Woodard, G. (1953) Tumors of the urinary bladder, gall bladder and liver in dogs fed o-aminoazotoluene or p-dimethylaminoazobenzene. J. nat. Cancer Inst., 13, 1497-1509

Odashima, S. (1959) Development of liver cancers in the rat by 20-methylcholanthrene painting following initial 4-dimethylaminoazobenzene feeding. Gann, 50, 321-345

Odashima, S. & Ishizawa, T. (1957) On the correlation between chemical carcinogens and their metabolism. II. The effect of sodium glucuronate or glucuronolactone on the development of liver cancer in rats fed DAB. Gann, 48, 583-585

Opie, E.L. (1947) Cytochondria of normal cells, of tumor cells and of cells with various injuries. J. exp. Med., 86, 45-54

Orr, J.W. (1940) The histology of the rat's liver during the course of carcinogenesis by butter-yellow (p-dimethylaminoazobenzene). J. Path. Bact., 50, 393-408

Orr, J.W. & Price, D.E. (1948) Observations on the hepatotoxic action of the carcinogen p-dimethylaminoazobenzene. J. Path. Bact., 60, 461-469

Poirier, L.A., Miller, J.A., Miller, E.C. & Sato, K. (1967) N-Benzoyloxy-N-methyl-4-aminoazobenzene: its carcinogenic activity in the rat and its reactions with proteins and nucleic acids and their constituents *in vitro*. Cancer Res., 27, 1600-1613

Rees, K.R., Rowland, G.F. & Varcoe, J.S. (1965) Intranuclear changes in rat liver during the early stages of feeding the hepatocarcinogens thioacetamide and 4-dimethylaminoazobenzene. Brit. J. Cancer, 19, 72-82

Roberts, J.J. & Warwick, G.P. (1966a) The covalent binding of metabolites of dimethylaminoazobenzene, β-naphthylamine and aniline to nucleic acids *in vivo*. Int. J. Cancer, 1, 179-196

Roberts, J.J. & Warwick, G.P. (1966b) Covalent binding of 4-dimethylaminophenylazo-^{3}H-benzene (butter yellow) metabolites with liver ribosomal RNA: the dissociation of the binding mechanism from the orotic acid incorporating system. Int. J. Cancer, 1, 573-578

Robinson, P.J., Ryan, A.J. & Wright, S.E. (1964) Metabolism of some dimethylaminoazobenzene derivatives. J. Pharm. Pharmacol., 16, 30T-82T

Roe, F.J.C., Warwick, G.P., Carter, R.L., Peto, R., Ross, W.C.J., Mitchley, B.C.V. & Barron, N.A. (1971) Liver and lung tumors in mice exposed at birth to 4-dimethylaminoazobenzene or its 2-methyl or 3'-methyl derivatives. J. nat. Cancer Inst., 47, 593-601

Roussy, G. & Guérin, M. (1946) Recherches sur l'action cancérogène de certaines substances colorantes. Bull. Acad. Med. (Paris), 130, 156-161

Scribner, J.D., Miller, J.A. & Miller, E.C. (1965) 3-Methylmercapto-N-methyl-4-aminoazobenzene: an alkaline degradation product of a labile protein-bound dye in the livers of rats fed N,N-dimethyl-4-aminoazobenzene. Biochem. Biophys. Res. Comm., 20, 560-565

Society of Dyers and Colourists (1971) Colour Index, 3rd ed., Vol. III, Bradford, Yorkshire, Deanhouse Piccadilly, p. 3566

Sorof, S. & Cohen, P.P. (1951) Electrophoretic and ultracentrifugal studies on the soluble proteins of various tumors and of livers from rats fed 4-dimethylaminoazobenzene. Cancer Res., 11, 376-382

Stevenson, E.S., Dobriner, K. & Rhoads, C.P. (1942) The metabolism of dimethylaminoazobenzene (butter yellow) in rats. Cancer Res., 2, 160-167

Sugiura, K. & Rhoads, C.P. (1941) Experimental liver cancer in rats and its inhibition by rice-bran extract, yeast and yeast extract. Cancer Res., 1, 3-16

Terayama, H. (1967) Aminoazo carcinogenesis - methods and biochemical problems. Methods Cancer Res., 1, 399-449

Terracini, B. & Della Porta, G. (1961) Feeding with aminoazo dyes, thioacetamide and ethionine. Arch. Path., 71, 566-575

Truhaut, R. (1955) Sur l'action cancérigène de certaines matières colorantes. Importance en hygiène alimentaire, en thérapeutique et en hygiène générale. Ann. pharm. fr., 13, 36-51

US Tariff Commission (1922) Census of Dyes and Other Synthetic Organic Chemicals, 1921, Tariff Information Series No. 26, Washington DC, US Government Printing Office, p. 63

US Tariff Commission (1974) Synthetic Organic Chemicals, US Production and Sales, 1972, TC Publication 681, Washington DC, US Government Printing Office, p. 64

duVigneaud, V., Spangler, J.M., Burk, D., Kensler, C.J., Sugiura, K. & Rhoads, C.P. (1942) The procarcinogenic effect of biotin in butter yellow tumour formation. Science, 95, 174-176

Walker, R. (1970) The metabolism of azo compounds: a review of the literature. Fd Cosmet. Toxicol., 8, 659-676

Warwick, G.P. & Roberts, J.J. (1967) Persistent binding of butter yellow metabolites to rat liver DNA. Nature (Lond.), 213, 1206-1207

White, J. & Edwards, J.E. (1942a) Effect of dietary cystine on the development of hepatic tumors in rats fed p-dimethylaminoazobenzene (butter yellow). J. nat. Cancer Inst., 2, 535-538

White, J. & Edwards, J.E. (1942b) Effect of supplementary methionine or choline plus cystine on the incidence of p-dimethylaminoazobenzene-induced hepatic tumors in the rat. J. nat. Cancer Inst., 3, 43-59

Yanai, R. & Kuretani, K. (1968) Effect of terephthalic acid on the activities of p-dimethylaminoazobenzene metabolizing enzymes in rat liver. Chem. pharm. Bull., 16, 136-141 *para*-DIMETHYLAMINOBENZENEDIAZO SODIUM SULPHONATE

1. Chemical and Physical Data

1.1 Synonyms and trade names

Chem. Abstr. Reg. Serial No.: 140-56-7

Chem. Abstr. Name: 4-[(Dimethylamino)phenyl]diazene sulphonic acid, sodium salt

For other names of which the Working Group was aware see index, p. 297.

1.2 Chemical formula and molecular weight

$(H_3C)_2N\text{-}C_6H_4\text{-}N=N^+\text{ }SO_3Na^-$

$C_8H_{10}N_3NaO_3S$ Mol. wt: 251.2

1.3 Chemical and physical properties of the pure substance

(a) Description: Yellowish-brown, odourless crystals

(b) Solubility: Soluble in water (3 g/100 ml at 25°C); soluble in dimethyl formamide and ethanol; insoluble in diethyl ether, benzene and petroleum oils

1.4 Technical products and impurities

No data were available to the Working Group.

2. Production, Use, Occurrence and Analysis

For important background information on this section, see preamble, p. 17.

2.1 Production and use

para-Dimethylaminobenzenediazo sodium sulphate can be synthesized by reacting diazotized *para*-dimethylaminoaniline with sodium sulphite (Martin, 1971); it is not known whether this method is used for commercial production.

Although commercial production of this chemical has not been reported to the US Tariff Commission, it is believed that approximately 11,500 kg were produced by one US company in 1973. Imports through the principal US customs districts from 1966 to 1969 reached a maximum of 14,500 kg in 1968 (US Tariff Commission, 1969); none have been reported in recent years.

To our knowledge *para*-dimethylaminobenzenediazo sodium sulphonate is not currently manufactured commercially in Western Europe or Japan.

This chemical is registered by the US Environmental Protection Agency for use as the active ingredient in several commercial fungicides used on ornamentals, sugarcane, avocados, lawns and turf. It is also permitted for the fungicidal treatment of the following seeds: beans, beets, corn, cotton, cucumbers, peas, sorghum, spinach and sugar beets (Carter *et al.*, 1973). Since these are non-food uses, tolerances for this chemical have not been established.

2.2 Occurrence

No data were available to the Working Group.

2.3 Analysis

See section, "General Remarks on the Substances Considered", p. 28.

3. Biological Data Relevant to the Evaluation of Carcinogenic Risk to Man

3.1 Carcinogenicity and related studies in animals

(a) Oral administration

Rat: Sprague-Dawley rats were fed a diet containing *para*-dimethylaminobenzenediazo sodium sulphonate (DAS) at a concentration of 1000 mg/kg of diet for 12 months; hepatomas described as 'similar to those produced by dimethylaminoazobenzene' were produced. Neither the number of rats used nor the tumour incidence were reported (Herrmann & DuBois, 1949a).

Groups of 20 Holtzman rats were fed a diet containing 1.35 or 4.0 millimoles DAS per kg of diet (339 or 1005 mg DAS/kg of diet) for 15 months. No liver tumours were observed in 12 and 14 rats examined at that time

(Miller et al., 1957). [In both studies the compound was synthesized according to the method given by Stolle (1912), but data on purity were not available.]

3.2 Other relevant biological data

(a) Animals

The LD_{50}'s for DAS in various species are as follows: mice, 70 mg/kg bw; rats, 15 mg/kg bw; guinea-pigs, 30 mg/kg bw; rabbits, 10-20 mg/kg bw; dogs, 5-10 mg/kg bw. The oral LD_{50} for rats was about 55 mg/kg bw (Herrmann & DuBois, 1949a). Either the addition of DAS to homogenates of rat, mouse or guinea-pig kidney or its administration in lethal doses to the animals causes a decrease in the aerobic phosphorylation of creatine (Herrmann & DuBois, 1949b).

3.3 Observations in man

No data were available to the Working Group.

4. Comments on Data Reported and Evaluation

4.1 Animal data

Contradictory results were obtained in two studies in which *para*-dimethylaminobenzenediazo sodium sulphonate was given orally to rats. The experiment suggesting hepatocarcinogenicity was inadequately reported, while the experiment suggesting lack of hepatocarcinogenicity was of too short duration. Therefore, no evaluation can be made.

4.2 Human data

No case reports or epidemiological studies were available to the Working Group.

5. References

Carter, L.J., Michell, J.G. & Wilson, D.J. (1973) *EPA Compendium of Registered Pesticides*, Vol. II, *Fungicides and Nematicides*, Technical Service Division, Office of Pesticides Programs, US Environmental Protection Agency, Washington DC, US Government Printing Office, Part I, p. S-56-50.01

Herrmann, R.C. & DuBois, K.P. (1949a) Studies on the toxicity and pharmacological action of p-dimethylaminobenzene diazo sodium sulfonate (DAS). *J. Pharmacol. exp. Ther.*, 95, 262-271

Herrmann, R.C. & DuBois, K.P. (1949b) The effect of p-dimethylaminobenzene diazo sodium sulfonate (DAS) on the enzymatic reactions of intermediate carbohydrate metabolism. *J. Pharmacol. exp. Ther.*, 95, 272-285

Martin, H., ed. (1971) *Pesticide Manual*, 2nd ed., Ombersley, British Crop Protection Council, p. 183

Miller, J.A., Miller, E.C. & Finger, G.C. (1957) Further studies on the carcinogenicity of dyes related to 4-dimethylaminoazobenzene. The requirement for an unsubstituted 2-position. *Cancer Res.*, 17, 387-398

Stolle, R. (1912) Über 4-Dimethylamido-diazobenzolchlorid. *Ber. dtsch. chem. Ges.*, 45, 2680-2685

US Tariff Commission (1969) *Imports of Benzenoid Chemicals and Products, 1968*, TC Publication 290, Washington DC, US Government Printing Office, p. 92

EVANS BLUE

1. Chemical and Physical Data

1.1 Synonyms and trade names

Colour Index No.: 23860

Colour Index Name: C.I. Direct Blue 53

Chem. Abstr. Reg. Serial No.: 314-13-6

Chem. Abstr. Name: 6,6'-{[3,3'-Dimethyl(1,1-biphenyl)-4,4'-diyl]bis(azo)}-bis(4-amino-5-hydroxy)-1,3-naphthalenedisulphonic acid, tetrasodium salt

For other names of which the Working Group was aware, see index, p. 297.

1.2 Chemical formula and molecular weight

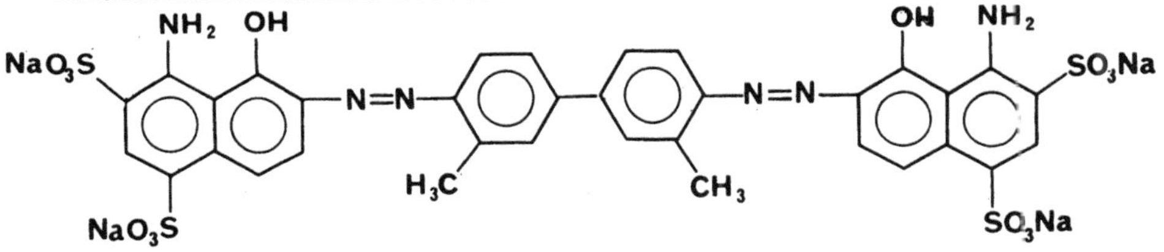

$C_{34}H_{24}N_6Na_4O_{14}S_4$ Mol. wt: 960.8

1.3 Chemical and physical properties of the pure substance

(a) Description: Blue crystals with bronze to green lustre

(b) Solubility: Soluble in water, ethanol, acids and alkalis

(c) Stability: Stable in aqueous solutions

1.4 Technical products and impurities

According to US industrial sources, Evans blue is not used in foods, drugs or cosmetics; thus its manufacture and testing do not conform to rigid chemical specifications, and its composition varies in order to meet customer shade and intensity requirements.

2. Production, Use, Occurrence and Analysis

For important background information on this section, see preamble, p. 17.

2.1 Production and use

Evans blue can be prepared by coupling tetrazotized *ortho*-tolidine with two equivalents of 1-amino-8-hydroxy-2,4-naphthalenedisulphonic acid (Chicago Acid) (Hartwell & Fieser, 1943); it is not known whether this method is used for commercial production, but in fact it is not believed to be manufactured on a large scale in the US, Western Europe or Japan.

Evans blue is reportedly used for dyeing textiles, leather and paper (Society of Dyers and Colourists, 1971) and as a diagnostic aid in blood volume determination (Merck & Co., 1968). According to the Deutsche Forschungsgemeinschaft (DFG, 1955, 1957) this colour was not approved for food use in any of the countries surveyed.

2.2 Occurrence

Evans blue is not known to occur in nature.

2.3 Analysis

See section, "General Remarks on the Substances Considered", p. 28.

3. Biological Data Relevant to the Evaluation of Carcinogenic Risk to Man

3.1 Carcinogenicity and related studies in animals

(a) Intraperitoneal administration

Rat: A group of 40 Wistar rats of both sexes, 3-4 months of age, received i.p. injections of 1 ml of a 1% aqueous solution of Evans blue every 2 weeks for 8 months. Commercial Evans blue from two sources was used. Early signs of toxicity were observed, and some animals were treated less frequently than indicated above. Ten animals developed histiocytic tumours of the liver, and 1 rat showed a reticulum-cell sarcoma of the mesenteric lymph nodes and peritoneum within 330 days after the start of treatment. No tumours occurred in 20 untreated controls after 340 days (Marshall, 1953).

Forty white rats weighing about 200 g were injected every 2 weeks with 1 ml of a 2% aqueous solution of commercial Evans blue (maximum, 17 injections/animal). The rats were sacrificed at regular intervals between the 14th and 475th day after the first injection; no tumours were found in 15 animals surviving 351-475 days (Rüttner & Brunner, 1956).

3.2 Other relevant biological data

(a) Animals

A dose of 200 mg Evans blue administered orally to dogs in which the intestinal flora had been eliminated by prior treatment with Nebacetin was found to be unabsorbed, 80-90% being recovered in the faeces; none was found in the tissues or plasma. Following i.v. injection of 2-3 mg/kg bw, 36-47% of the injected dose was recovered from the liver, kidney, spleen and bile; no colour was excreted in the urine (although 3% was found in the faeces of dogs with ligated bile ducts); only small amounts were found in the reticuloendothelial system; and the remainder of the colour was unaccounted for (Stoelinga & Van Munster, 1967). Very little Evans blue appears in dog urine after its i.v. injection for blood volume determination (Allen & Orahovats, 1948).

Evans blue and ^{131}I-labelled human serum albumin were injected intravenously into hamsters. During the first two minutes, the colour was removed from the circulation more rapidly than the albumin; afterwards they left the blood at the same rate, probably through binding of the colour to albumin (Wilde *et al.*, 1971).

Evans blue is teratogenic in rats following i.p. injection of 50-250 mg/kg bw on the 8th day of pregnancy (Beaudoin, 1968; Beaudoin & Pickering, 1960; Wilson, 1955).

(b) Man

Evans blue is excreted from the body at a lower rate than is trypan blue (Gregerson & Rawson, 1943). Although these colours are bound to protein, electrophoretic studies show that most binding occurs with Evans blue (Rawson, 1943; Schwarzkopf, 1963). *In vitro*, low concentrations of Evans blue (5-25 mg/100 ml of saline) were bound to α_1-lipoprotein and higher concentrations to albumin (Schen *et al.*, 1967).

3.3 Observations in man

No data were available to the Working Group.

Some suspicion of carcinogenicity of *ortho*-tolidine, a starting material and possible impurity of Evans blue, has been suggested (Scott, 1962), but supporting evidence is not available (IARC, 1972).

4. Comments on Data Reported and Evaluation[1]

4.1 Animal data

Evans blue was carcinogenic in one study in rats when administered intraperitoneally, the only species and route tested. It produced sarcomas of the reticuloendothelial system in the liver.

4.2 Human data

No case reports or epidemiological studies were available to the Working Group.

---

[1] See also the section, "Animal Data in Relation to the Evaluation of Risk to Man" in the introduction to this volume, p. 15.

5. References

Allen, T.H. & Orahovats, P.D. (1948) Spectrophotometric measurement of traces of dye T-1824 by extraction with cellophane from both blood serum and urine of normal dogs. Amer. J. Physiol., 154, 27-37

Beaudoin, A.R. (1968) Teratogenic activity of six disazo dyes in the Wistar albino rat. Proc. Soc. exp. Biol. (N.Y.), 127, 215-219

Beaudoin, A.R. & Pickering, M.J. (1960) Teratogenic activity of several synthetic compounds structurally related to trypan blue. Anat. Rec., 137, 297-305

DFG (Deutsche Forschungsgemeinschaft) (1955) Kommission zur Bearbeitung des Lebensmittelfarbstoffproblems, Toxikologische Daten von Farbstoffen und ihre Zulassung für Lebensmittel in verschiedenen Ländern, Mitt. 6(1), Wiesbaden, Steiner Verlag

DFG (Deutsche Forschungsgemeinschaft) (1957) Farbstoff-Kommission, Toxikologische Daten von Farbstoffen und ihre Zulassung für Lebensmittel in verschiedenen Ländern, Mitt. 6(2), Wiesbaden, Steiner Verlag, p. 51

Gregerson, M.I. & Rawson, R.A. (1943) The disappearance of T-1824 and structurally related dyes from the blood stream. Amer. J. Physiol., 138, 698-707

Hartwell, J.L. & Fieser, L.F. (1943) In: Blatt, A.H., ed., Organic Synthesis, Vol. II, New York, John Wiley & Sons, p. 145

IARC (1972) IARC Monographs on the Evaluation of Carcinogenic Risk of Chemicals to Man, 1, 87-91

Marshall, A.H.E. (1953) The production of tumours of the reticular tissue by di-azo vital dyes. Acta path. microbiol. scand., 33, 1-9

Merck & Co. (1968) The Merck Index, 8th ed., Rahway, N.J., p. 446

Rawson, R.A. (1943) The binding of T-1824 and structurally related diazo dyes by the plasma proteins. Amer. J. Physiol., 138, 708-717

Rüttner, J.R. & Brunner, H.E. (1956) Zur Frage einer cancerogenen Wirkung der Azofarbstoffe Evans Blue und Trypanblau auf das retikuloendotheliale System der Leber. Schweiz. Z. Path. Bact., 19, 436-455

Schen, R.J., Rabinovitz, M., Goldschmid, A. & Tenne, M. (1967) The affinity of Evans blue for the α-1-lipoprotein of human serum. Clin. Chim. Acta, 16, 445-448

Schwartzkopff, W. (1963) Zur Bindung von Azofarbstoffen (Evans Blue, Trypanblau, Trypanrot) an Plasmaalbumin und ihre Verweildauer in Blutserum. Proteines biol. Fluids, 10, 255-262

Scott, T.S. (1962) *Carcinogenic and chronic toxic hazards of aromatic amines*, Amsterdam, New York, Elsevier, p. 55

Society of Dyers and Colourists (1971) *Colour Index*, 3rd ed., Bradford, Yorkshire, Deanhouse Piccadilly

Stoelinga, G.B.A. & Van Munster, P.J.J. (1967) The behavior of Evans blue (azodye T-1824) in the body after intravenous injection. *Acta physiol. pharmacol. neerl.*, 14, 391-409

Wilde, W.S., Hill, J.H., Wilson, E. & Schielke, G.P. (1971) Exchange of free and albumin-bound Evans blue in interstitium of hamster kidney. *Amer. J. Physiol.*, 220, 1991-1999

Wilson, J.G. (1955) Teratogenic activity of several azo dyes chemically related to trypan blue. *Anat. Res.*, 123, 313-333

4-HYDROXYAZOBENZENE

1. Chemical and Physical Data

1.1 Synonyms and trade names

Colour Index No.: 11800

Colour Index Name: C.I. Solvent Yellow 7

Chem. Abstr. Reg. Serial No.: 1689-82-3

Chem. Abstr. Name: 4-(Phenylazo) phenol

For other names of which the Working Group was aware see index, p. 297.

1.2 Chemical formula and molecular weight

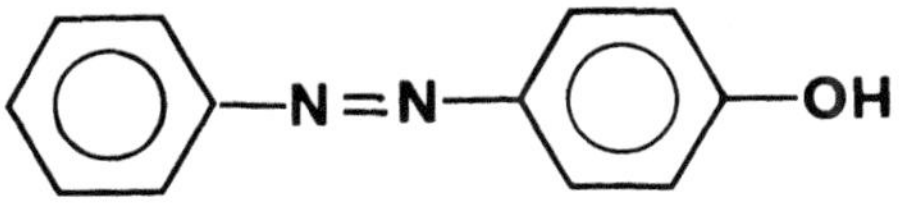

$$\text{C}_6\text{H}_5-\text{N}=\text{N}-\text{C}_6\text{H}_4-\text{OH}$$

$C_{12}H_{10}N_2O$ Mol. wt: 198.2

1.3 Chemical and physical properties of the pure substance

(a) Description: Orange prisms

(b) Melting-point: 155-156°C

(c) Boiling-point: 220-230°C (at 20 mm Hg)

(d) Solubility: Soluble in acetone, ethanol, benzene and ether; slightly soluble in hot water

1.4 Technical products and impurities

No data were available to the Working Group.

2. Production, Use, Occurrence and Analysis

For important background information on this section, see preamble, p. 17.

2.1 Production and use

4-Hydroxyazobenzene was first prepared by P. Griess in 1864 (Society of

Dyers and Colourists, 1971). It can be made by coupling diazotized aniline with phenol (Oddo & Puxeddu, 1905); it is not known whether this method is used for commercial production. It is not believed to be produced on a large-scale, however, in either the US or Western Europe. In Japan, this chemical was first produced in 1953, and one manufacturer reported production of 2000 kg in 1972. Separate data on exports were not available.

4-Hydroxyazobenzene has reportedly been used to colour varnishes, fats, waxes, resins and soaps (Society of Dyers and Colourists, 1971).

2.2 Occurrence

4-Hydroxyazobenzene is not known to occur in nature.

2.3 Analysis

See section, "General Remarks on the Substances Considered", p. 28.

3. Biological Data Relevant to the Evaluation of Carcinogenic Risk to Man

3.1 Carcinogenicity and related studies in animals

(a) Oral administration

Rat: Nine albino rats were fed a diet containing 4-hydroxyazobenzene (concentration not given); 4/5 rats dying between 159-284 days developed multiple papillomas of the forestomach (Kinosita & Harada, 1938).

A group of 12 male Sprague-Dawley rats was fed a diet containing 4-hydroxyazobenzene at a concentration of 53 mg/kg of diet for 9 months. No tumours were observed (Miller & Miller, 1948). [Although the duration of this experiemnt was inadequate, it was noted that 4-dimethylaminoazobenzene fed at a concentration of 60 mg/kg of diet to a similar group of rats produced a 100% incidence of liver tumours within 6 months.]

3.2 Other relevant biological data

(a) Animal

The urine of rabbits given 4-hydroxyazobenzene contained 2-acetamidophenol, 4 acetamidophenol, conjugated 4-aminophenol, conjugated 2-aminophenol (Bray *et al.*, 1951), and 4-hydroxyazobenzene glucuronide (Smith & Williams, 1951).

Doses of 500 and 700 mg 4-hydroxyazobenzene, which did not produce toxic effects, were completely absorbed from the diet of rabbits and were excreted mainly in the urine as glucuronide (Salant & Bengis, 1916).

The compound has been reported to be non-mutagenic when tested in *Drosophila* for the production of X-linked recessive lethals (the purity was not defined) (Demerec *et al.*, 1949).

3.3 <u>Observations in man</u>

No data were available to the Working Group.

4. <u>Comments on Data Reported and Evaluation</u>

4.1 <u>Animal data</u>

4-Hydroxyazobenzene was tested in rats by the oral route. An evaluation of its carcinogenicity was not possible due to the inadequate duration or inadequacy of reporting of the studies.

4.2 <u>Human data</u>

No case reports or epidemiological studies were available to the Working Group.

5. References

Bray, H.G., Clowes, R.C. & Thorpe, W.V. (1951) The metabolism of azobenzene and p-hydroxyazobenzene in the rabbit. Biochem. J., 49, lxv

Demerec, M., Wallace, B., Witkin, E.M. & Bertani, G. (1949) The Gene. In: Carnegie Institution of Washington Yearbook, 1948-1949, No. 48, Washington DC, pp. 154-166

Kinosita, R. & Harada, M. (1938) Production of multiple papillomas in the stomach of the rat by the oral administration of 4-oxyazobenzene. Gann, 32, 225-229

Miller, J.A. & Miller, E.C. (1948) The carcinogenicity of certain derivatives of p-dimethylaminoazobenzene in the rat. J. exp. Med., 87, 139-156

Oddo, G. & Puxeddu, E. (1905) Reduktion der Oxyazoverbindungen zu Aminophenolen vermittelst Phenylhydrazin. Ber. dtsch. chem. Ges., 38, 2752-2755

Salant, W. & Bengis, R. (1916) Physiological and pharmacological studies on coal-tar colors. I. Experiments with fat-soluble dyes. J. biol. Chem., 27, 403-427

Smith, J.N. & Williams, R.T. (1951) Studies in detoxication. 36. A note on the glucuronides of benzeneazophenol and benzeneazoresorcinol. Biochem. J., 48, 546-547

Society of Dyers and Colourists (1971) Colour Index, 3rd ed., Vol. III, Bradford, Yorkshire, Deanhouse Piccadilly, p. 3566

METHYL RED

1. Chemical and Physical Data

1.1 Synonyms and trade names

Colour Index No.: 13020

Colour Index Name: C.I. Acid Red 2

Chem. Abstr. Reg. Serial No.: 493-52-7

Chem. Abstr. Name: 2-[(4-Dimethylamino)phenylazo]benzoic acid

For other names of which the Working Group was aware see index, p. 297.

1.2 Chemical formula and molecular weight

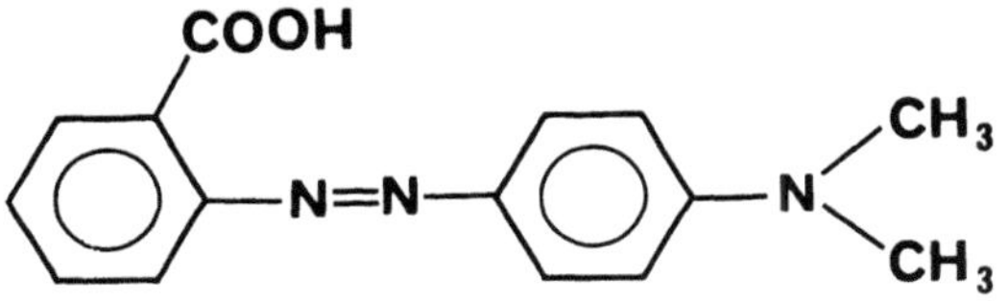

$C_{15}H_{15}N_3O_2$

Mol. wt: 269.3

1.3 Chemical and physical properties of the pure substance

(a) Description: Glistening violet crystals from toluene

(b) Melting-point: 181-182°C

(c) Absorption spectroscopy: λ_{max} 490 nm

(d) Solubility: Almost insoluble in water; moderately soluble in ethanol (0.1 g/100 ml warm ethanol); soluble in acetic acid, chloroform and lipids

1.4 Technical products and impurities

No data were available to the Working Group.

2. Production, Use, Occurrence and Analysis

For important background information on this section, see preamble, p. 17.

2.1 Production and use

Methyl red was first synthesized by E. Rupp & R. Loose in 1908 (Society of Dyers and Colourists, 1971). It can be made by coupling diazotized anthranilic acid with N,N-dimethylaniline (Howard & Pope, 1911), but it is not known whether this method is used for commercial production.

Production of methyl red in the US was first reported in 1921 (US Tariff Commission, 1922), but it is not now produced in that country and separate data on imports are not available. It is probably not currently produced on a large scale in Western Europe or Japan.

Methyl red is used as a pH indicator (Society of Dyers and Colourists, 1971).

The Deutsche Forschungsgemeinschaft (DFG, 1955, 1957) reported that it was not approved for food use in any of the countries surveyed.

2.2 Occurrence

Methyl red is not known to occur in nature.

2.3 Analysis

See section, "General Remarks on the Substances Considered", p. 28.

3. Biological Data Relevant to the Evaluation of Carcinogenic Risk to Man

A review on azo compounds, including methyl red, and their carcinogenic action has been published (Truhaut, 1955).

3.1 Carcinogenicity and related studies in animals

(a) Oral administration

Rat[*]: No tumours of the alimentary tract were observed in 5 male and 5 female Wistar rats fed a diet containing 40,000 mg methyl red per kg of

---

[*] Two articles by Kinosita (1936, 1937) have frequently been cited. The first study, in which liver tumours were reported, did not refer to methyl red but to a compound called "3-dimethylaminoazobenzol-1'-carbonsäure". The second article is a review briefly mentioning a 165-day feeding experiment, without reference to tumour production.

diet for up to 2 years. The median survival time was not reported (Willheim & Ivy, 1953).

3.2 Other relevant biological data

(a) Animals

Methyl red is bound to bovine serum albumin (Burkhard et al., 1961). Its azo link was reduced by a number of different strains of rat bacteria: the products of reduction are anthranilic acid (ortho-aminobenzoic acid) and dimethyl-para-phenylenediamine (Scheline, 1968; Soleim & Scheline, 1972).

3.3 Observations in man

No data were available to the Working Group.

4. Comments on Data Reported and Evaluation

4.1 Animal data

Methyl red was tested only by the oral route in rats. The inadequacy of the experiment does not allow an evaluation of the data with regard to the carcinogenicity of this compound.

4.2 Human data

No case reports or epidemiological studies were available to the Working Group.

5. References

Burkhard, R.K., Moore, F.A. & Louloudes, S.J. (1961) The interactions of the methyl reds and bovine serum albumin. Arch. Biochem. Biophys., 94, 291-300

DFG (Deutsche Forschungsgemeinschaft) (1955) Kommission zur Bearbeitung des Lebensmittelfarbstoffproblems, Toxikologische Daten von Farbstoffen und ihre Zulassung für Lebensmittel in verschiedenen Ländern, Mitt. 6(1), Wiesbaden, Steiner Verlag

DFG (Deutsche Forschungsgemeinschaft) (1957) Farbstoff-Kommission, Toxikologische Daten von Farbstoffen und ihre Zulassung für Lebensmittel in verschiedenen Ländern, Mitt. 6(2), Wiesbaden, Steiner Verlag, p. 43

Howard, H. & Pope, F.G. (1911) Indicators of the methyl red type. J. chem. Soc., 99, 1334-1336

Kinosita, R. (1936) Researches on the cancerogenesis of the various chemical substances. Gann, 30, 423-426

Kinosita, R. (1937) Special report. Studies on the cancerogenic chemical substances. Tr. Jap. Path. Soc., 27, 665-727

Scheline, R.R. (1968) The metabolism of drugs and other organic compounds by the intestinal microflora. Acta pharmacol. toxicol., 26, 332-342

Society of Dyers and Colourists (1971) Colour Index, 3rd ed., Vol. I, Bradford, Yorkshire, Deanhouse Piccadilly, p. 1123

Soleim, H.A. & Scheline, R.R. (1972) Metabolism of xenobiotics by strains of intestinal bacteria. Acta pharmacol. toxicol., 31, 471-480

Truhaut, R. (1955) Sur l'action cancérigène de certaines matières colorantes. Importance en hygiène alimentaire, en thérapeutique et en hygiène générale. Ann. pharm. fr., 13, 36-51

Willheim, R. & Ivy, A.C. (1953) A preliminary study concerning the possibility of dietary carcinogenesis. Gastroenterology, 23, 1-19

US Tariff Commission (1922) Census of Dyes and Other Synthetic Organic Chemicals, 1921, Tariff Information Series No. 26, Washington DC, US Government Printing Office, p. 68

OIL ORANGE SS

1. Chemical and Physical Data

1.1 Synonyms and trade names

Colour Index No.: 12100

Colour Index Name: C.I. Solvent Orange 2

Chem. Abstr. Reg. Serial No.: 2646-17-5

Chem. Abstr. Name: 1-[(2-Methylphenyl)azo]-2-naphthalenol

For other names of which the Working Group was aware see index, p. 297.

1.2 Chemical formula and molecular weight

$C_{17}H_{14}N_2O$

Mol. wt: 262.3

1.3 Chemical and physical properties of the pure substance

(a) Description: Red needles crystallized from glacial acetic acid

(b) Melting-point: 131°C (recrystallized from glacial acetic acid)

(c) Solubility: Insoluble in water; slightly soluble in ethanol, chloroform and benzene

(d) Absorption spectroscopy: λ_{max} 492 nm (in chloroform)

1.4 Technical products and impurities

Specifications for oil orange SS given by the Japan Food Hygiene Association (1974) require it to contain a minimum of 98% pure dye. When used as a colour reference standard, it must contain 99.9% of the pure chemical (Fujii et al., 1965).

According to US industrial sources, when oil orange SS is not used in foods, drugs or cosmetics, its manufacture and testing do not conform to rigid chemical specifications, and its composition varies in order to meet customer shade and intensity requirements.

2. Production, Use, Occurrence and Analysis

For important background information on this section, see preamble, p. 17.

2.1 Production and use

Oil orange SS was first prepared by Z. Roussin & A. Poirrier in 1878 (Society of Dyers and Colourists, 1971). It can be synthesized by coupling diazotized *ortho*-toluidine with 2-naphthol (Zinke, 1866), but it is not known whether this is the method used for commercial production.

Large-scale production of oil orange SS in the US was first reported in 1940 (US Tariff Commission, 1941). In 1972, since only one US manufacturer reported production of this colour, separate data were not published, and it was included in a miscellaneous category containing at least 11 other colours, with a total combined production of 236,000 kg (US Tariff Commission, 1974). Separate data on US imports and exports were not available.

There may be as many as five producers of oil orange SS in Western Europe, but current production is believed to be small. In 1972, there were believed to be four Japanese producers, who manufactured 4100 kg of this colour. Separate data on Japanese imports and exports were not available.

Oil orange SS is reportedly used for colouring varnishes, oils, fats and waxes (Society of Dyers and Colourists, 1971); in Japan, it is probably used as a colour in petroleum products, cosmetics and drugs applied externally (except on lips and mucous membrane).

The Deutsche Forschungsgemeinschaft (DFG, 1955) reported that this substance had been approved for use as a general food colouring in Canada, Greece, Japan, Mexico, New Zealand, Norway, Peru and South Africa. A later edition (DFG, 1957) reported approval in Cuba, the Dominican Republic, Guatemala and Venezuela, but indicated that approval had been withdrawn in Canada, New Zealand and Norway. Approval for its use in food was withdrawn in Japan prior to 1966; however, it is permitted for certain non-food uses (Japan Food Hygiene Association, 1974).

Oil orange SS was added to the US approved list of food, drug and cosmetic colours in 1939; however in 1956, on the basis of toxicological data, it was removed from the list for use in food but was permitted in externally applied drugs and cosmetics. In 1963, it was removed for even these uses (National Research Council, 1971).

2.2 Occurrence

Oil orange SS is not known to occur in nature.

2.3 Analysis

See section, "General Remarks on the Substances Considered", p. 28.

3. Biological Data Relevant to the Evaluation of Carcinogenic Risk to Man

3.1 Carcinogenicity and related studies in animals

(a) Oral administration

Mouse: A group of 15 male and 15 female stock albino mice was fed a diet containing 1000 mg oil orange SS per kg of diet for 52 weeks (weekly intake, 14 mg/mouse; total intake, 728 mg/mouse). Only 12 males and 10 females survived 20 or more weeks, and the experiment was terminated at 90 weeks. Of 19 animals examined between 20-89 weeks, 9 males had developed benign intestinal tumours and 1 male a carcinoma of the intestine; 1/13 controls injected with arachis oil and dying at 50-90 weeks developed a benign intestinal tumour. Treatment with the colour did not significantly raise the lymphoma incidence (Bonser et al., 1956).

Rat: Groups of 20 male and 20 female rats, 5-6 weeks of age, received oil orange SS daily in the diet at levels of 300, 7500 or 15,000 mg/kg of diet. Twenty rats in the low dose group survived up to 44 weeks; all rats of the middle dose group died within 20 weeks; and all rats of the high dose group died within 12 weeks. Two animals of the low dose group developed tumours, one an ovarian fibroma and the other an ovarian cystadenoma. No tumours occurred in 20 controls killed at 44 weeks (Allmark et al., 1956). [The Working Group noted the short duration of the experiment.]

(b) Subcutaneous and/or intramuscular administration

Mouse: Albino mice were injected subcutaneously twice weekly with 3 mg oil orange SS (purified by chromatography on alumina) as a 3% solution in arachis oil for 50 weeks. Thirteen mice survived more than 46 weeks, and the experiment was terminated at 84 weeks. Spindle-cell sarcomas at the injection site were observed in 3 mice at 46, 53 and 61 weeks, and in 3 other mice tumours of the intestine (1 adenocarcinoma, 1 adenocarcinomatous polyp and 1 adenomatous polyp) were found at 62, 65 and 69 weeks. The incidence of lymphomas, lung adenomas and mammary cancer was comparable with that of controls dying between 46-80 weeks (Bonser et al., 1954).

In a later paper it was reported that a group of 15 male and 15 female stock albino mice received twice weekly s.c. injections of 0.1 ml of a 1.5% suspension of oil orange SS in arachis oil for 52 weeks (weekly dose, 3 mg/mouse; total dose, 156 mg/mouse). Only 4 males and 11 females survived 20 or more weeks, and the experiment was terminated after 89 weeks. Three females developed injection site spindle-cell sarcomas, 1 female and 1 male, carcinomas of the intestine and 1 female, a benign tumour of the intestine. No subcutaneous sarcomas and 1/13 benign intestinal tumours were observed in controls autopsied between 50-90 weeks. Treatment with the colour did not significantly raise the lymphoma incidence (Bonser et al., 1956). [These tumours appear to be the same as those described in Bonser et al. (1954).]

Rat: A group of 18 Osborne-Mendel rats was given s.c. injections of 0.5-1 mg oil orange SS as a 1% suspension in glycerol once a week for 13 months, when the experiment was terminated. No tumours were observed by the end of the treatment (Nelson & Davidow, 1957). [The Working Group noted the short duration of the experiment.]

(c) Other experimental systems

Bladder implantation and/or instillation: Pellets of cholesterol containing 12.5% oil orange SS were implanted into the urinary bladders of a group of 32 stock albino mice. The experiment was terminated at 40 weeks. Bladder carcinomas developed in 12 mice, and benign tumours of the bladder in another 2. In comparison, 5/55 control mice implanted with cholesterol pellets developed bladder carcinomas, and 1 animal showed a benign tumour of the bladder. The results are statistically significant (P<0.01) (Clayson et al., 1958).

3.2 Other relevant biological data

(a) Animals

Rats fed diets containing 7500 and 15,000 mg oil orange SS per kg of diet showed changes in food consumption, food efficiency and growth rate, while those fed 300 mg/kg of diet showed no such effects. Rats fed 7500 mg/kg of diet showed 100% mortality in 20 weeks, and rats fed 15,000 mg/kg of diet reached 100% mortality in 12 weeks. Oral doses of 200 and 400 mg/kg bw caused a decrease in haemoglobin production (Allmark et al., 1956). Rats fed 40,000 mg/kg of diet live at most only a few months (Willheim & Ivy, 1953). Oral doses of 100 and 200 mg of the colour had a cathartic effect in dogs (Radomski & Deichmann, 1956).

3.3 Observations in man

No data were available to the Working Group.

4. Comments on Data Reported and Evaluation[1]

4.1 Animal data

Oil orange SS is carcinogenic in mice following its oral and subcutaneous administration, producing intestinal and local tumours; it also produced carcinomas of the bladder in mice following its administration by bladder implantation. Tests by the oral and subcutaneous routes in rats were either inadequately reported or of too short duration to be evaluated.

4.2 Human data

No case reports or epidemiological studies were available to the Working Group.

---

[1] See also the section, "Animal Data in Relation to the Evaluation of Risk to Man" in the introduction to this volume, p. 15.

5. References

Allmark, M.G., Grice, H.C. & Mannell, W.A. (1956) Chronic toxicity studies on food colours. II. Observations on the toxicity of FD & C Green No. 2 (light green SF yellowish), FD & C Orange No. 2 (orange SS) and FD & C Red No. 32 (oil red XO) in rats. J. Pharm. Pharmacol., 8, 417-424

Bonser, G.M., Clayson, D.B. & Jull, J.W. (1954) Induction of tumours with 1-(2-tolylazo)-2-naphthol (oil orange TX). Nature (Lond.), 174, 879-880

Bonser, G.M., Clayson, D.B. & Jull, J.W. (1956) The induction of tumours of the subcutaneous tissues, liver and intestine in the mouse by certain dyestuffs and their intermediates. Brit. J. Cancer, 10, 653-667

Clayson, D.B., Jull, J.W. & Bonser, G.M. (1958) The testing of *ortho*-hydroxyamines and related compounds by bladder implantation and a discussion of their structural requirements for carcinogenic activity. Brit. J. Cancer, 12, 222-230

DFG (Deutsche Forschungsgemeinschaft) (1955) Kommission zur Bearbeitung des Lebensmittelfarbstoffproblems, Toxikologische Daten von Farbstoffen und ihre Zulassung für Lebensmittel in verschiedenen Ländern, Mitt. 6(1), Wiesbaden, Steiner Verlag

DFG (Deutsche Forschungsgemeinschaft) (1957) Farbstoff-Kommission, Toxikologische Daten von Farbstoffen und ihre Zulassung für Lebensmittel in verschiedenen Ländern, Mitt. 6(2), Wiesbaden, Steiner Verlag, p. 12

Fujii, S., Kamikura, M. & Oka, N. (1965) Dye standards of National Institute of Hygienic Sciences, oil orange SS standard, naphthol yellow S standard and ponceau 3R standard. Bull. Nat. Inst. Hyg. Sci. (Tokyo), 83, 72-74

Japan Food Hygiene Association (1974) Japanese Standards of Food Additives, 3rd ed., Tokyo, Ministry of Health and Welfare

National Research Council (1971) Food Colors, Washington DC, National Academy of Sciences, p. 43

Nelson, A.A. & Davidow, B. (1957) Injection site fibrosarcoma production in rats by food colors. Fed. Proc., 16, 367

Radomski, J.L. & Deichmann, W.B. (1956) Cathartic action and metabolism of certain coal-tar food dyes. J. Pharmacol. exp. Ther., 118, 322-327

Society of Dyers and Colourists (1971) Colour Index, 3rd ed., Vol. III, Bradford, Yorkshire, Deanhouse Piccadilly, p. 3580

US Tariff Commission (1941) Synthetic Organic Chemicals, US Production and Sales, 1940, Report No. 148, Second Series, Washington DC, US Government Printing Office, p. 25

US Tariff Commission (1974) Synthetic Organic Chemicals, US Production and Sales, 1972, TC Publication 681, Washington DC, US Government Printing Office, p. 84

Willheim, R. & Ivy, A.C. (1953) A preliminary study concerning the possibility of dietary carcinogenesis. Gastroenterology, 23, 1-19

Zinke, Th. (1886) Untersuchungen über β-Naphtochinon. I. Ber. dtsch. chem. Ges., 19, 2493-2502

ORANGE I

1. Chemical and Physical Data

1.1 Synonyms and trade names

Colour Index No.: 14600

Colour Index Name: C.I. Acid Orange 20

Chem. Abstr. Reg. Serial No.: 523-44-4

Chem. Abstr. Name: 4-[(4-Hydroxy-1-naphthalenyl)azo]benzenesulphonic acid, monosodium salt

For other names of which the Working Group was aware see index, p. 297.

1.2 Chemical formula and molecular weight

$NaO_3S-\underset{}{\bigcirc}-N=N-\underset{}{\bigcirc\!\!\bigcirc}-OH$

$C_{16}H_{11}N_2NaO_4S$　　　　　　Mol. wt: 350.3

1.3 Chemical and physical properties of the pure substance

(a) Description: Reddish-brown crystals

(b) Absorption spectroscopy: λ_{max} 476 nm (in 0.02N ammonium acetate solution). Red in alkaline solutions

(c) Solubility: Soluble in water; generally insoluble in organic solvents, but slightly soluble in ethanol and acetone

1.4 Technical products and impurities

Specifications for orange I given by FAO/WHO (1966) and by the Japan Food Hygiene Association (1974) require that the product contain a minimum of 85% pure colour. Specifications given for a colour reference standard require that it contain a minimum of 96.5% pure colour (Inoue *et al.*, 1967).

2. Production, Use, Occurrence and Analysis

For important background information on this section, see preamble, p. 17.

2.1 Production and use

Orange I was first synthesized by P. Griess & Z. Roussin in 1876 (Society of Dyers and Colourists, 1971). It can be made by diazotizing sulphanilic acid, followed by coupling with 1-naphthol (Fieser, 1943), but it is not known whether this is the method used for commercial production.

Large-scale production of orange I in the US was first reported in 1914. In 1921, a total of 13,000 kg was manufactured by three producers (US Tariff Commission, 1922); however, US production of this colour was last reported in 1961, when it was manufactured by one company and was included in a group of at least 22 other dyes or colours, with a total production of 160,000 kg (US Tariff Commission, 1962).

In Western Europe there may have been as many as 11 producers of orange I in the past, but it is believed that present production is small. The production of this colour in Japan was stopped in 1966.

Orange I is used for dyeing textiles and leather and as an indicator (Society of Dyers and Colourists, 1971). It was one of the seven original colours permitted under the US Pure Food and Drugs Act of 1906, and the Deutsche Forschungsgemeinschaft (1955) reported that it was approved for use as a general food colouring in many countries throughout the world; known exceptions at that time were the Federal Republic of Germany, Finland, Spain, Turkey, the United Kingdom, the USSR and Yugoslavia. A later edition (DFG, 1957) indicated that it was not permitted in Bulgaria, Canada, Denmark, India, The Netherlands, New Zealand, Norway, Protugal, South Africa, Sweden or the US. In Japan, approval for its use in food was withdrawn prior to 1966, although it was retained for certain non-food uses (Japan Food Hygiene Association, 1974). It was removed from the approved list for food use in the US in 1956, but was permitted in externally applied drugs and cosmetics; however, in 1968, approval for these latter uses was also discontinued, on the basis of toxicological evidence (National Research Council, 1971).

2.2 Occurrence

Orange I is not known to occur in nature.

2.3 Analysis

See section, "General Remarks on the Substances Considered", p. 28.

3. Biological Data Relevant to the Evaluation of Carcinogenic Risk to Man

Two reviews on azo compounds, including orange I, and their carcinogenic activity have been published (Radomski, 1974; Truhaut, 1955).

3.1 Carcinogenicity and related studies in animals

(a) Oral administration

Mouse: No liver tumours were observed in a group of 20 mice (sex and strain unspecified) which received weekly doses of 15-20 mg orange I for life, given over 5 days a week in the form of a solution in tap-water added to 20 g brown bread. The last surviving mouse died 409 days after the start of treatment; the median lifespan was not reported. Autopsies were carried out on 14 mice and sections examined for 7 mice (Cook *et al.*, 1940). [The short duration of the experiment was noted by the Working Group.]

Rat: Groups of 12 male and 12 female rats were fed diets containing 0 (control), 5000, 10,000 or 20,000 mg orange I per kg of diet for 2 years. All animals administered the highest level died within 5 weeks. No tumours were reported in the four groups (Bourke *et al.*, 1956).

Eighty-five rats (sex and strain unspecified) were fed 1000 mg orange I per kg of diet for 400 days. No tumours were reported (Klinke, unpublished study quoted in DFG, 1957).

Dog: Fourteen dogs were fed the colour at four levels, ranging from 5 mg/kg bw/day by capsule (equivalent to 200 mg/kg of diet) to 2000-10,000 mg/kg of diet. The 3 dogs fed 5 mg/kg bw/day survived for 5 years. No tumours were reported (Bourke *et al.*, 1956).

(b) Subcutaneous and/or intramuscular administration

Rat: Injection site fibrosarcomas were observed in 6/18 young Osborne-Mendel rats given weekly s.c. injections of 20 mg orange I as a 2% aqueous solution for 2 years. Similar groups of saline- or glycerine-injected controls developed no injection site tumours (Nelson & Davidow, 1957).

3.3 Other relevant biological data

(a) Animals

The i.p. LD$_{50}$ in rats is 1000 mg/kg bw (Truhaut, 1958). Concentrations of 10,000 mg orange I per kg of diet caused some deaths, spleen enlargement, leucocytosis, anaemia, diarrhoea and growth depression in rats; 5000 mg/kg of diet increased the incidence of nephritis and enlargement of the spleen with hyperplasia and increased pigmentation (Bourke et al., 1956).

The urine of a dog given 5 g orange I contained a little of the unchanged colour together with sulphanilic acid and 4-amino-1-naphthol after 48 hours (Sisley & Porcher, 1911).

The carthartic action of 200 mg orange I administered orally in dogs is responsible for 22-41% being excreted in the faeces of animals with diarrhoea. The colour induces catharsis in the rat at a concentration of 20 mg/kg bw. Low excretion of orange I in animals not showing diarrhoea is due to its degradation by intestinal flora, as demonstrable by *in vitro* tests, rather than to its absorption through the intestinal wall. Oral administration of 100 mg to a dog with a bile fistula results in the recovery of only 0.4% in the bile, compared to a 47% recovery after its s.c. administration (Radomski & Deichmann, 1956).

(b) Man

Single doses of 80 mg orange I produced diarrhoea (catharsis) in 4-8 hours in several volunteers (Radomski & Deichmann, 1956).

3.3 Observations in man

No data were available to the Working Group.

4. Comments on Data Reported and Evaluation

4.1 Animal data

Orange I has been tested by the oral route in mice, rats and dogs, but the studies could not be evaluated due to inadequate reporting. It was also tested by the subcutaneous route in rats, producing injection site tumours (see also preamble, p. 21).

4.2 Human data

No case reports or epidemiological studies were available to the Working Group.

5. References

Bourke, A.R., Nelson, A.A. & Fitzhugh, O.G. (1956) Chronic toxicity of FD & C Orange No. 1. Fed. Proc., 15, 404

Cook, J.W., Hewett, C.L., Kennaway, E.L. & Kennaway, N.M. (1940) Effects produced in the livers of mice by azonaphthalenes and related compounds. Amer. J. Cancer, 40, 62-77

DFG (Deutsche Forschungsgemeinschaft) (1955) Kommission zur Bearbeitung des Lebensmittelfarbstoffproblems, Toxikologische Daten von Farbstoffen und ihre Zulassung für Lebensmittel in verschiedenen Ländern, Mitt. 6(1), Wiesbaden, Steiner Verlag

DFG (Deutsche Forschungsgemeinschaft) (1957) Farbstoff-Kommission, Toxikologische Daten von Farbstoffen und ihre Zulassung für Lebensmittel in verschiedenen Ländern, Mitt. 6(2), Wiesbaden, Steiner Verlag, p. 25

FAO/WHO (1966) Joint Expert Committee on Food Additives. Specifications for identity and purity and toxicological evaluation of food colours, FAO Nutr. Mtgs Rep. Ser. No. 38B; WHO/Food Add./66.25, p. 68

Fieser, L.F. (1943) In: Blatt, A.H., ed., Organic Synthesis, Vol. II, New York, John Wiley & Sons, p. 39

Inoue, T., Kamikura, M. & Murakami, N. (1967) Dye standards of National Institute of Hygienic Sciences. Orange I standard and ponceau R standard. Bull. Nat. Inst. Hyg. Sci. (Tokyo), 85, 150-152

Japan Food Hygiene Association (1974) Japanese Standard of Food Additives, 3rd ed., Tokyo, Ministry of Health and Welfare

National Research Council (1971) Food Colors, Washington DC, National Academy of Sciences, p. 6

Nelson, A.A. & Davidow, B. (1957) Injection site fibrosarcoma production in rats by food colors. Fed. Proc., 16, 367

Radomski, J.L. (1974) Toxicology of food colors. Ann. Rev. Pharmacol., 14, 127-137

Radomski, J.L. & Deichmann, W.B. (1956) Cathartic action and metabolism of certain coal-tar food dyes. J. Pharmacol. exp. Ther., 118, 322-327

Sisley, P. & Porcher, C. (1911) Du sort des matières colorantes dans l'organisme animal. C.R. Acad. Sci. (Paris), 152, 1062-1064

Society of Dyers and Colourists (1971) Colour Index, 3rd ed., Vol. I, Bradford, Yorkshire, Deanhouse Piccadilly, p. 1079

Truhaut, R. (1955) Sur l'action cancérigène de certaines matières colorantes. Importance en hygiène alimentaire, en thérapeutique et en hygiène générale. <u>Ann. pharm. fr.</u>, <u>13</u>, 36-51

Truhaut, R. (1958) Sur l'utilisation des colorants en thérapeutique et les dangers qui peuvent en résulter pour la santé humaine. <u>Chimie moderne</u>, <u>3</u>, 337-350

US Tariff Commission (1922) <u>Census of Dyes and Other Synthetic Chemicals, 1921</u>, Tariff Information Series No. 26, Washington DC, US Government Printing Office, p. 63

US Tariff Commission (1962) <u>Synthetic Organic Chemicals, US Production and Sales, 1969</u>, TC Publication 72, Washington DC, US Government Printing Office, p. 15

ORANGE G

1. Chemical and Physical Data

1.1 Synonyms and trade names

Colour Index No.: 16230

Colour Index Name: C.I. Acid Orange 10

Chem. Abstr. Reg. Serial No.: 1936-15-8

Chem. Abstr. Name: 7-Hydroxy-8-(phenylazo)-1,3-naphthalenedisulphonic acid, disodium salt

For other names of which the Working Group was aware see index, p. 297.

1.2 Chemical formula and molecular weight

$C_{16}H_{10}N_2Na_2O_7S_2$

Mol. wt: 452.4

1.3 Chemical and physical properties of the pure substance

(a) Description: Yellowish-red crystals or leaflets

(b) Absorption spectroscopy: λ_{max} 474 nm (in 0.02N ammonium acetate solution)

(c) Solubility: Soluble in water; generally insoluble in organic solvents, but slightly soluble in ethanol and cellosolve

1.4 Technical products and impurities

Specifications for orange G are given by the British Standards Institution (1960), together with appropriate analytical methods: the product must contain a minimum of 85% of the colour (Society of Dyers and Colourists, 1973).

The FAO/WHO (1966) standard also requires a minimum of 85% pure colour.

According to US industrial sources, when orange G is not used in foods, drugs or cosmetics, its manufacture and testing do not conform to rigid chemical specifications, and its composition may vary in order to meet customer shade and intensity requirements.

2. Production, Use, Occurrence and Analysis

For important background information on this section, see preamble, p. 17.

2.1 Production and use

Orange G was first synthesized by H. Baum in 1878 (Society of Dyers and Colourists, 1971). It can be made by diazotizing aniline and coupling the resulting diazonium salt with 2-naphthol-6,8-disulphonic acid (Conant & Pratt, 1926), but it is not known whether this method is used for commercial production.

Production of orange G in the US was first reported in 1914, and in 1921 a total of about 42,000 kg was produced (US Tariff Commission, 1922). In 1972, eight manufacturers reported production of 131,000 kg (US Tariff Commission, 1974); separate data on US imports and exports were not available.

In Western Europe, there may be as many as 19 producers of orange G, and it is believed that current annual production is in the order of several hundred thousand kg. In Japan in 1973, two manufacturers produced approximately 19,000 kg of the colour.

In the US, this colour was used as a drug and cosmetic colourant until October 1966, when its use for these applications was cancelled (US Code of Federal Regulations, 1974). Its use in cosmetics was reported to be permitted in the Federal Republic of Germany (DFG, 1968).

Orange G is used in staining biological materials, paper and wood, in inks and coloured pencils (Society of Dyers and Colourists, 1971), and for dyeing textiles (mainly wool) and leather.

The Deutsche Forschungsgemeinschaft (DFG, 1955) reported that it was approved for use in food colouring in Belgium, the German Democratic Republic, Norway, South Africa, Sweden and the United Kingdom. A later edition (DFG, 1957) reported additional approvals in Australia, Bulgaria, Denmark and Uruguay, and more recently DeGiacomi (1974) reported that in Denmark, South Africa and the United Kingdom it is still used as a general purpose food colour.

2.2 Occurrence

Orange G is not known to occur in nature.

2.3 Analysis

See section, "General Remarks on the Substances Considered", p. 28.

3. Biological Data Relevant to the Evaluation of Carcinogenic Risk to Man

3.1 Carcinogenicity and related studies in animals

One review on azo compounds, including orange G, and their carcinogenic activity has been published (Truhaut, 1955).

(a) Oral administration

Mouse: No liver tumours occurred in a group of 20 mice (sex and strain unspecified) which received weekly doses of 15-20 mg orange G for life, given over 5 days a week, in the form of a solution in tap-water added to 20 g brown bread. The last surviving mouse died 538 days after the start of treatment; the median lifespan was not reported. Autopsies were carried out on 10 mice and sections examined for 4 mice (Cook et al., 1940).

Male and female mice of a type B heterozygous strain were administered 1 mg orange G per animals (as a 2% solution in water added to the laboratory diet) daily for 500-700 days. Tumours developed in 12/113 males and in 15/78 females, including 8 lymphomas, 5 mammary tumours, 10 lung tumours, 2 endotheliomas and 2 papillomas of the stomach. Of the controls, 7/109 males and 11/59 females developed a total of 18 tumours, including 8 lymphomas 6 mammary tumours, 3 lung tumours and 1 papilloma of the forestomach. Of the treated mice, 70 males and 59 females were alive at 400 days, compared with 92 male and 51 female control mice. The last treated mouse died at 712 days, compared with 684 days in the control group (Waterman & Lignac, 1958).

Rat: No tumours were observed after oral administration of 2000 mg orange G per kg of diet to 10 rats (sex and strain unspecified) for 245 days, or 1000 mg orange G per kg of diet to 75 rats for 400 days (Klinke, unpublished study quoted in DFG, 1957). [No further details were reported.]

3.2 Other relevant biological data

(a) Animals

Administration of levels of 2500, 5000, 10,000, 20,000 or 50,000 mg orange G per kg of diet to groups of 10 albino rats for 90 days caused enlargement of the spleen (Hansen et al., 1960). Administration of a diet containing 50 mg orange G per kg of diet (approximately equivalent to 2.5 mg/kg bw/day) for 15 weeks to CFE rats had no effect on behaviour, growth rate, food or water consumption, blood and urine analyses, organ weights or histopathology (Gaunt et al., 1971).

Of 500 mg/kg bw orange G fed to rabbits, 40% is excreted in the urine as *para*-aminophenol, 3% as *ortho*-aminophenol and 0.6% as free aniline (Daniel, 1962). In the urine of rats given single oral doses of 250 mg/kg bw, 61% appears as *para*-aminophenol, and aniline is found in the faeces. No unchanged dye is found in either the urine or the faeces (Walker et al., unpublished study quoted in Gaunt et al., 1973).

The azo linkage of orange G is reduced by bacteria present in rat faeces (Roxon et al., 1967) and by rat-liver homogenates (Daniel, 1967). *In vivo* cleavage of orange G is presumably effected by azoreductases of the gut flora or of the liver; *in vitro* tests suggest that there is much greater activity in the flora (Ryan et al., 1968).

Heinz bodies are formed in red blood cells of rats fed diets containing 9000 mg/kg of diet (Rofe, 1957) or 5000 mg/kg of diet (Gaunt et al., 1971).

(b) Man

The urine of humans given 20 mg/kg bw orange G contained 95% as *para*-aminophenol, 0.5% as aniline and 1.3% as unchanged colour (Walker *et al.*, unpublished study quote in Gaunt *et al.*, 1973).

3.3 Observations in man

No data were available to the Working Group.

4. Comments on Data Reported and Evaluation

4.1 Animal data

Orange G was only tested in mice and rats by the oral route. The available studies in mice do not allow an evaluation, since in one study the adequacy of the dose could not be assessed and in the other information on pathology and survival rates was insufficient. The study in rats cannot be evaluated due to limited reporting.

4.2 Human data

No case reports or epidemiological studies were available to the Working Group.

5. References

British Standards Institution (1960) Methods for the analysis of water-soluble coal-tar dyes permitted for use in foods. BS 3210:1960, London

Conant, J.B. & Pratt, M.F. (1926) The irreversible reduction of organic compounds. III. The reduction of azo dyes. J. Amer. chem. Soc., 48, 2468-2485

Cook, J.W., Hewett, C.L., Kennaway, E.L. & Kennaway, N.M. (1940) Effects produced in the livers of mice by azonaphthalenes and related compounds. Amer. J. Cancer, 40, 62-77

Daniel, J.W. (1962) The excretion and metabolism of edible food colours. Toxicol. appl. Pharmacol., 4, 572-594

Daniel, J.W. (1967) Enzymic reduction of azo food colourings. Fd Cosmet. Toxicol., 5, 533-534

DeGiacomi, R., ed. (1974) Food Processing and Packaging Directory 1974, 13th ed., London, IPC Consumer Industries Press Ltd, pp. 797-802

DFG (Deutsche Forschungsgemeinschaft) (1955) Kommission zur Bearbeitung des Lebensmittelfarbstoffproblems, Toxikologische Daten von Farbstoffen und ihre Zulassung fur Lebensmittel in verschiedenen Landern, Mitt. 6(1), Wiesbaden, Steiner Verlag, p. 9

DFG (Deutsche Forschungsgemeinschaft) (1957) Farbstoff-Kommission, Toxikologische Daten von Farbstoffen und ihre Zulassung fur Lebensmittel in verschiedenen Landern, Mitt. 6(2), Wiesbaden, Steiner Verlag, p. 9

DFG (Deutsche Forschungsgemeinschaft) (1968) Farbstoff-Kommission, Toxikologische Daten von Farbstoffen und ihre Zulassung fur Lebensmittel in verschiedenen Landern, Mitt. 6, Wiesbaden, Steiner Verlag

FAO/WHO (1966) Joint Expert Committee on Food Additives. Specifications for identity and purity and toxicological evaluation of food colours, FAO Nutr. Mtgs Rep. Ser. No. 38B; WHO/Food Add./66.25, p. 131

Gaunt, I.F., Wright, M., Grasso, P. & Gangolli, S.D. (1971) Short-term toxicity of orange G in rats. Fd Cosmet. Toxicol., 9, 329-342

Gaunt, I.F., Kiss, I.S., Grasso, P. & Gangolli, S.D. (1973) Short-term toxicity of orange G in pigs. Fd Cosmet. Toxicol., 11, 367-374

Hansen, W.H., Wilson, D.C. & Fitzhugh, O.G. (1960) Subacute oral toxicity of ten D & C coal-tar colors. Fed. Proc., 19, 390

Rofe, P. (1957) Azo dyes and Heinz bodies. Brit. J. industr. Med., 14, 275-280

Roxon, J.J., Ryan, A.J. & Wright, S.E. (1967) Reduction of water-soluble azo dyes by intestinal bacteria. Fd Cosmet. Toxicol., 5, 367-369

Ryan, A.J., Roxon, J.J. & Sivayavirojana, A. (1968) Bacterial azo reduction: a metabolic reaction in mammals. Nature (Lond.), 219, 854-855

Society of Dyers and Colourists (1971) Colour Index, 3rd ed., Vol. I, Bradford, Yorkshire, Deanhouse Piccadilly, p. 1076

Truhaut, R. (1955) Sur l'action cancérigène de certaines matières colorantes. Importance en hygiène alimentaire, en thérapeutique et en hygiène générale. Ann. pharm. fr., 13, 36-51

US Code of Federal Regulations (1974) Food and Drugs, Title 21, part 8.510, Washington DC, US Government Printing Office, p. 181

US Tariff Commission (1922) Census of Dyes and Other Synthetic Organic Chemicals, 1921, Tariff Information Series No. 26, Washington DC, US Government Printing Office, pp. 47, 63

US Tariff Commission (1974) Synthetic Organic Chemicals, US Production and Sales, 1972, TC Publication 681, Washington DC, US Government Printing Office, p. 57

Waterman, N. & Lignac, G.O.E. (1958) The influence of the feeding of a number of food colours on the occurrence of tumours in mice. Acta physiol. pharmacol. neerl., 7, 35-55

PONCEAU MX

1. Chemical and Physical Data

1.1 Synonyms and trade names

Colour Index No.:   16150

Colour Index Name: C.I. Food Red 5

Chem. Abstr. Reg. Serial No.:   3761-53-3

Chem. Abstr. Name: 4-[(2,4-Dimethylphenyl)azo]-3-hydroxy-2,7-naphthalenedisulphonic acid, disodium salt

For other names of which the Working Group was aware see index, p. 297.

1.2 Chemical formula and molecular weight

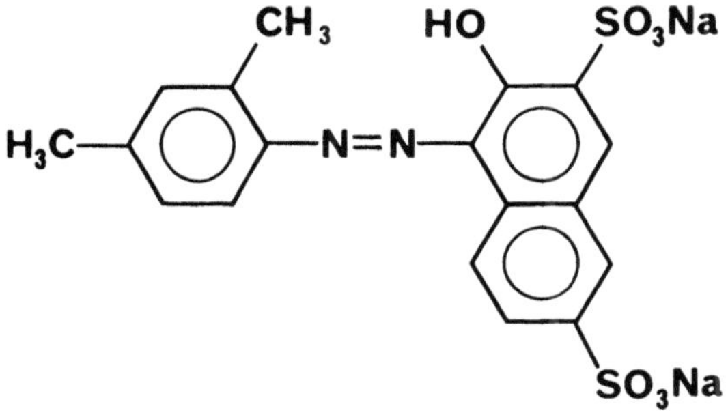

$C_{18}H_{14}N_2Na_2O_7S_2$ Mol. wt: 480.4

1.3 Chemical and physical properties of the pure substance

(a) Description: Dark-red crystals

(b) Absorption spectroscopy: λ_{max} 506 nm (in 0.02N ammonium acetate solution)

(c) Solubility: Soluble in water; very slightly soluble in ether, ethanol and acetone; insoluble in oil

1.4 Technical products and impurities

Specifications for ponceau MX are given by the British Standards Institution (1960), together with appropriate analytical methods; the product must contain a minimum of 85% of the colour. The FAO/WHO (1966) standard requires a minimum of 82%. Specifications for its use as a colour reference standard require that it contains a minimum of 96% pure colour (Inoue et al., 1967).

According to US industrial sources, when ponceau MX is not used in foods, drugs or cosmetics, its manufacture and testing do not conform to rigid chemical specifications, and its composition may vary in order to meet customer shade and intensity requirements.

2. Production, Use, Occurrence and Analysis

For important background information on this section, see preamble, p. 17.

2.1 Production and use

Ponceau MX was first synthesized by H. Baum in 1878 (Society of Dyers and Colourists, 1971); it is produced commercially by coupling diazotized 2,4-dimethylaniline with 2-naphthol-3,6-disulphonic acid (R acid) (King, 1929; Zuckerman, 1964).

Large-scale production of ponceau MX in the US was first reported in 1914, and in 1921 a total of 81,000 kg was produced (US Tariff Commission, 1922). In 1972, three US producers manufactured 17,000 kg (US Tariff Commission, 1974); separate data on US imports and exports were not available.

In Western Europe, there may be as many as 15 producers of ponceau MX. Total production data are not available, but it is believed that at least several thousand kg per year are manufactured in the United Kingdom.

One Japanese manufacturer reported the production of 3000 kg of this colour in 1972 and 4000 kg in 1973; it was not imported or exported in Japan at that time.

In the US, ponceau MX is used principally as a textile and leather dye. It is also used to colour inks, paper, pigment, wood stains and (specifically in the United Kingdom) in fruit, confectionary and meat products (Society of Dyers and Colourists, 1971).

Approval for its use in drugs and cosmetics in the US was cancelled in October, 1966 (US Code of Federal Regulations, 1974). In Japan, it is believed to be used in soaps and face lotions, but its use in pills, capsules and dental creams is prohibited (Pharmacopoeia of Japan, 1971).

The Deutsche Forschungsgemeinschaft (DFG, 1955) reported that ponceau MX was approved for food use in the following countries: Argentina, Australia, Belgium, Brazil, Chile, Colombia, Denmark, Egypt, France, Italy, Japan, Mexico, New Zealand, Norway, Poland, South Africa, Sweden, Switzerland, Uruguay and for limited use in the United Kingdom. A later edition (DFG, 1957) reported additional approvals in Bolivia, Cambodia, Colombia, Lebanon, Morocco, Tunisia, Turkey, the United Kingdom and Vietnam, but indicated that approval had been withdrawn in New Zealand, Norway and Sweden. Although the EEC does not recommend the use of ponceau MX in foodstuffs, DeGiacomi (1974) has reported recently that it is so used, at least in Denmark. Approval for its use in food was withdrawn in Japan prior to 1966, although it was retained for certain non-food uses (Japan Food Hygiene Association, 1974).

2.2 Occurrence

Ponceau MX is not known to occur in nature.

2.3 Analysis

See section, "General Remarks on the Substances Considered", p. 28.

3. Biological Data Relevant to the Evaluation of Carcinogenic Risk to Man

Two reviews on azo dyes, including ponceau MX, and their carcinogenic activity have been published (Radomski, 1974; Truhaut, 1955).

3.1 Carcinogenicity and related studies in animals

(a) Oral administration

Mouse: Twenty mice (sex and strain unspecified) were given weekly doses of 15-20 mg ponceau MX as a solution in tap-water added to brown bread over 5 days per week for lifespan. Survival rates were not reported, but the last mouse died 773 days after the start of the experiment.

Autopsies performed on 15 mice and sections examined from 11 showed an abdominal epithelial tumour of doubtful nature metastasizing to the lung and a "patch of cholangioma in the liver" (Cook et al., 1940).

A group of 15 mice of each sex (strain unknown) was given the colour (purity unspecified) in drinking-water for 52 weeks at a concentration of 0.05%; the weekly and total intakes were reported to be 17 mg and 884 mg/mouse, respectively. Early mortality was high. Lymphomas were observed in 6/8 males and 1/5 females, compared with 1/9 males and 4/9 females in a control group given s.c. injections of arachis oil and dying between 20-90 weeks. Benign intestinal tumours occurred in 4/6 surviving animals, compared with 1/13 in controls (Bonser et al., 1956). [P<0.05.]

No increased incidence of tumours over that in 168 controls was found in 126 mice of a type B heterozygous strain which received a solution of 2% ponceau MX in water added to food, corresponding to an intake of about 1 mg/mouse/day: 8 lymphomas, 6 mammary tumours, 3 lung tumours and 1 papilloma of the stomach occurred in controls, compared with 2 lymphomas, 3 mammary tumours and 6 lung tumours in treated mice. Treatment lasted for up to 700 days. The colour used was partly commercial ponceau MX and partly a sample purified by steaming or by recrystallization: the two samples showed no difference in their effects (Waterman & Lignac, 1958).

In later studies, groups of 50 male and 50 female ddY mice were fed diets containing 2000, 10,000 or 50,000 mg ponceau MX per kg of diet for 19 months. A group of 80 males and 80 females served as controls. After 4 and 12 months 5 animals from each group were killed for pathological examination, and all survivors were killed after 19 months. In mice dying between 12-19 months, the incidences of liver tumours (hepatocellular adenomas and carcinomas) were as follows:

Concentration (mg/kg of diet)	Male	Female
0	1/31	1/34
2000	1/8	6/27
10,000	5/6	5/11
50,000	9/12	7/12

Hyperplastic nodules of the liver occurred frequently in non-tumour-bearing treated mice and occurred in all tumour-bearing treated mice (Ikeda et al., 1968).[1]

Rat: In a group of 5 male and 5 female Wistar rats fed 40,000 mg ponceau MX (purity unspecified) per kg of diet for up to 2 years, no cirrhosis of the liver and no tumours were seen (Willheim & Ivy, 1953).

Groups of 20 male Wistar rats were fed a diet containing 0, 2000, 10,000 or 50,000 mg ponceau MX per kg of diet for 15 months. The incidences of liver tumours observed macroscopically in rats dying after the 10th month of treatment were 0/12 in controls and 4/15, 4/12 and 6/14 at the three feeding levels, respectively. Histological examination of the livers of animals killed at the end of the study showed "adenomatous alterations" in 1/4 controls, in 4/5 rats given 2000 mg/kg of diet and in 6/6 rats given 50,000 mg ponceau MX per kg of diet (Ikeda et al., 1966). [No histological examination was carried out in rats fed 10,000 mg/kg of diet.]

Groups of 30 male and 30 female CFE rats were fed a diet containing 0, 1250, 2500, 5000 or 10,000 mg ponceau MX per kg of diet for 2 years. Over half of the animals survived for 80 weeks or longer; in males receiving the two highest dose levels mortality was increased after week 88 of treatment. Liver nodules up to 1 cm in diameter, which the authors considered to be "morphologically similar to the pre-adenomatous nodules reported by Ikeda et al. (1966)", were seen in a number of rats, with an obvious dose-response effect, as indicated in the following table:

---

[1]The sample of ponceau MX used was reported to contain more than 85% pure chemical. The remaining components were water, sodium sulphate and sodium chloride.

	Males		Females	
Concentration (mg/kg of diet)	Nodules of enlarged hepatocytes	Nodular hyperplasia	Nodules of enlarged hepatocytes	Nodular hyperplasia
0	0/30	0/30	0/30	0/30
1250	5/30	0/30	3/30	1/30
2500	11/29	1/29	6/29	0/29
5000	8/30	1/30	18/28	5/28
10,000	17/29	3/29	21/25	14/25

Other tumours found in treated animals did not differ from those found in controls. The colour used in this experiment complied with the specifications laid down by the British Standards Institution (Grasso et al., 1969).

3.2 **Other relevant biological data**

(a) Animals

The i.p. LD_{50} for ponceau MX is greater than 1 g/kg bw in rats; it has been estimated to be 2 g/kg bw in mice (Hall et al., 1966). Oral doses of 2 g/kg bw are well tolerated in both species.

In 90-day tests in rats, administration of 5000, 10,000 or 20,000 mg ponceau MX per kg of diet had no apparent effect, except for initial growth retardation due to unpalatability (Hall et al., 1966). However, rats fed diets containing 10,000 or 15,000 mg ponceau MX per kg of diet for 15 months had decreased growth and enlarged liver and kidneys (Ikeda, 1966; Ikeda et al., 1966).

When rabbits are fed the colour their urine contains 2.5% unchanged colour, 35% 2,4-dimethylaniline, 6% 3-methyl-4-acetamidobenzoic acid, 3-methyl-4-aminobenzoic acid and 2,4-dimethylphenylsulphamate. Ponceau MX is not hydroxylated by rabbits (Daniel, 1962). 2,4-Dimethylaniline (2,4-xylidine) is metabolized by rats to 3-methyl-4-aminobenzoic acid; no aminophenol derivatives are formed (Lindstrom, 1960).

Experiments with the oral administration to rats of ^{35}S-labelled ponceau MX showed that it is accumulated in the liver. After oral administration most of it is found in faeces, but after i.v. injection most is excreted in urine; in both cases, 50% of unchanged colour was found (Urakubo, 1967). When ponceau MX was injected intravenously into rats with cannulated bile ducts, 42% was excreted in bile; the excretion rate was independent of the dose (Iga et al., 1970). In a similar experiment, Ryan & Wright (1961) reported that only 15% was excreted unchanged in the bile.

Ponceau MX did not induce Heinz bodies (Rofe, 1957).

3.3 Observations in man

No data were available to the Working Group.

4. Comments on Data Reported and Evaluation[1]

4.1 Animal data

Ponceau MX is carcinogenic, producing liver-cell tumours in mice and rats and possibly intestinal tumours in mice, following its administration by the oral route. A dose-response effect was noted in the mouse and rat studies.

4.2 Human data

No case reports or epidemiological studies were available to the Working Group.

---

[1] See also the section, "Animal Data in Relation to the Evaluation of Risk to Man" in the introduction to this volume, p. 15.

5. References

Bonser, G.M., Clayson, D.B. & Jull, J.W. (1956) The induction of tumours of the subcutaneous tissues, liver and intestine in the mouse by certain dyestuffs and their intermediates. Brit. J. Cancer, 10, 653-667

British Standards Institution (1960) Methods for the analysis of water-soluble coal-tar dyes permitted for use in foods. BS3210:1960, London

Cook, J.W., Hewett, C.L., Kennaway, E.L. & Kennaway, N.M. (1940) Effects produced in the livers of mice by azonaphthalenes and related compounds. Amer. J. Cancer, 40, 62-77

Daniel, J.W. (1962) The excretion and metabolism of edible food colors. Toxicol. appl. Pharmacol., 4, 572-594

DeGiacomi, R., ed. (1974) Food Processing and Packaging Directory, 1974, 13th ed., London, IPC Consumer Industries Press Ltd, pp. 797-802

DFG (Deutsche Forschungsgemeinschaft) (1955) Kommission zur Bearbeitung des Lebensmittelfarbstoffproblems, Toxikologische Daten von Farbstoffen und ihre Zulassung für Lebensmittel in verschiedenen Ländern, Mitt. 6(1), Wiesbaden, Steiner Verlag

DFG (Deutsche Forschungsgemeinschaft) (1957) Farbstoff-Kommission, Toxikologische Daten von Farbstoffen und ihre Zulassung für Lebensmittel in verschiedenen Ländern, Mitt. 6(2), Wiesbaden, Steiner Verlag, p. 14

FAO/WHO (1966) Joint Expert Committee on Food Additives. Specifications for identity and purity and toxicological evaluation of food colours. FAO Nutr. Mtgs Rep. Ser. No. 38B, WHO/Food Add./66.25, p. 136

Grasso, P., Lansdown, A.B.G., Kiss, I.S. & Gaunt, I.F. (1969) Nodular hyperplasia in the rat liver following prolonged feeding with Ponceau MX. Fd Cosmet. Toxicol., 7, 425-442

Hall, D.E., Lee, F.S. & Fairweather, F.A. (1966) Acute (mouse and rat) and short-term (rat) toxicity studies on ponceau MX. Fd Cosmet. Toxicol., 4, 375-382

Iga, T., Awazu, S., Hanano, M. & Nogami, H. (1970) Pharmacokinetic studies of biliary secretion. I. Comparison of the excretion behaviour in azo dyes and indigo carmine. Chem. Pharm. Bull., 18, 2431-2440

Ikeda, Y. (1966) Long-term study of ponceau MX in rats and mice. Fd Cosmet. Toxicol., 4, 361-363

Ikeda, Y., Horiuchi, S., Furuya, T. & Omori, Y. (1966) Chronic toxicity of ponceau MX in the rat. Fd Cosmet. Toxicol., 4, 485-492

Ikeda, Y., Horiuchi, S., Kobayashi, K., Furuya, T. & Kohgo, K. (1968) Carcinogenicity of ponceau MX in the mouse. Fd Cosmet. Toxicol., 6, 591-598

Inoue, T., Kamikura, M. & Murakami, N. (1967) Dye standards of National Institute of Hygienic Sciences. Orange I standard and ponceau R standard. Bull. Nat. Inst. Hyg. Sci. (Tokyo), 85, 150-152

Japan Food Hygiene Association (1974) Japanese Standards of Food Additives, 3rd ed., Tokyo, Ministry of Health and Welfare

King, A.T. (1929) Constitutional influences on the conversion of azo-naphthols into their azo-sulphites and their bearing on the structure of α- and β-naphthol. J. chem. Soc., 117, 601-609

Lindstrom, H.V. (1960) The metabolism of FD and C Red No. 1. I. The fate of 2,4-meta-xylidine in rats. Fed. Proc., 19, 183

Pharmacopoeia of Japan (1971) 8th ed., Tokyo, Ministry of Health and Welfare

Radomski, J.L. (1974) Toxicology of food colors. Ann. Rev. Pharmacol., 14, 127-137

Rofe, P. (1957) Azo dyes and Heinz bodies. Brit. J. industr. Med., 14, 275-280

Ryan, A.J. & Wright, S.E. (1961) The excretion of some azo dyes in rat bile. J. Pharm. Pharmacol., 13, 492-495

Society of Dyers and Colourists (1971) Colour Index, 3rd ed., Vol. I, Bradford, Yorkshire, Deanhouse Piccadilly, p. 1131

Truhaut, R. (1955) Sur l'action cancérigène de certaines matières colorantes. Importance en hygiène alimentaire, en thérapeutique et en hygiène générale. Ann. pharm. fr., 13, 36-51

Urakubo, G. (1967) Distribution (in experimental animals) and excretion of sulfur-35-labelled ponceau MX. Shokuhin Eiseigaku Zasshi, 8, 489-493

US Code of Federal Regulations (1974) Food and Drugs, Title 21, part 8.510, Washington DC, US Government Printing Office, p. 181

US Tariff Commission (1922) Census of Dyes and Other Synthetic Organic Chemicals, 1921, Tariff Information Series No. 26, Washington DC, US Government Printing Office, p. 63

US Tariff Commission (1974) Synthetic Organic Chemicals, US Production and Sales, 1972, TC Publication 681, Washington DC, US Government Printing Office, p. 57

Waterman, N. & Lignac, G.O.E. (1958) The influence of the feeding of a number of food colours on the occurrence of tumours in mice. Acta physiol. pharmacol. neerl., 7, 35-55

Willheim, R. & Ivy, A.C. (1953) A preliminary study concerning the possibility of dietary carcinogenesis. Gastroenterology, 23, 1-19

Zuckerman, S. (1964) Colors for Foods, Drugs and Cosmetics. In: Kirk, R.E. & Othmer, D.F., eds, Encyclopedia of Chemical Technology, 2nd ed., Vol. 5, New York, John Wiley & Sons, p. 869

PONCEAU 3R

1. Chemical and Physical Data

1.1 Synonyms and trade names

Colour Index No.: 16155

Colour Index Name: C.I. Food Red 6 (in Society of Dyers and Colourists, 1956, but deleted in 1971 edition)

Chem. Abstr. Reg. Serial No.: 3564-09-8

Chem. Abstr. Name: 3-Hydroxy-4-[(2,4,5-trimethylphenyl)azo]-2,7-naphthalenedisulphonic acid, disodium salt

For other names of which the Working Group was aware see index, p. 297.

1.2 Chemical formula and molecular weight

$C_{19}H_{16}N_2Na_2O_7S_2$ Mol. wt: 494.5

1.3 Chemical and physical properties of the pure substance

(a) Description: Dark-red crystals

(b) Absorption spectroscopy: λ_{max} 508 nm (in 0.02N ammonium acetate solution)

(c) Solubility: Very soluble in water; slightly soluble in ethanol; insoluble in vegetable oils

1.4 Technical products and impurities

One specification for ponceau 3R requires that the product include a minimum of 85% of the colour (Japan Food Hygiene Association, 1974). Used as a colour reference standard, it must contain a minimum of 98% ponceau 3R (Fujii *et al.*, 1965).

2. Production, Use, Occurrence and Analysis

For important background information on this section, see preamble, p. 17.

2.1 Production and use

Ponceau 3R was first prepared by H. Baum in 1878 (Society of Dyers and Colourists, 1971). It can be synthesized by coupling diazotized pseudocumidine with 2-naphthol-3,6-disulphonic acid (R acid) and neutralizing with an alkali.

Large-scale production of ponceau 3R in the US was first reported in 1914 (US Tariff Commission, 1922). In 1959, four US manufacturers reported a total production of 26,000 kg (US Tariff Commission, 1960), but the last report of US commercial production was in 1960, when it was produced by four manufacturers; separate production data were not given (US Tariff Commission, 1961). It is not believed to be produced commercially in either Western Europe or Japan at the present time.

Ponceau 3R has been used to dye wool (Merck & Co., 1968). It was one of the seven original food colours permitted under the US Food and Drug Act of 1906; however, on the basis of animal toxicity studies, it was removed from the list of approved substances for use in foodstuffs in November 1960, although it was permitted in externally applied drugs and cosmetics. In 1966, it was removed from the list of approved substances (National Research Council, 1971).

The Deutsche Forschungsgemeinschaft (DFG, 1955) reported that this material was approved for use as a general food colouring in Australia, Canada, Denmark, France, Greece, Italy, Japan, Mexico, New Zealand, Norway, Peru, Poland, Portugal, Rumania, South Africa, Sweden, Switzerland, Turkey, Venezuela and Yugoslavia, and for limited use in the United Kingdom. A later edition (DFG, 1957) reported additional approvals in Brazil, Costa Rica, Cuba, the Dominican Republic, Guatemala, Israel, Lebanon, Morocco, the Philippines, Tunisia, the United Kingdom, Uruguay and Vietnam, but indicated that approval had been withdrawn in France, New Zealand, Norway, Sweden, Switzerland and Yugoslavia. By 1960, it was no longer permitted in Morocco, Turkey or Uruguay, but was approved for use in Bulgaria and Thailand (Nieman, 1961). It is believed to have been used in foods in Japan from 1948 until 1965 when approval was retained only for certain non-food uses (Japan Food Hygiene Association, 1974).

2.2 Occurrence

Ponceau 3R is not known to occur in nature.

2.3 Analysis

See section, "General Remarks on the Substances Considered", p. 28.

3. Biological Data Relevant to the Evaluation of Carcinogenic Risk to Man

Two reviews on azo compounds, including ponceau 3R, and their carcinogenic properties have been published (Radomski, 1974; Truhaut, 1955).

3.1 Carcinogenicity and related studies in animals

(a) Oral administration

Mouse: Groups of 50 male and 50 female C3HeB/Fe mice were fed a diet containing 10,000 or 20,000 mg commercial ponceau 3R per kg of diet. None of the mice survived longer than 68 weeks. Of 67 mice examined which had received the 20,000 mg/kg level, 36 had hepatic adenomas and 16 had hepatic carcinomas, 4 of which metastasized to the lungs (Hansen et al., 1963). An untreated group of 217 C3HeB/Fe mice, divided approximately equally by sex and with an average survival time of 60 weeks, was observed in the same institution at approximately the same period. Nine animals developed liver tumours (Davis & Fitzhugh, 1962). [The Working Group noted the poor survival rate, lack of detailed pathology, loss of information due to inability to autopsy a large percentage of animals and failure to treat the results in males and females separately.]

Rat: In a group of 5 male and 5 female Wistar rats fed ponceau 3R (purity unspecified) at a concentration of 40,000 mg per kg of diet for up to 19 months, cirrhosis of the liver with hyperplasia of the bile ducts occurred in 3/8 rats surviving longer than 12 months; one of these rats also had a lesion of the liver described as "resembling early hepatoma". No cirrhosis occurred in 50 control animals surviving for 20 or more months (Willheim & Ivy, 1953).

Three groups of 15 male and 15 female rats (strain unspecified) were fed a diet containing 3000, 10,000 or 30,000 mg ponceau 3R per kg of diet for 65 weeks. A group of 90 rats of both sexes served as controls. Among the treated animals, bile-duct adenomas were found in 1/20, 5/24 and 7/23 rats, respectively, and hepatic carcinomas were found in 0/20, 2/24 and 7/23 rats, respectively. No liver tumours occurred in controls (Grice et al., 1961).

Groups of 25 male and 25 female Osborne-Mendel rats were fed a diet containing 0 (control), 5000, 10,000, 20,000 or 50,000 mg commercial ponceau 3R per kg of diet for 2 years. Similar groups of Bethesda Black rats received a diet containing 0 (control) or 20,000 mg commercial ponceau 3R per kg of diet. A small number of treated animals of both sexes and about 40% of control animals survived for 2 years. In treated Osborne-Mendel rats, hepatic carcinomas were found in 1, 2, 4 and 9 rats, respectively, the incidence increasing with the dose, compared with none in the controls. Benign hepatomas occurred in 12, 17, 22 and 25 rats in the treated groups, compared with 1 in controls; nodular hyperplasia of the liver was also observed in 12, 18, 9 and 4 treated animals, compared with none in the controls. In Bethesda Black rats hepatic carcinomas and benign hepatomas were found in 11 and 8 treated rats, respectively, compared with none in controls; nodular hyperplasia of the liver was observed in 10 treated rats and in 1 control (Hansen et al., 1963).

Hepatic-cell carcinomas were also observed in 6/29 and 5/29 male and female Wistar rats fed either a diet containing 30,000 mg ponceau 3R per kg of diet or a similar diet containing 5% corn oil in addition to the ponceau 3R for up to 70 weeks. In control animals killed after 70 weeks, no liver tumours occurred in 29 receiving the basal diet alone or in 30 receiving the basal diet plus 5% corn oil (Mannell, 1964).

Although the amounts of amines obtained by reduction of the samples of ponceau 3R used by Grice *et al.* (1961), Hansen *et al.* (1963) and Mannell (1964) differed, the incidences of liver tumours were similar (Mannell, 1964).

Liver tumours have also been reported in Wistar rats fed diets containing 5000, 10,000 or 20,000 mg ponceau 3R per kg of diet for up to 105 weeks. Among 16 rats at the highest dose level killed at 105 weeks, 1 female rat had developed a hepatocellular carcinoma and 2 females, liver-cell adenomas; of rats receiving the medium dose level, 1 male, and of those at the lowest dose level, 1 female and 1 male, had liver-cell adenomas. No liver tumours were found in 3 controls (Aiso *et al.*, 1966).

(b) Other experimental systems

Bladder implantation and/or instillation: Of 33 stock mice given single bladder implantations of a 15-17 mg pellet of a 12.5% suspension of ponceau 3R in crushed paraffin wax and surviving for 25 weeks, 5 developed carcinomas of the bladder, compared with 1/82 controls implanted with paraffin wax pellets (Bonser *et al.*, 1963). [P<0.01.]

3.2 Other relevant biological data

(a) Animals

Rats fed dietary levels of 5000-50,000 mg ponceau 3R per kg of diet developed enlarged livers and kidneys, growth inhibition and high mortality. The dye was also toxic to dogs and mice (Hansen *et al.*, 1963). The livers of rats fed 30,000 mg/kg of diet showed damage characterized by fatty change, cirrhosis, focal haemorrhage and focal necrosis (Grice *et al.*, 1961); there were no changes in other organs (Kanisawa *et al.*, 1965). At levels of 3000-30,000 mg/kg of diet, female rats showed weight loss, while male rats did not (Grice *et al.*, 1961).

Following its oral administration to rabbits, 0.4% unchanged dye and 44% 2,4,5-trimethylaniline were excreted in urine (Daniel, 1962). 2,4,5-Trimethylaniline (4-cumidine or pseudocumidine) caused pathological changes in the livers of rats but was less toxic than 2,4,6-trimethylaniline (mesidine); both isomers were oxidized *in vivo* to dimethyl aminobenzoic acids: three isomers were formed from 4-cumidine and two from mesidine

(Lindstrom et al., 1963). 2,4,6-Trimethylaniline has been reported to produce transplantable hepatomas in rats when fed in the diet at a level of 150 mg/kg of diet for 18 months (Mannell, 1964; Morris & Wagner, 1962).

3.3 Observations in man

No data were available to the Working Group.

4. Comments on Data Reported and Evaluation[1]

4.1 Animal data

Ponceau 3R is carcinogenic in rats following its oral administration, producing liver-cell tumours. It also produced bladder tumours in mice following its implantation in the urinary bladder. The oral study in mice was considered inadequate for evaluation.

4.2 Human data

No case reports or epidemiological studies were available to the Working Group.

---

[1] See also the section, "Animal Data in Relation to the Evaluation of Risk to Man" in the introduction to this volume, p. 15.

5. References

Aiso, K., Kanisawa, M., Okamoto, T. & Chujo, T. (1966) Chronic oral toxicity and carcinogenicity of ponceau 3R. Shokuhin Eiseigaku Zasshi, 7, 211-221

Bonser, G.M., Boyland, E., Busby, E.R., Clayson, D.B., Grover, P.L. & Jull, J.W. (1963) A further study of bladder implantation in the mouse as a means of detecting carcinogenic activity: use of crushed paraffin wax or stearic acid as the vehicle. Brit. J. Cancer, 17, 127-136

Daniel, J.W. (1962) The excretion and metabolism of edible food colors. Toxicol. appl. Pharmacol., 4, 572-594

Davis, K.J. & Fitzhugh, O.G. (1962) Tumorigenic potential of aldrin and dieldrin for mice. Toxicol. appl. Pharmacol., 4, 187-189

DFG (Deutsche Forschungsgemeinschaft) (1955) Kommission zur Bearbeitung des Lebensmittelfarbstoffproblems, Toxikologische Daten von Farbstoffen und ihre Zulassung für Lebensmittel in verschiedenen Ländern, Mitt. 6(1), Wiesbaden, Steiner Verlag

DFG (Deutsche Forschungsgemeinschaft) (1957) Farbstoff-Kommission, Toxikologische Daten von Farbstoffen und ihre Zulassung für Lebensmittel in verschiedenen Ländern, Mitt. 6(2), Wiesbaden, Steiner Verlag, p. 16

Fujii, S., Kamikura, M. & Oka, N. (1965) Dye standards of National Institute of Hygienic Sciences. Oil orange SS standard, naphthol yellow S standard and ponceau 3R standard. Bull. Nat. Inst. Hyg. Sci. (Tokyo), 83, 72-74

Grice, H.C., Mannell, W.A. & Allmark, M.G. (1961) Liver tumors in rats fed ponceau 3R. Toxicol. appl. Pharmacol., 3, 509-520

Hansen, W.H., Davis, K.J., Fitzhugh, O.G. & Nelson, A.A. (1963) Chronic oral toxicity of ponceau 3R. Toxicol. appl. Pharmacol., 5, 105-118

Japan Food Hygiene Association (1974) Japanese Standards of Food Additives, 3rd ed., Tokyo, Ministry of Health and Welfare

Kanisawa, M., Okamoto, T., Chujo, T. & Aiso, K. (1965) Histopathological observations in rats fed ponceau 3R (food red No. 1). Ann. Rep. Inst. Food Microbiol. Chiba Univ., 18, 45-54

Lindstrom, H.V., Wallace, W.C., Hansen, W.H., Nelson, A.A. & Fitzhugh, O.G. (1963) The metabolism of FD & C Red No. 1. IV. The metabolism and toxicity of pseudocumidine and mesidine in rats. Fed. Proc., 22, 188

Mannell, W.A. (1964) Further investigations on the production of liver tumours in rats by ponceau 3R. Fd Cosmet. Toxicol., 2, 169-174

Merck & Co. (1968)　The Merck Index, 8th ed., Rahway, N.J., p. 850

Morris, H.P. & Wagner, B.P. (1962)　Development of 'minimum deviation' hepatomas. In: Wolfson, K.G., ed., Proceedings of the VIIIth International Cancer Congress, Moscow, 1962, Moscow, Medgiz, p. 143

National Research Council (1971)　Food Colors, Washington DC, National Academy of Sciences, p. 43

Nieman, C. (1961)　Food Colours Recently Authorized in 43 Countries, Amsterdam, Consudel

Radomski, J.L. (1974)　Toxicology of food colors. Ann. Rev. Pharmacol., 14, 127-137

Society of Dyers and Colourists (1956)　Colour Index, 2nd ed., Bradford, Yorkshire, Deanhouse Piccadilly

Society of Dyers and Colourists (1971)　Colour Index, 3rd ed., Vol. III, Bradford, Yorkshire, Deanhouse Piccadilly, p. 4092

Truhaut, R. (1955)　Sur l'action cancérigène de certaines matières colorantes. Importance en hygiène alimentaire, en thérapeutique et en hygiène générale. Ann. pharm. fr., 13, 36-51

US Tariff Commission (1922)　Census of Dyes and Other Synthetic Organic Chemicals, 1921, Tariff Information Series No. 26, Washington DC, US Government Printing Office, p. 47

US Tariff Commission (1960)　Synthetic Organic Chemicals, US Production and Sales, 1959, Report No. 206, Second Series, Washington DC, US Government Printing Office, p. 21

US Tariff Commission (1961)　Synthetic Organic Chemicals, US Production and Sales, 1960, TC Publication 34, Washington DC, US Government Printing Office, p. 101

Willheim, R. & Ivy, A.C. (1953)　A preliminary study concerning the possibility of dietary carcinogenesis. Gastroenterology, 23, 1-19

PONCEAU SX

1. Chemical and Physical Data

1.1 Synonyms and trade names

Colour Index No.: 14700

Colour Index Name: C.I. Food Red I

Chem. Abstr. Reg. Serial No.: 4548-53-2

Chem. Abstr. Name: 3-[(2,4-Dimethyl-5-sulphophenyl)azo]-4-hydroxy-1-naphthalenesulphonic acid, disodium salt

For other names of which the Working Group was aware see index, p. 297.

1.2 Chemical formula and molecular weight

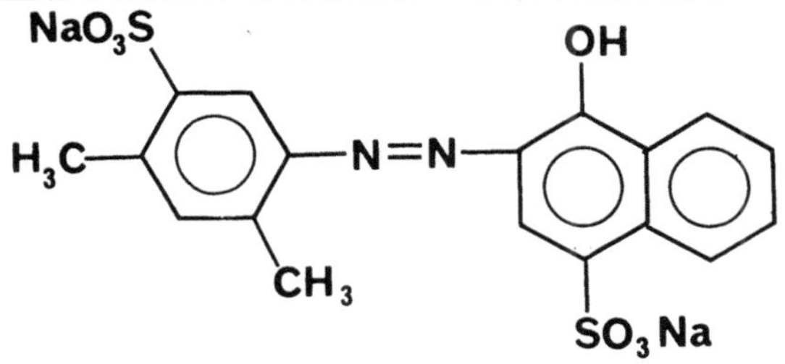

$C_{18}H_{14}N_2Na_2O_7S_2$ Mol. wt: 480.4

1.3 Chemical and physical properties of the pure substance

(a) Description: Red crystals

(b) Absorption spectroscopy: λ_{max} 500 nm (in 0.02N ammonium acetate solution)

(c) Solubility: Soluble in water; slightly soluble in ethanol; insoluble in vegetable oils

1.4 Technical products and impurities

Specifications for ponceau SX in foods, drugs and cosmetics require that the product contain a minimum of 85% pure colour (US Code of Federal Regulations, 1974a). When used as a colour reference standard it must contain a minimum of 99.9% (Inoue et al., 1967).

2. Production, Use, Occurrence and Analysis

For important background information on this section, see preamble, p. 17.

2.1 Production and use

The preparation of ponceau SX was first reported in 1886 by Nölting & Kohn (1886), and it is believed that the method used for the commercial production of ponceau SX involves their original route of synthesis, in which diazotized 5-amino-2,4-xylenesulphonic acid is coupled with 4-hydroxy-1-naphthalenesulphonic acid (Zuckerman, 1964).

Large-scale production was first reported in the US in 1929 (US Tariff Commission, 1930), and increased to a maximum of 181,000 kg in 1961 (US Tariff Commission, 1962). In 1972, ponceau SX was manufactured by two companies and was included in a group of at least six other colours, with a total production of 530,000 kg (US Tariff Commission, 1974). Separate data on US imports and exports were not available.

In Western Europe there may be as many as five producers of ponceau SX, but current production is believed to be small. It is not produced commercially in Japan at present.

The Deutsche Forschungsgemeinschaft (DFG, 1955) reported that ponceau SX was approved for food use in Australia, Canada, Greece, Japan, Mexico, The Netherlands, New Zealand, Norway, Peru, South Africa, the United Kingdom and the US. A later edition (DFG, 1957) reported additional approvals in Cuba, Denmark, the Dominican Republic, Finland, Guatemala, Israel, the Philippines, Sweden and Uruguay, but indicated that approval had been withdrawn in The Netherlands. More recently, it has been reported that its use in foods has been approved in Austria (DeGiacomi, 1974; Nieman, 1961). In Japan, ponceau SX was permitted in foodstuffs from 1948 until 1966, when it was approved only for certain non-food uses.

In the US, it was on the list of food colours approved under the US Pure Food and Drug Act of 1906 (National Research Council, 1971), and

Zuckerman (1964) reported that ponceau SX was used as a colouring in the following products: gelatin desserts, maraschino cherries, frozen desserts, carbonated beverages, dry drink powders, confectionary products, spaghetti, puddings, aqueous drug solutions, tablets, capsules, ointments, bath salts and hair rinses.

However, its general use in foods, drugs and cosmetics has not been permitted since June 1965, because of adverse toxicological evidence (US Code of Federal Regulations, 1974b) and at present it is only permitted in the US for use in the colouring of maraschino cherries at a level not exceeding 150 mg/kg by weight of the cherries. It may be used in ingested drugs, provided that the labelling does not recommend or suggest continuous administration (maximum, 6 weeks) and that the amount of ponceau SX used is such that not more than 5 mg are consumed per day; it may be used in externally applied drugs and cosmetics without restriction. This colour is now listed provisionally and its status reviewed every six months (US Code of Federal Regulations, 1974c).

2.2 Occurrence

Ponceau SX is not known to occur in nature.

2.3 Analysis

See section, "General Remarks on the Substances Considered", p. 28.

3. Biological Data Relevant to the Evaluation of Carcinogenic Risk to Man

3.1 Carcinogenicity and related studies in animals

(a) Oral administration

Mouse: Groups of 50 male and 50 female C57BL/He mice and similar groups of C3Heb/Jax mice were fed a diet containing 10,000 or 20,000 mg commercial ponceau SX per kg of diet for 2 years. Two groups of 100 male and 100 female mice of each strain were fed a control diet. In C57BL/He mice fed the 10,000 mg/kg or 20,000 mg/kg levels, tumours occurred in 8/47 (6 hepatomas, 1 reticulum-cell sarcoma and 1 other) and 12/56 (1 mammary tumour, 9 hepatomas and 2 others), respectively, compared with 13/91 (12 hepatomas and 1 reticulum-cell sarcoma) in controls. No tumours were reported in 50 and 28 C3Heb/Jax mice fed ponceau SX at each level, respectively, compared with 5/66 in controls (the numbers of animals given are those examined for pathology). In treated animals, 56-67% survived 52 weeks, compared with 91% of control C57BL/He and 58% of control C3Heb/Jax mice (Davis et al., 1966).

Rat: A group of 5 male and 5 female Wistar rats was fed a diet containing 40,000 mg ponceau SX per kg of diet for up to 18 months. In 1/7 rats living to a tumour-bearing age, a mesenteric lymphosarcoma was observed. No tumours occurred in 50 controls surviving for 20 months or more (Willheim & Ivy, 1953). [The limited number of animals used was noted by the Working Group.]

Five groups, each containing 12 male and 12 female Osborne-Mendel rats, were fed a diet containing 0 (control), 5000, 10,000, 20,000 or 50,000 mg commercial ponceau SX per kg of diet for 2 years. Benign and malignant tumours, mainly pulmonary lymphosarcomas, mammary fibroadenomas and mammary adenocarcinomas, occurred in 10/19, 8/23, 10/22 and 5/24 rats in the respective treatment groups, compared with 7/16 controls (the numbers of animals given are those whose organs were examined microscopically). Additional experiments, using groups of 200, 100 and 100 Osborne-Mendel rats of both sexes and 200, 100 and 100 Sprague-Dawley rats of both sexes fed a diet containing 0, 10,000 or 20,000 mg ponceau SX per kg of diet, resulted in tumour incidences of 67/171 (39%), 23/89 (26%) and 32/89 (36%) in Osborne-Mendel rats and 38/147 (26%), 16/83 (19%) and 14/74 (19%) in Sprague-Dawley rats in the respective groups (the numbers of animals given are those examined for pathology). Survival rates at 80 weeks were 79, 75 and 78%, respectively, in Osborne-Mendel rats and 61, 66 and 54%, respectively, in Sprague-Dawley rats (Davis et al., 1966).

In a group of 50 non-inbred rats given ponceau SX in the diet at a concentration of 20,000 mg/kg of diet on 6 days a week for 33 months (total dose, 107-139 g), 4/38 rats surviving at the appearance of the first tumour developed tumours, including 3 subcutaneous sarcomas and 1 hepatoma. No tumours were reported to have occurred in 50 controls surviving up to 33 months (Andrianova, 1970). [$P>0.05$.]

Dog: Commercial ponceau SX was fed at a level of 20,000 mg/kg of diet to 5 female beagle dogs for up to 7 years; 3 dogs died at 6, 9½ and 64 months of treatment. A second group of 5 females received ponceau SX at a level of 10,000 mg/kg of diet for 7 years, while 9 females served as controls. Thus, 2, 5 and 9 dogs, respectively, survived the 7 years of treatment. Of dogs fed the 20,000 mg/kg level, 2 had adrenal cortical adenomas and 1 had a follicular-cell adenoma of the ovary. Of the dogs fed the 10,000 mg/kg level, 1 had an adrenal medullary adenoma and 1 had a mammary adenocarcinoma. Adrenal cortical adenomas occurred in 2 controls (Davis *et al.*, 1966).

(b) *Subcutaneous and/or intramuscular injection*

Mouse: Groups of 50 male and 50 female C57BL/He mice and similar groups of C3Heb/Jax mice received monthly s.c. injections of either 0.5 ml of a 2% aqueous solution of commercial ponceau SX or 0.5 ml of saline. About 60% of both control and experimental animals survived 52 weeks or more. In C57BL/He mice, 3/59 controls and 1/59 test animals developed tumours (2 mammary tumours and 1 hepatoma in controls, 1 other tumour in treated animals), whereas in C3Heb/Jax mice, 0/69 controls and 2/66 treated mice developed tumours (Davis *et al.*, 1966).

Rat: Groups of 50 male and 50 female Osborne-Mendel rats and similar groups of Sprague-Dawley rats received weekly s.c. injections of either 1 ml of a 2% aqueous solution of commercial ponceau SX or 1 ml of saline. Survivors at 80 weeks were 70% and 82% for control and test rats of the Osborne-Mendel strain and 61% and 56% for the Sprague-Dawley rats, respectively. No tumours at the site of injection occurred in 98 and 99 controls, compared with 1/100 and 2/98 in treated animals. The total tumour incidence was 29/98 in controls, compared with 33/100 in treated Osborne-Mendel rats, and 18/99 in controls, compared with 20/98 in treated Sprague-Dawley rats. Tumours were mainly mammary fibroadenomas, adenocarcinomas and lymphosarcomas of the lung. No tumours occurred in controls which were not found in treated animals, other than tumours at the site of injection (Davis *et al.*, 1966).

3.2 Other relevant biological data

(a) Animals

The oral LD_{50} in male Wistar rats was >2 g/kg bw (Lu & Lavellée, 1964). Rats fed diets containing 5000-50,000 mg ponceau SX per kg of diet for 2 years showed no changes in growth, survival, haematological values or organ weights at autopsy. The colour fed to dogs at a level of 20,000 mg/kg of diet caused some deaths, together with moderate to marked atrophy of adrenal zona glomerulosa, chronic follicular cystitis with haematomatous projections into the urinary bladder and small haemosiderotic foci in the liver (Davis et al., 1966).

When ponceau SX was given orally in doses of 100 mg to rats, only 2% of unchanged dye was found in the faeces. When it was administered slowly by intrasplenic infusion to rats with cannulated bile ducts, 82.3% of the administered dose was excreted in the bile and 4% in the urine (Radomski & Mellinger, 1962). Products of reductive cleavage of ponceau SX, 2-amino-1-hydroxy-4-naphthalenesulphonic acid, 1-amino-2,4-dimethyl-5-benzene-sulphonic acid and 2-acetamino-1-hydroxy-4-naphthalenesulphonic acid, were found in the urine of rats fed the colour (Radomski & Mellinger, 1962). It is not reduced by rat liver homogenates (Ryan et al., 1968), but in vitro it is rapidly reduced by bacteria obtained from the intestines of rats. Three amines were detected by thin-layer chromatography of the incubation mixture (Roxon et al., 1967).

Like amaranth and sunset yellow FCF, but unlike certain other azo dyes, ponceau SX fed to dogs in amounts of 200 mg is not cathartic (Radomski & Deichmann, 1956).

3.3 Observations in man

No data were available to the Working Group.

4. Comments on Data Reported and Evaluation

4.1 Animal data

Ponceau SX was tested by the oral route in mice, rats and dogs and by subcutaneous injection in mice and rats. The experiments did not indicate a carcinogenic effect.

4.2 Human data

No case reports or epidemiological studies were available to the Working Group.

5. References

Andrianova, M.M. (1970) Carcinogenous properties of red food pigments - amaranth, SX purple and 4R purple. Vop. Pitan., 29, 61-65

Davis, K.J., Nelson, A.A., Zwickey, R.E., Hansen, W.H. & Fitzhugh, O.G. (1966) Chronic toxicity of ponceau SX to rats, mice and dogs. Toxicol. appl. Pharmacol., 8, 306-317

DeGiacomi, R., ed. (1974) Food Processing & Packaging Directory, 1974, 13th ed., London, IPC Consumer Industries Press Ltd, pp. 797-802

DFG (Deutsche Forschungsgemeinschaft) (1955) Kommission zur Bearbeitung des Lebensmittelfarbstoffproblems, Toxikologische Daten von Farbstoffen und ihre Zulassung für Lebensmittel in verschiedenen Ländern, Mitt. 6(1), Wiesbaden, Steiner Verlag

DFG (Deutsche Forschungsgemeinschaft) (1957) Farbstoff-Kommission, Toxikologische Daten von Farbstoffen und ihre Zulassung für Lebensmittel in verschiedenen Ländern, Mitt. 6(2), Wiesbaden, Steiner Verlag, p. 33

Inoue, T., Kamikura, M. & Murikami, Y. (1967) Dye standards of National Institute of Hygienic Sciences. Orange I standard and ponceau R standard. Bull. Nat. Inst. Hyg. Sci. (Tokyo), 85, 150-152

Lu, F.C. & Lavallée, A. (1964) The acute toxicity of some synthetic colours used in drugs and foods. Canad. pharm. J., 97, 30

National Research Council (1971) Food Colors, Washington DC, National Academy of Sciences, p. 7

Nieman, C. (1961) Food Colors Recently Authorized in 43 Countries, Amsterdam, Consudel

Nölting, E. & Kohn, O. (1886) Uber Xylidinsulfonsaure. Ber. dtsch. chem. Ges., 19, 137-144

Radomski, J.L. & Deichmann, W.B. (1956) Cathartic action and metabolism of certain coal-tar food dyes. J. Pharmacol. exp. Ther., 118, 322-327

Radomski, J.L. & Mellinger, T.J. (1962) The absorption, fate and excretion in rats of the water-soluble azo dyes, FD & C Red No. 2, FD & C Red No. 4 and FD and C Yellow No. 6. J. Pharmacol. exp. Ther., 136, 259-266

Roxon, J.J., Ryan, A.J. & Wright, S.E. (1967) Reduction of water-soluble azo dyes by intestinal bacteria. Fd Cosmet. Toxicol., 5, 367-369

Ryan, A.J., Roxon, J.J. & Sivayavirojana, A. (1968) Bacterial azo reduction: a metabolic reaction in mammals. Nature (Lond.), 219, 854-855

US Code of Federal Regulations (1974a) *Food and Drugs*, Title 21, part 9.63, Washington DC, US Government Printing Office, p. 195

US Code of Federal Regulations (1974b) *Food and Drugs*, Title 21, part 8.502, Washington DC, US Government Printing Office, p. 178

US Code of Federal Regulations (1974c) *Food and Drugs*, Title 21, part 8.503, Washington DC, US Government Printing Office, p. 180

US Tariff Commission (1930) *Census of Dyes and Other Synthetic Organic Chemicals, 1929*, Tariff Information Series No. 39, Washington DC, US Government Printing Office, p. 71

US Tariff Commission (1962) *Synthetic Organic Chemicals, US Production and Sales, 1961*, TC Publication 72, Washington DC, US Government Printing Office, p. 21

US Tariff Commission (1974) *Synthetic Organic Chemicals, US Production and Sales, 1972*, TC Publication 681, Washington DC, US Government Printing Office, p. 63

Willheim, R. & Ivy, A.C. (1953) A preliminary study concerning the possibility of dietary carcinogenesis. *Gastroenterology*, 23, 1-19

Zuckerman, S. (1964) *Colors for Foods, Drugs and Cosmetics*. In: Kirk, R.E. & Othmer, D.F., eds, *Encyclopedia of Chemical Technology*, 2nd ed., Vol. 2, New York, John Wiley & Sons, p. 867

SCARLET RED

1. Chemical and Physical Data

1.1 Synonyms and trade names

Colour Index No.: 26105

Colour Index Name: C.I. Solvent Red 24

Chem. Abstr. Reg. Serial No.: 85-83-6

Chem. Abstr. Name: 1-{{2-Methyl-4-[(2-methylphenyl)azo]phenyl}azo}-2-naphthalenol

For other names of which the Working Group was aware see index, p. 297.

1.2 Chemical formula and molecular weight

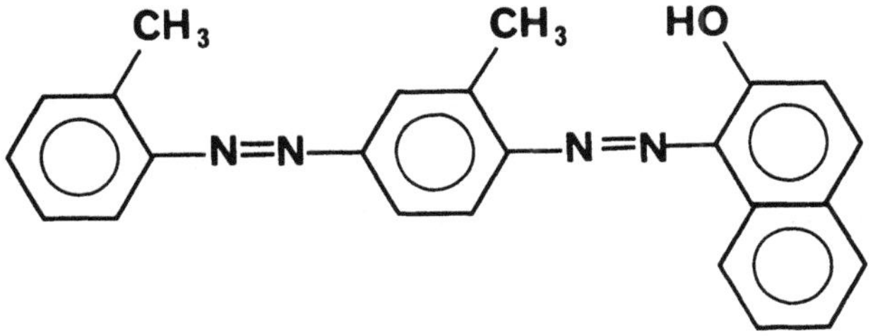

$C_{24}H_{20}N_4O$ Mol. wt: 380.4

1.3 Chemical and physical properties of the pure substance

(a) Description: Dark-reddish-brown, odourless crystals

(b) Melting-point: 181-188°C

(c) Boiling-point: 260°C (decomposition)

(d) Solubility: Practically insoluble in water; 1 g dissolves in 15 ml chloroform; soluble in oils, fats, warm petroleum, paraffin, phenol; slightly soluble in acetone, ethanol and benzene

1.4 Technical products and impurities

Specifications for scarlet red given by the Japan Food Hygiene Association (1974) require that the product contain a minimum of 85% pure chemical.

According to US industrial sources, when scarlet red is not used in foods, drugs or cosmetics, its manufacture and testing do not conform to rigid chemical specifications, and its composition varies in order to meet customer shade and intensity requirements.

2. Production, Use, Occurrence and Analysis

For important background information on this section, see preamble, p. 17.

2.1 Production and use

Scarlet red can be synthesized by coupling diazotized 4-*ortho*-tolylazo-*ortho*-toluidine with 2-naphthol (Zincke & Lawson, 1887), but it is not known whether this method is used for commercial production.

Large-scale production of scarlet red in the US was first reported in 1914 (US Tariff Commission, 1922). In 1972, there were three manufacturers of this colour, but separate data were not reported, and it was included in a miscellaneous category with 20 other red solvent colours with a combined total production of 1,075, 000 kg (US Tariff Commission, 1974). In 1972, about 300 kg of scarlet red were imported into the US (US Tariff Commission, 1973); separate data on exports were not available.

In Western Europe, there may be as many as 17 manufacturers of this substance but it is believed that production is small. In Japan, seven producers manufactured 41,000 kg of scarlet red in 1972; separate data on imports and exports were not available.

This colour has reportedly found use in veterinary and human medicine as a 4 to 8% ointment for stimulating wound healing (Merck & Co., 1968); dressings containing scarlet red and allantoin have been used in the management of indolent ulcers; and a 5% suspension in castor oil containing 1% stropine has been used in the treatment of corneal ulcers (Blacow,

1972). The Colour Index (Society of Dyers and Colourists, 1971) has reported that it is used to colour hydrocarbon solvents, oils, fats and waxes for shoe and floor polishes, in petroleum oils and greases, in wood stains, polystyrene, soap, cellulose acetate and acrylic resins, lacquers and varnishes and as an indicator.

In Japan, scarlet red has approval for certain non-food usages (Japan Food Hygiene Association, 1974) and is believed to be used in paint colourants, printing inks, plastics, gasoline, petroleum products, cosmetics and drugs applied externally (except on lips and mucous membrane).

The Deutsche Forschungsgemeinschaft (DFG, 1955) reported that scarlet red was approved in France for use in food colouring (e.g., of cheese rinds) prior to 1955; a later edition (DFG, 1957) indicated that this approval had been withdrawn.

2.2 Occurrence

Scarlet red is not known to occur in nature.

2.3 Analysis

See section, "General Remarks on the Substances Considered", p. 28.

3. Biological Data Relevant to the Evaluation of Carcinogenic Risk to Man

Two reviews on azo compounds, including scarlet red, and their carcinogenic properties have been published (Terayama, 1967; Truhaut, 1955).

3.1 Carcinogenicity and related studies in animals

(a) Oral administration

Mouse: Male and female mice of a heterozygous type B strain were given 2 mg scarlet red per animal per day as a 1% solution in rapeseed or beechnut oil. The animals were killed after 500-700 days. Tumours (mainly of the lung and lymphomas) developed in 2/81 males and 7/25 females, compared with 7/109 male and 11/59 female controls. One multiple adenoma of the liver was seen in a treated female (Waterman & Lignac, 1958). [Part of the material used was purified; however, since no evidence was found for a difference in effect between the purified and the original sample, the data were pooled.]

Rat: A group of 20 rats was fed a diet containing 1000 mg scarlet red per kg of diet for life. Three rats survived longer than 1 year, but only 1 longer than 2 years. Hepatomas were found in 2 rats, 1 dying after 272 days (total dose, 2.8 g) and the other after 763 days (total dose, 4 g). Although controls were used, data were not reported (Hackmann, 1951). [The Working Group noted the short survival time and the small number of animals used.]

(b) Skin application and subcutaneous injection

Mouse: A group of 161 white mice was painted thrice-weekly with a 2.5% solution of scarlet red in olive oil (129 times) and were simultaneously given a total of 7 s.c. injections of 0.5-0.75 ml of the same solution in the same area. No tumours were seen in 64 mice alive at 312 days after the start of treatment. Hyperplasia of the epithelial layer was found in 18 animals (Echert et al., 1935).

(c) Subcutaneous and/or intramuscular injection

Mouse: A group of 90 male and female mice was given repeated s.c. injections of scarlet red as a saturated solution in olive oil in the area of the mammary glands at intervals of 1-2 weeks for up to 86 weeks. No tumours developed, but "atypical epithelial proliferation" was noted at the site of injection. In addition, 3 male mice had "cystadenomatous proliferation" of the mammary glands at the injected area (Takeuchi, 1918).

Rat: Of 24 male and female albino rats of the Saitama strain given weekly s.c. injections of 0.2 ml of a 2% solution of scarlet red in Tween 80, 8 survived the 403 days of treatment (total doses, 128-188 mg/animal). Of these survivors, 4 developed sarcomas at the injection site at 403, 427, 428 and 463 days. No controls injected with Tween 80 alone were used, although the author made reference to possible physical effects of Tween-type, non-ionic, long-chain fatty acid solvents (Umeda, 1957, 1958).

Rabbit: Some of the rabbits used in the original study of Fischer (1906) received scarlet red in olive oil subcutaneously into the ears; epithelial growths "similar to carcinomas" were reported. This finding was confirmed in other early studies, with the common observation that such epithelial proliferation could be observed a few weeks after treatment (Jores, 1907; Meyer, 1909). In one report, 6/6 rabbits which received scarlet red subcutaneously showed epithelial proliferation characterized by "penetration of pavement epithelium recalling carcinoma" (Huguenin, 1910), whereas in another report only 1/108 rabbits developed an epithelioma (Bullock & Rohdenburg, 1918).

(d) Other experimental systems

Bladder implantation and/or instillation: No tumours were observed in 5 rabbits 95-715 days after single injections into the wall of the urinary bladder of 0.5 ml of a 1% emulsion of scarlet red in peach oil. However, when the same treatment was carried out in association with the deposition into the bladder lumen of two beads of wax dental cement, 1/6 survivors at 600 days developed a bladder carcinoma and 4 developed bladder papillomas. Of 15 rabbits receiving the wax dental cement beads only, 3 survivors at 583 days developed bladder papillomas (Podilchak, 1962).

3.2 Other relevant biological data

(a) Animals

In a group of 5 male and 5 female Wistar rats fed a diet containing 40,000 mg scarlet red per kg of diet, cirrhotic changes were observed in 1/4 rats surviving 12-18 months (Willheim & Ivy, 1953). S.c. injection of the colour into normal or benzene-pretreated rabbits caused epithelial proliferation (Vasiliev & Cheung, 1962).

I.p. injection of scarlet red into rats caused the induction of 7,12-dimethylbenz(a)anthracene metabolizing enzymes in the liver (Levin & Conney, 1967).

No colour was found in urine and very little in the faeces of rats injected intraperitoneally with scarlet red (Ryan & Welling, 1967).

(b) Man

Scarlet red has been used as a wound-healing agent, probably by stimulating tissue proliferation; however, ointments containing 8% of the colour can be irritating to the skin (Blacow, 1972).

3.3 Observations in man

No data were available to the Working Group.

4. Comments on Data Reported and Evaluation

4.1 Animal data

Scarlet red induced local sarcomas in rats following its subcutaneous injection; however, no data are reported for controls given the solvent alone (see also preamble, p. 21). Another experiment in which mice were treated orally gave a negative result, but the adequacy of the dose could not be assessed. Other experiments were considered inadequate for evaluation.

4.2 Human data

No case reports or epidemiological data were available to the Working Group.

5. References

Blacow, N.W. ed. (1972) Martindale, The Extra Pharmacopoeia, 26th ed., London, The Pharmaceutical Press, p. 208

Bullock, F.D. & Rohdenburg, G.L. (1918) Experimental "carcinomata" of animals and their relation to true malignant tumors. J. Cancer Res., 3, 227-273

DFG (Deutsche Forschungsgemeinschaft) (1955) Kommission zur Bearbeitung des Lebensmittelfarbstoffproblems, Toxikologische Daten von Farbstoffen und ihre Zulassung für Lebensmittel in verschiedenen Ländern, Mitt. 6(1), Wiesbaden, Steiner Verlag

DFG (Deutsche Forschungsgemeinschaft) (1957) Farbstoff-Kommission, Toxikologische Daten von Farbstoffen und ihre Zulassung für Lebensmittel in verschiedenen Ländern, Mitt. 6(2), Wiesbaden, Steiner Verlag, p. 55

Echert, C.T., Cooper, Z.K. & Seelig, M.G. (1935) Scarlet red as a possible carcinogenic agent. Arch. Path., 19, 83-90

Fischer, B. (1906) Die experimentelle Erzeugung atypischer Epithelwucherungen und die Entstehung bösartiger Geschwülste. Münch. med. Wschr., 53, 2041-2047

Hackmann, C. (1951) Untersuchungen über die cancerogene Wirkung einiger fettlöslicher Azofarbstoffe. Z. Krebsforsch., 57, 530-541

Huguenin, B. (1910) Contribution à l'étude des hétérotopies épithéliales actives non carcinomateuses spontanées et expérimentales. Arch. Med. exp., 22, 422-432

Japan Food Hygiene Association (1974) Japanese Standards of Food Additives, 3rd ed., Tokyo, Ministry of Health and Welfare

Jores, L. (1907) Über Art und Zustandekommen der von B. Fischer mittels "Scharlachöl" erzeugten Epithelwucherungen. Münch. med. Wschr., 54, 879-881

Levin, W. & Conney, A.H. (1967) Stimulatory effect of polycyclic hydrocarbons and aromatic azo derivatives on the metabolism of 7,12-dimethylbenz(a)anthracene. Cancer Res., 27, 1931-1938

Merck & Co. (1968) The Merck Index, 8th ed., Rahway, N.J., p. 936

Meyer, A.W. (1909) Experimentelle Epithelwucherungen. Beitr. path. Anat., 46, 437-451

Podilchak, M. (1962) Cancerogenesis and chronic inflammation. Acta biol. med. germ., 8, 559-572

Ryan, A.J. & Welling, P.G. (1967) Some observations on the metabolism and excretion of the bisazo dyes Sudan III and Sudan IV. Fd Cosmet. Toxicol., 5, 755-761

Society of Dyers and Colourists (1971) Colour Index, 3rd ed., Vol. III, Bradford, Yorkshire, Deanhouse Piccadilly, p. 3594

Takeuchi, M. (1918) Über die Veränderungen der Milchdrüse der Maus nach Scharlachrotolivenölinjektion. Mitt. med. Fak. Kais. Univ. Tokyo, 20, 47-60

Terayama, H. (1967) Aminoazo carcinogenesis - methods and biochemical problems. Methods Cancer Res., 1, 399-449

Truhaut, R. (1955) Sur l'action cancérigène de certaines matières colorrantes. Importance en hygiène alimentaire, en thérapeutique et en hygiène générale. Ann. pharm. fr. 13, 36-51

Umeda, M. (1957) Production of rat sarcoma by injections of Tween 80 solution of scarlet red. Gann, 48, 579-580

Umeda, M. (1958) Production of rat sarcoma by injections of Tween 80 solution of scarlet red. Gann, 49, 27-31

US Tariff Commission (1922) Census of Dyes and Other Synthetic Organic Chemicals, 1921, Tariff Information Series No. 26, Washington DC, US Government Printing Office, p. 47

US Tariff Commission (1973) Imports of Benzenoid Chemicals and Products, 1972, TC Publication 601, Washington DC, US Government Printing Office, p. 68

US Tariff Commission (1974) Synthetic Organic Chemicals, US Production and Sales, 1972, TC Publication 681, Washington DC, US Government Printing Office, p. 64

Vasiliev, J.M. & Cheung, A.B. (1962) Evolution of epithelial proliferation induced by scarlet red in the skin of normal and carcinogen-treated rabbits. Brit. J. Cancer, 16, 238-245

Waterman, N. & Lignac, G.O.E. (1958) The influence of the feeding of a number of food colours on the occurrence of tumours in mice. Acta physiol. pharmacol. neerl., 7, 35-55

Willheim, R. & Ivy, A.C. (1953) A preliminary study concerning the possibility of dietary carcinogenesis. Gastroenterology, 23, 1-19

Zincke, T. & Lawson, A.T. (1887) Untersuchungen über Orthoamidoazoverbindungen und Hydrazimidoverbindungen. II. Ber. dtsch. chem. Ges., 20, 1176-1183

SUDAN I

1. Chemical and Physical Data

1.1 Synonyms and trade names

Colour Index No.: 12055

Colour Index Name: C.I. Solvent Yellow 14

Chem. Abstr. Reg. Serial No.: 842-07-9

Chem. Abstr. Name: 1-(Phenylazo)-2-naphthalenol

For other names of which the Working Group was aware, see index, p. 297.

1.2 Chemical formula and molecular weight

$C_{16}H_{12}N_2O$ Mol. wt: 248.3

1.3 Chemical and physical properties of the pure substance

(a) *Description*: Brick-red crystals (leaflets from ethanol)

(b) *Melting-point*: 134°C (recrystallized from ethanol)

(c) *Absorption spectroscopy*: λ_{max} 514-516 nm (in ethanol)

(d) *Solubility*: Soluble in ethanol, acetone, ether and benzene; insoluble in water

1.4 Technical products and impurities

According to US industrial sources, when Sudan I is not used in foods, drugs or cosmetics, its manufacture and testing do not conform to rigid chemical specifications, and its composition may vary in order to meet customer shade and intensity requirements.

2. Production, Use, Occurrence and Analysis

For important background information on this section, see preamble, p. 17.

2.1 Production and use

Sudan I was first prepared by C. Liebermann in 1883 (Society of Dyers and Colourists, 1971). It can be made by coupling diazotized aniline with 2-naphthol (Hauser & Breslow, 1941).

Production of Sudan I in the US was first reported in 1914, and in 1921 four manufacturers reported sales of 11,500 kg (US Tariff Commission, 1922). In 1972, six US manufacturers reported production of about 270,000 kg (US Tariff Commission, 1974); imports were about 600 kg in that year (US Tariff Commission, 1973).

In Western Europe, there may be as many as 16 producers of Sudan I, with a total current production estimated at 100,000 kg per year. In Japan in 1972, six manufacturers reported production of 46,000 kg of this colour. Sudan I is reportedly used for colouring hydrocarbon solvents, oils, fats, waxes, shoe and floor polishes, cellulose ether varnishes, styrene resins, petrol, soap and coloured smokes (Society of Dyers and Colourists, 1971). Most current Western European production is probably consumed in the colouring of plastics.

The Deutsche Forschungsgemeinschaft (DFG, 1955) reported that this material was approved for use in food colouring in Belgium, Egypt, Italy, Norway, Poland, Portugal, Rumania, South Africa, Switzerland and Turkey. A later edition (DFG, 1957) indicated that such approval had subsequently been withdrawn in Belgium, Norway, Portugal and South Africa.

The Joint FAO/WHO Expert Committee on Food Additives, which provides information to those concerned with regulating the use of chemical substances in food, considers Sudan I, on the basis of toxicological evidence, to be unsafe for use in food (FAO/WHO, 1973).

2.2 Occurrence

Sudan I is not known to occur in nature.

2.3 Analysis

See section, "General Remarks on the Substances Considered", p. 28.

3. Biological Data Relevant to the Evaluation of Carcinogenic Risk to Man

Several review articles on azo compounds, including Sudan I, and their carcinogenic activity have been published (Druckrey, 1955; Miller & Miller, 1953; Truhaut, 1955).

3.1 Carcinogenicity and related studies in animals

(a) Oral administration

Mouse: Groups of 47 CBA and 35 stock mice of both sexes, 10 weeks old, received a diet containing Sudan I at a concentration of 1000 mg/kg of diet for 12 months (total dose, 1400 mg/animal). Ten treated CBA mice survived 99 weeks and 18 treated stock mice survived 79 weeks. The incidence of hepatomas after 120 weeks in CBA mice and after 99 weeks in stock mice was lower in treated than in untreated mice (1/44 and 1/35 compared with 9/123 and 4/49, respectively). In the CBA group 2 mice developed reticulum-cell tumours of the ovary and 5 animals developed leukaemia; the tumours were not considered by the authors to be related to the treatment (Clayson et al., 1965).

Rat: A group of 20 rats weighing about 100 g was fed a diet containing Sudan I at a concentration of 1000 mg/kg of diet for lifespan. In all, 17 rats survived for more than 1 year, 8 for more than 2 years and 1 rat for more than 3 years. No tumours were found (Hackmann, 1951).

(b) Subcutaneous and/or intramuscular administration

Mouse: A group of 18 male and 18 female stock mice, 2-3 months of age, was given 17-20 s.c. injections of 0.25 ml of a 3% solution of Sudan I in arachis oil at 3-week intervals. Between the 305th and 615th day after the start of treatment 8/12 males had developed tumours: 6 hepatomas, 1 adenocarcinoma of the lung and 1 squamous carcinoma at the injection site. Between the 460th and 500th day, 3 females developed tumours: 1 hepatoma, 1 adenoma of the lung and 1 adenocarcinoma of the lung. Exact data for controls are not given, but the authors report the results to be significantly different from those in untreated mice (Kirby & Peacock, 1949).

(c) Other experimental systems

Bladder implantation and/or instillation: Paraffin wax pellets weighing 10-18 mg and containing 12% Sudan I were implanted into the urinary bladders of 32 albino mice for 40 weeks. Eight mice developed carcinomas of the bladder, 6 mice had benign tumours and 5 showed squamous metaplasia of the bladder. In 56 control animals, 2 carcinomas, 9 squamous metaplasia and 3 benign tumours were found (Bonser, 1962; Bonser et al., 1956, 1963).

Paraffin wax pellets containing 12.5% Sudan I were implanted into the urinary bladders of female (C57xIF)F_1 mice; 14/100 mice surviving 25 or more weeks developed carcinomas of the bladder, and 2 mice showed squamous metaplasia of the bladder. The incidence of bladder carcinoma in controls surviving the same time was 4/89, and no squamous metaplasia, papillomas or adenomas were seen (Clayson & Bonser, 1965).

A group of 61 (C57xIF)F_1 mice, 10-12 weeks of age, received implants into the urinary bladder of pellets of paraffin wax weighing 15-17 mg and containing 12.5% Sudan I. At 40 weeks, when the experiment was terminated, 13/56 mice had carcinomas of the bladder, compared with 6/142 controls which had received implants of paraffin wax pellets only (Clayson et al., 1968).

3.2 Other relevant biological data

(a) Animals

The s.c. LD_{50} of Sudan I in rabbits is <500 mg/kg bw (Truhaut, 1958).

Following its oral administration in rabbits, 1.2% was excreted unchanged, 1.5% as 1-*para*-hydroxyphenylazo-2-naphthol, 44% as free and conjugated *para*-aminophenol, 24% as *para*-aminophenylglucuronide, 0.5% as *ortho*-aminophenol and 1.1% as aniline; *para*-acetamidophenyl glucuronide, 1-*para*-hydroxyphenylazo-2-naphthol glucuronide and 1-amino-2-naphthol were also found in the urine (Daniel, 1962).

Other investigators found that glucuronides of 4',6-dihydroxy-1-phenylazo-2-naphthol and 4'- and 6-hydroxy-1-phenylazo-2-naphthol were present in both bile and urine of rabbits. The urine also contained 1-amino-2-naphthyl hydrogen sulphate, 1-amino-2-naphthyl glucuronide and the N-glucuronides of 1-phenylhydrazo-2-naphthol and of 4'-hydroxy-1-phenylhydrazo-2-naphthol and other metabolites which were not identified (Childs & Clayson, 1966).

Sudan I was reduced on incubation with intestinal contents, intestinal tissue or clones of bacteria isolated from rat intestine; and the bile and urine of rats contained the same metabolites as found in rabbits by Childs & Clayson (1966), although the presence of N-glucuronide of 4'-hydroxy-1-phenylhydrazo-2-naphthol was not established with certainty. After its oral administration more unchanged dye was present in faeces and less 1-amino-2-naphthyl hydrogen sulphate was found in urine than when the colour was given by i.p. injection (Childs et al., 1967).

3.3 Observations in man

No data were available to the Working Group.

4. Comments on Data Reported and Evaluation[1]

4.1 Animal data

Sudan I is carcinogenic in mice following its subcutaneous administration, producing tumours of the liver. It also produced bladder tumours in mice following its implantation into the urinary bladder. Tests by oral administration in mice and rats were negative, but the adequacy of the dose level used could not be assessed.

4.2 Human data

No case reports or epidemiological studies were available to the Working Group.

---

[1] See also the section, "Animal Data in Relation to the Evaluation of Risk to Man" in the introduction to this volume, p. 15.

5. References

Bonser, G.M. (1962) The experimental induction of cancer of the bladder. Acta Un. int. Cancr, 18, 538-544

Bonser, G.M., Bradshaw, L., Clayson, D.B. & Jull, J.W. (1956) A further study of the carcinogenic properties of *ortho* hydroxy-amines and related compounds by bladder implantation in the mouse. Brit. J. Cancer, 10, 539-546

Bonser, G.M., Clayson, D.B. & Jull, J.W. (1963) The potency of 20-methylcholanthrene relative to other carcinogens on bladder implantation. Brit. J. Cancer, 17, 235-241

Childs, J.J. & Clayson, D.B. (1966) The metabolism of 1-phenylazo-2-naphthol in the rabbit. Biochem. Pharmacol., 15, 1247-1258

Childs, J.J., Nakajima, C. & Clayson, D.B. (1967) The metabolism of 1-phenylazo-2-naphthol in the rat with reference to the action of the intestinal flora. Biochem. Pharmacol., 16, 1555-1561

Clayson, D.B. & Bonser, G.M. (1965) The induction of tumours of the mouse bladder epithelium by 4-ethylsulphonylnaphthalene-1-sulphonamide. Brit. J. Cancer, 19, 311-316

Clayson, D.B., Lawson, T.A., Santana, S. & Bonser, G.M. (1965) Correlation between the chemical induction of hyperplasia and of malignancy in the bladder epithelium. Brit. J. Cancer, 19, 297-310

Clayson, D.B., Pringle, J.A.S., Bonser, G.M. & Wood, M. (1968) The technique of bladder implantation: further results and an assessment. Brit. J. Cancer, 22, 825-832

Daniel, J.W. (1962) The excretion and metabolism of edible food colors. Toxicol. appl. Pharmacol., 4, 572-594

DFG (Deutsche Forschungsgemeinschaft) (1955) Kommission zur Bearbeitung des Lebensmittelfarbstoffproblems, Toxikologische Daten von Farbstoffen und ihre Zulassung für Lebensmittel in verschiedenen Ländern, Mitt. 6(1), Wiesbaden, Steiner Verlag

DFG (Deutsche Forschungsgemeinschaft) (1957) Farbstoff-Kommission, Toxikologische Daten von Farbstoffen und ihre Zulassung für Lebensmittel in verschiedenen Ländern, Mitt. 6(2), Wiesbaden, Steiner Verlag, p. 6

Druckrey, H. (1955) Schädliche und unschädliche Farbstoffe für Lebensmittel. Z. Krebsforsch., 60, 344-360

FAO/WHO (1973) List of Additives Evaluated for their Safety-in-Use in Food, First Series, CAC/FAL 1-1973, p. 45

Hackmann, C. (1951) Untersuchungen über die cancerogene Wirkung einiger fettlöslicher Azofarbstoffe. Z. Krebsforsch., 57, 530-541

Hauser, C.R. & Breslow, D.S. (1941) Condensations. XV. The electronic mechanism of the diazo coupling reaction. J. Amer. chem. Soc., 63, 418-420

Kirby, A.H.M. & Peacock, P.R. (1949) Liver tumours in mice injected with commercial food dyes. Glasgow med. J., 30, 364-372

Miller, J.A. & Miller, E.C. (1953) The carcinogenic aminoazo dyes. Advanc. Cancer Res., 1, 339-396

Society of Dyers and Colourists (1971) Colour Index, 3rd ed., Vol. III, Bradford, Yorkshire, Deanhouse Piccadilly, p. 3566

Truhaut, R. (1955) Sur l'action cancérigène de certaines matières colorantes. Importance en hygiène alimentaire, en thérapeutique et en hygiène générale. Ann. pharm. fr., 13, 36-51

Truhaut, R. (1958) Sur l'utilisation des colorants en thérapeutique et les dangers qui peuvent en résulter pour la santé humaine. Chimie moderne, 3, 337-350

US Tariff Commission (1922) Census of Dyes and Other Synthetic Organic Chemicals, 1921, Tariff Information Series No. 26, Washington DC, US Government Printing Office, p. 63

US Tariff Commission (1973) Imports of Benzenoid Chemicals and Products, 1972, TC Publication 601, Washington DC, US Government Printing Office, p. 66

US Tariff Commission (1974) Synthetic Organic Chemicals, US Production and Sales, 1972, TC Publication 681, Washington DC, US Government Printing Office, p. 64

SUDAN II

1. Chemical and Physical Data

1.1 Synonyms and trade names

Colour Index No.: 12140

Colour Index Name: C.I. Solvent Orange 7

Chem. Abstr. **Reg.** Serial No.: 3118-97-6

Chem. Abstr. Name.: 1-[(2,4-Dimethylphenyl)azo]-2-naphthalenol

For other names of which the Working Group was aware see index, p. 297.

1.2 Chemical formula and molecular weight

$C_{18}H_{16}N_2O$

Mol. wt: 276.3

1.3 Chemical and physical properties of the pure substance

(a) Description: Brown-red crystals; red needles

(b) Melting-point: 166°C (recrystallized); 133°C (from glacial acetic acid)

(c) Absorption spectroscopy: λ_{max} (in ethanol) varies from 492-531 nm

(d) Solubility: Soluble in ethanol, acetone, benzene and ether; insoluble in water

1.4 Technical products and impurities

According to US industrial sources, when Sudan II is not used in foods, drugs or cosmetics, its manufacture and testing do not conform to rigid chemical specifications, and its composition may vary in order to meet customer shade and intensity requirements.

2. Production, Use, Occurrence and Analysis

For important background information on this section, see preamble, p. 17.

2.1 Production and use

Sudan II can be synthesized by coupling diazotized 2,4-dimethylaniline with 2-naphthol (Richter, 1958), but it is not known whether this method is used for commercial production.

Large-scale production of Sudan II in the US was first reported in 1921 (US Tariff Commission, 1922). In 1971, three manufacturers reported production of 34,500 kg (US Tariff Commission, 1973); in 1972, it was also produced by three manufacturers, but separate production data were not published, and it was included in a miscellaneous category containing at least 11 other colours, with a total production of 236,000 kg (US Tariff Commission, 1974). Separate data on US imports and exports were not available.

In Western Europe, there may be as many as eight producers of Sudan II; one producer in the United Kingdom manufactures some several thousand kg per year. In Japan, three producers manufactured 3300 kg of this colour in 1972; separate data on imports and exports were not available.

Sudan II is reportedly used for colouring oils, waxes, hydrocarbon solvents for polishes, candles and polystyrene resins (Society of Dyers and Colourists, 1971). In Japan it is used to colour petroleum products, plastics, shoe polish, cosmetics and drugs applied externally (except on mucous membrane).

The Deutsche Forschungsgemeinschaft (DFG, 1955) reported that Sudan II was approved for use as a general food colouring in Canada, Greece, Japan, Mexico, Norway and Peru. A later edition (DFG, 1957) reported approval in Cuba, the Dominican Republic and Guatemala, but indicated that approval had been withdrawn in Canada and Norway. Approval for its use in food in Japan was withdrawn prior to 1966, although it was retained for certain non-food uses (Japan Food Hygiene Association, 1974).

Sudan II was added to the US approved list of food, drug and cosmetic colours in 1939, but in 1956, on the basis of toxicological data, it was removed from this list for use in food but permitted in externally applied drugs and cosmetics. In 1963, it was removed for even these uses (National Research Council, 1971).

2.2 Occurrence

Sudan II is not known to occur in nature.

2.3 Analysis

See section, "General Remarks on the Substances Considered", p. 28.

3. Biological Data Relevant to the Evaluation of Carcinogenic Risk to Man

3.1 Carcinogenicity and related studies in animals

(a) Oral administration

Mouse: A group of 15 male and 15 female stock albino mice was fed a diet containing 1000 mg Sudan II per kg of diet for 52 weeks (weekly intake, 14 mg/mouse; total dose, 728 mg/mouse). Only 11 males and 10 females survived longer than 20 weeks, and the experiment was terminated at 90 weeks. Of 15 animals examined during 20-89 weeks, 3 males and 1 female had developed benign intestinal tumours, compared with 1/13 controls. The treatment did not significantly raise the lymphoma incidence (Bonser *et al.*, 1956).*

Rat: In a 2-year experiment, an unspecified number of weanling rats were fed a diet containing 1000 or 2500 mg Sudan II per kg of diet. Both doses caused an increase in mortality, but no tumour development was described (Fitzhugh *et al.*, 1956). [No further details were given.]

A group of 20 male and 20 female rats, 5-6 weeks of age, received 300, 7500 or 15,000 mg Sudan II per kg of diet. Only 13/40 animals of the low dose group survived to 44 weeks; all rats of the middle dose group died

---

* Bonser *et al.* (1956) give the formula of 1-(2,5-xylylazo)-2-naphthol and refer to it as xylylazo-2-naphthol; but in a following paper (Clayson *et al.*, 1968), the same authors refer to their previous paper and describe the substance used as oil orange KB, which is identical with Sudan II and 1-(2,4-xylylazo)-2-naphthol.

within 40 weeks; and all rats of the high dose group died within 20 weeks. No tumours were found (Allmark et al., 1956). [The Working Group noted the short duration of the experiment.]

(b) Subcutaneous and/or intramuscular administration

Mouse: A group of 15 male and 15 female stock albino mice received twice weekly s.c. injections of 0.1 ml of a 3% suspension of Sudan II in arachis oil for 52 weeks (6 mg/week/mouse; total dose, 312 mg/mouse). Only 7 males and 3 females survived longer than 20 weeks; the duration of the experiment was 89 weeks. A hepatoma occurred in 1 male; none were found in 18 control mice treated with arachis oil and surviving from 20-90 weeks. Treatment with the colour did not significantly raise the lymphoma incidence (Bonser et al., 1956).* [The Working Group noted the limited number of surviving animals.]

Rat: A group of 18 Osborne-Mendel rats received weekly s.c. injections of 0.5-1 mg Sudan II as a 1% suspension in glycerol for 13 months, when the experiment was terminated. No tumours occurred (Nelson & Davidow, 1957). [The Working Group noted the short duration of the experiment.]

(c) Other experimental systems

Bladder implantation and/or instillation: A group of 60 (C57xIF)F$_1$ mice, 10-12 weeks old, received pellets of paraffin wax weighing 15-17 mg and containing 12.5% Sudan II implanted into the urinary bladder. The experiment was terminated at 40 weeks, and bladder carcinomas were found to have occurred in 43/44 surviving animals. In additional groups of similarly treated mice, 40/62 females killed at 40 weeks and 6/9 females surviving 61 weeks developed bladder carcinomas; 9 males surviving 61 weeks showed no tumours. Bladder carcinomas developed in 6/142 control mice given implants of paraffin wax alone (Clayson et al., 1968).

---

*Bonser et al. (1956) give the formula of 1-(2,5-xylylazo)-2-naphthol and refer to it as xylylazo-2-naphthol; but, in a following paper (Clayson et al., 1968), the same authors refer to their previous paper and describe the substance used as oil orange KB, which is identical with Sudan II and 1-(2,4-xylylazo)-2-naphthol.

3.2 Other relevant biological data

(a) Animals

Rats fed a diet containing 300 mg Sudan II per kg of diet showed no change in food consumption, growth or haemoglobin production; rats given levels of 7500 mg/kg of diet died within 40 weeks; and all rats given 15,000 mg/kg of diet died within 20 weeks. Oral doses of 200-400 mg/kg bw caused a decline in haemoglobin levels (Allmark et al., 1956). The maximum tolerated dose of Sudan II, when administered to rats by stomach tube, is about 40 mg (Radomski, 1962). Single oral doses of 100 or 200 mg are cathartic in dogs (Radomski & Deichmann, 1956).

The colour was easily reduced by intestinal bacteria; after its administration to rats in corn oil by stomach tube, 1-amino-2-naphthyl sulphate and eight other metabolites, five of which were red-coloured, were excreted in urine. When $8\text{-}^{14}C$-labelled 1-xylylazo-2-naphthol was administered, the urine was found to contain 14% and the faeces 86% of the total radioactivity (Radomski, 1961)*; 11 metabolites were identified, including 1-amino-2-naphthyl sulphate and 1-amino-2-naphthyl glucuronide (Radomski, 1962).

Sudan II fed continuously to rats at a concentration of 6000 mg/kg of diet induces Heinz bodies (Rofe, 1957).

3.3 Observations in man

No data were available to the Working Group.

4. Comments on Data Reported and Evaluation

4.1 Animal data

Sudan II was tested in mice and rats by the oral and subcutaneous routes. Results of these studies cannot be evaluated because of the inadequacy either of the number of animals used, the duration of the experiment or the degree of reporting.

Sudan II was also tested in mice by bladder implantation, resulting in a high incidence of bladder carcinomas (see also preamble, p. 21).

---

* The 2,5-isomer was used.

4.2 Human data

No case reports or epidemiological studies were available to the Working Group.

5. References

Allmark, M.G., Grice, H.C. & Mannell, W.A. (1956) Chronic toxicity studies on food colours. II. Observations on the toxicity of FD & C Green No. 2 (light green SF yellowish), FD & C Orange No. 2 (orange SS) and FD & C Red No. 32 (oil red XO) in rats. J. Pharm. Pharmacol., 8, 417-424

Bonser, G.M., Clayson, D.B. & Jull, J.W. (1956) The induction of tumours of the subcutaneous tissues, liver and intestine in the mouse by certain dyestuffs and their intermediates. Brit. J. Cancer, 10, 653-667

Clayson, D.B., Pringle, J.A.S., Bonser, G.M. & Wood, M. (1968) The technique of bladder implantation: further results and an assessment. Brit. J. Cancer, 22, 825-832

DFG (Deutsche Forschungsgemeinschaft) (1955) Kommission zur Bearbeitung des Lebensmittelfarbstoffproblems, Toxikologische Daten von Farbstoffen und ihre Zulassung für Lebensmittel in verschiedenen Ländern, Mitt. 6(1), Wiesbaden, Steiner Verlag

DFG (Deutsche Forschungsgemeinschaft) (1957) Farbstoff-Kommission, Toxikologische Daten von Farbstoffen und ihre Zulassung für Lebensmittel in verschiedenen Ländern, Mitt. 6(2), Wiesbaden, Steiner Verlag, p. 13

Fitzhugh, O.G., Nelson, A.A. & Bourke, A.R. (1956) Chronic toxicities of two food colors, FD & C Red No. 32 and FD & C Orange No. 2. Fed. Proc., 15, 422

Japan Food Hygiene Association (1974) Japanese Standards of Food Additives, 3rd ed., Tokyo, Ministry of Health and Welfare

National Research Council (1971) Food Colors, Washington DC, National Academy of Sciences, p. 43

Nelson, A.A. & Davidow, B. (1957) Injection site fibrosarcoma production in rats by food colors. Fed. Proc., 16, 367

Radomski, J.L. (1961) The absorption, fate and excretion of citrus red No. 2 (2,5-dimethoxyphenyl-azo-2-naphthol) and Ext. D & C Red No. 14 (1-xylylazo-2-naphthol). J. Pharmacol. exp. Ther., 134, 100-109

Radomski, J.L. (1962) 1-Amino-2-naphthyl glucuronide, a metabolite of 2,5-dimethoxyphenylazo-2-naphthol and 1-xylyl-2-naphthol. J. Pharmacol. exp. Ther., 136, 378-385

Radomski, J.L. & Deichmann, W.B. (1956) Cathartic action and metabolism of certain coal-tar food dyes. J. Pharmacol. exp. Ther., 118, 322-327

Richter, F. (1958) Beilstein's Handbuch der Organischen Chemie, Berlin, Springer Verlag, Vol. 16, 168, p. I-260

Rofe, P. (1957) Azo dyes and Heinz bodies. *Brit. J. industr. Med.*, __14__, 275-280

Society of Dyers and Colourists (1971) *Colour Index*, 3rd ed., Vol. III, Bradford, Yorkshire, Deanhouse Piccadilly, p. 3580

US Tariff Commission (1922) *Census of Dyes and Other Synthetic Organic Chemicals, 1921*, Tariff Information Series No. 26, Washington DC, US Government Printing Office, p. 63

US Tariff Commission (1973) *Synthetic Organic Chemicals, US Production and Sales, 1971*, TC Publication 614, Washington DC, US Government Printing Office, p. 64

US Tariff Commission (1974) *Synthetic Organic Chemicals, US Production and Sales, 1972*, TC Publication 681, Washington DC, US Government Printing Office, p. 85

SUDAN III

1. Chemical and Physical Data

1.1 Synonyms and trade names

Colour Index No.: 26100

Colour Index Name: C.I. Solvent Red 23

Chem. Abstr. Reg. Serial No.: 85-86-9

Chem. Abstr. Name: 1-{[4-(Phenylazo)phenyl]azo}-2-naphthalenol

For other names of which the Working Group was aware, see index, p. 297.

1.2 Chemical formula and molecular weight

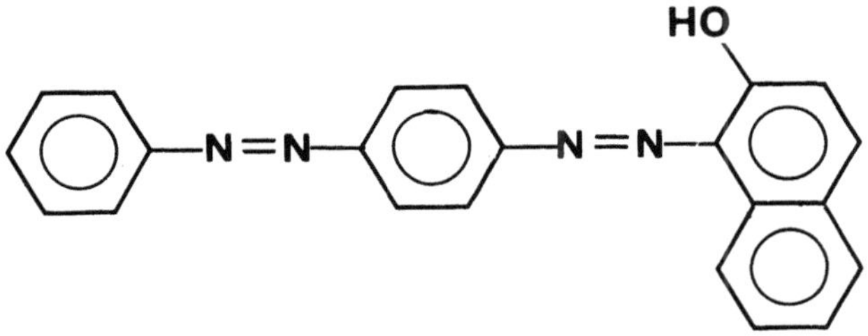

$C_{22}H_{16}N_4O$ Mol. wt: 352.4

1.3 Chemical and physical properties of the pure substance

(a) Description: Reddish-brown or yellowish-red crystals; brown crystals with green, metallic glimmer (crystallized from glacial acetic acid)

(b) Melting-point: 195°C (recrystallized from glacial acetic acid)

(c) Solubility: Soluble in chloroform, glacial acetic acid; moderately soluble in ethanol (3% at room temperature), ether, acetone, petrol ether, oils and waxes; very soluble in benzene; insoluble in water

1.4 Technical products and impurities

Specifications for Sudan III are given for drug and cosmetic applications, in which the product must contain a minimum of 85% pure colour (US Code of Federal Regulations, 1974a).

2. Production, Use, Occurrence and Analysis

For important background information on this section, see preamble, p. 17.

2.1 Production and use

Sudan III was first prepared by F. Grässler in 1879 (Society of Dyers and Colourists, 1971). It is manufactured commercially by coupling diazotized aniline with an excess of aniline to produce *para*-phenylazoaniline, which is then condensed with 2-naphthol (Nietzki, 1880; Zuckerman, 1964).

Large-scale production of Sudan III in the US was first reported in 1914 (US Tariff Commission, 1922). In 1972, only one US manufacturer reported production; separate production data were not published and it was included in a miscellaneous category with 20 other colours, with a combined production of 70,000 kg (US Tariff Commission, 1974). Separate data on US imports and exports were not available.

There may be as many as 14 producers of Sudan III in Western Europe, but production is believed to be small. In Japan, four producers manufactured 3400 kg of this colour in 1972; separate data on imports and exports were not available.

Zuckerman (1964) reported that Sudan III was used in oil-based drug solutions, ointments, soap, suntan oils, hair oils and pomades. Another source has reported its use in the colouring of oils and alcohol lacquers and as a stain for zoological, pathological and vegetable materials (Merck & Co., 1968). In Japan, it is believed to be used for colouring oils, fats, waxes, solvents, paints, gasoline, plastics, cosmetics and drugs applied externally (except on mucous membrane).

According to the Deutsche Forschungsgemeinschaft (DFG, 1955) Sudan III was approved for general food use in the USSR prior to 1955, but approval had been withdrawn by 1957 (DFG, 1957). In the US, on December 31, 1968, Sudan III and all mixtures containing it were cancelled for use in ingested products (US Code of Federal Regulations, 1974b); at present it is permitted for use in certain non-food applications, at least in the US and Japan (Japan Food Hygiene Association, 1974).

2.2 Occurrence

Sudan III is not known to occur in nature.

2.3 Analysis

See section, "General Remarks on the Substances Considered", p. 28.

3. Biological Data Relevant to the Evaluation of Carcinogenic Risk to Man

A review article on aromatic azo compounds, including Sudan III, and their carcinogenic activity has been published (Truhaut, 1955).

3.1 Carcinogenicity and related studies in animals

(a) Oral administration

Mouse: Eighty-three male and 54 female type B mice were given Sudan III in the food as a 1% oil solution at the rate of 2 mg/animal/day. At 200, 400, 600 and 724 (or 752) days, survival rates in males and females were 83, 75, 53 and 29 and 54, 45, 37 and 13 mice, respectively. In males 9 lung tumours and 2 forestomach papillomas, and in females 6 mammary and 7 lung tumours were observed. The authors did not consider the number of lung tumours to be significantly greater than that in controls, due to the heterogenous background of the mice (Waterman & Lignac, 1958).

Rat: In a group of 5 male and 5 female Wistar rats fed a diet containing 40,000 mg Sudan III per kg of diet for 18 months, no tumours were observed (Willheim & Ivy, 1953). [No individual data on survival were given.]

(b) Subcutaneous and/or intramuscular administration

Mouse: No tumours were observed in two groups of 10 female stock mice given repeated s.c. injections of 0.25 ml of a saturated solution of Sudan III in lard or about 5 mg of crystals injected subcutaneously; and none were found in a group of 10 A strain mice injected subcutaneously with Sudan III in lard. The duration of the experiment was 24 months (Shear & Stewart, 1941). [No further details were available.]

3.2 **Other relevant biological data**

(a) Animals

The i.p. LD_{50} of Sudan III in rats was about 0.5 g/kg bw. This was the most effective of the Sudan colours in producing hyaline, fatty and hydropic lesions of the liver in rabbits and fatty and hydropic lesions of the liver in rats and mice (Carrol, 1964). However, it did not appear to be toxic to rats when fed at a level of 40,000 mg/kg of diet (Willheim & Ivy, 1953).

Three rabbits given 1.7 g/kg bw of Sudan III by i.p. injection died after 1-3 weeks; 2 had congested kidneys (Salant & Bengis, 1916). All of 16 rabbits injected intrapleurally with a single dose of approximately 9% Sudan III in 10 ml olive oil and sodium tauroglycocholate showed cellular metaplasia or hyperplasia or both of the serosal epithelium of the visceral pleura or in the pulmonary epithelium between 10 and 47 days later (Young, 1928).

Sudan III was found to be an active inducer of 7,12-dimethylbenz(a)-anthracene (DMBA)-metabolizing enzymes (Conney & Levin, 1966; Levin & Conney, 1967). It was the most active of several azo compounds in preventing adrenal necrosis and mammary cancer in rats tested with DMBA (Huggins & Pataki, 1965; Wheatley & Sims, 1969).

Following oral administration to rats of 50 mg Sudan III suspended in methylcellulose, 95% was excreted unchanged in the faeces; when it was suspended in olive oil, 84% was excreted (Ryan & Welling, 1967). None of the anticipated metabolites, *para*-aminophenol, *para*-phenylenediamine, 1-amino-2-naphthol or 1-(4-aminophenylazo)-2-naphthol, were detectable in the urine or bile. After i.p. injection of 20 mg Sudan III in olive oil to rats, only a little unchanged colour was found in the faeces, and no metabolites were seen in the urine or bile. However, the distribution of radioactivity in a male rat after a single i.p. dose of 2.72 mg ^{3}H-labelled Sudan III dissolved in dimethyl sulphoxide was 5.1% in the faeces, 15.8% in the urine, 0.3% in the bile and 27.8% in the body, leaving 51% unaccounted for. Most of the radioactivity present in the urine was represented by *para*-aminophenol (Ryan & Welling, 1967).

3.3 Observations in man

No data were available to the Working Group.

4. Comments on Data Reported and Evaluation

4.1 Animal data

The Working Group considered the results of tests in which Sudan III was administered to mice and rats by the oral route and to mice by the subcutaneous route. All experiments were inadequate with regard to either the dose administered, the degree of reporting or the number of animals used.

4.2 Human data

No case reports or epidemiological studies were available to the Working Group.

5. References

Carroll, R. (1964) Lesions of the liver produced by Sudan dyes. J. Path. Bact., 87, 317-324

Conney, A.H. & Levin, W. (1966) Induction of hepatic 7,12-dimethylbenz(a)-anthracene metabolism by polycyclic aromatic hydrocarbons and aromatic azo derivatives. Life Sci., 5, 465-471

DFG (Deutsche Forschungsgemeinschaft) (1955) Kommission zur Bearbeitung des Lebensmittelfarbstoffproblems, Toxikologische Daten von Farbstoffen und ihre Zulassung für Lebensmittel in verschiedenen Ländern, Mitt. 6(1), Wiesbaden, Steiner Verlag

DFG (Deutsche Forschungsgemeinschaft) (1957) Farbstoff-Kommission, Toxikologische Daten von Farbstoffen und ihre Zulassung für Lebensmittel in verschiedenen Ländern, Mitt. 6(2), Wiesbaden, Steiner Verlag, p. 53

Huggins, C. & Pataki, J. (1965) Aromatic azo derivatives preventing mammary cancer and adrenal injury from 7,12-dimethylbenz(a)anthracene. Proc. nat. Acad. Sci., 53, 791-796

Japan Food Hygiene Association (1974) Japanese Standards of Food Additives, 3rd ed., Tokyo, Ministry of Health and Welfare

Levin, W. & Conney, A.H. (1967) Stimulatory effect of polycyclic hydrocarbons and aromatic azo derivatives on the metabolism of 7,12-dimethylbenz(a)anthracene. Cancer Res., 27, 1931-1938

Merck & Co. (1968) The Merck Index, 8th ed., Rahway, N.J., p. 993

Nietzki, R. (1880) Uber biebucher Scharlach. Ber. dtsch. chem. Ges., 13, 1838-1840

Ryan, A.J. & Welling, P.G. (1967) Some observations on the metabolism and excretion of the bisazo dyes Sudan III and Sudan IV. Fd Cosmet. Toxicol., 5, 755-761

Salant, W. & Bengis, R. (1916) Physiological and pharmacological studies on coal-tar colors. I. Experiments with fat-soluble dyes. J. biol. Chem., 27, 403-427

Shear, M.J. & Stewart, H.L. (1941) In: Hartwell, J.L., Survey of compounds which have been tested for carcinogenic activity, Washington DC, US Government Printing Office (Public Health Service Publication No. 149)

Society of Dyers and Colourists (1971) Colour Index, 3rd ed., Bradford, Yorkshire, Deanhouse Piccadilly

Truhaut, R. (1955) Sur l'action cancérigène de certaines matières colorantes. Importance en hygiène alimentaire, en thérapeutique et en hygiène générale. Ann. pharm. fr., 13, 36-51

US Code of Federal Regulations (1974a) Food and Drugs, Title 21, part 9.162, Washington DC, US Government Printing Office, p. 199

US Code of Federal Regulations (1974b) Food and Drugs, Title 21, part 8.510, Washington DC, US Government Printing Office, p. 181

US Tariff Commission (1922) Census of Dyes and Other Synthetic Organic Chemicals, 1921, Tariff Information Series No. 26, Washington DC, US Government Printing Office, p. 47

US Tariff Commission (1974) Synthetic Organic Chemicals, US Production and Sales, 1972, TC Publication 681, Washington DC, US Government Printing Office, p. 64

Waterman, N. & Lignac, G.O.E. (1958) The influence of the feeding of a number of food colours on the occurrence of tumours in mice. Acta physiol. pharmacol. neerl., 7, 35-55

Wheatley, D.N. & Sims, P. (1969) Comparison of the efficacy of pretreatment protection against adrenal necrosis induced by 7-hydroxymethyl-12-methylbenz(a)anthracene and by 7-methyl-12-methylbenz(a)anthracene in rats. Biochem. Pharmacol., 18, 2583-2587

Willheim, R. & Ivy, A.C. (1953) A preliminary study concerning the possibility of dietary carcinogenesis. Gastroenterology, 23, 1-19

Young, J.S. (1928) The experimental production of metaplasia and hyperplasia in the serosal endothelium and of hyperplasia in the alveolar epithelium of the lung of the rabbit. J. Path. Bact., 31, 265-275

Zuckerman, S. (1964) Colors for Foods, Drugs and Cosmetics. In: Kirk, R.E. & Othmer, D.F., eds, Encyclopedia of Chemical Technology, 2nd ed., Vol. 5, New York, John Wiley & Sons, p. 870

SUDAN BROWN RR

1. **Chemical and Physical Data**

1.1 Synonyms and trade names

Colour Index No.: 11285

Colour Index Name: C.I. Solvent Brown I

Chem. Abstr. Reg. Serial No.: 6416-57-5

Chem. Abstr. Name: 4-(1-Naphthylazo)-1,3-phenylenediamine

For other names of which the Working Group was aware see Index, p. 297.

1.2 Chemical formula and molecular weight

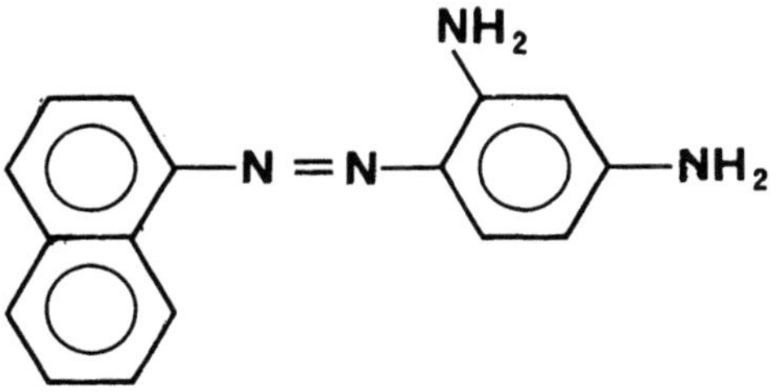

$C_{16}H_{14}N_4$ Mol. wt: 262.3

1.3 Chemical and physical properties of the pure substance

(a) Melting-point: 155-160°C

(b) Solubility: Soluble in ethanol, acetone and benzene; insoluble in water

1.4 Technical products and impurities

No data were available to the Working Group.

2. Production, Use, Occurrence and Analysis

For important background information on this section, see preamble, p. 17.

2.1 Production and use

Sudan brown RR can be synthesized by coupling diazotized 1-naphthylamine with *meta*-phenylenediamine (Society of Dyers and Colourists, 1971), but to our knowledge it has not been produced commercially in either the US or Japan; production data were not available for Western Europe.

Sudan brown RR is reportedly used to colour alcoholic solvents, oils, fats, waxes, printing inks and spirit lacquers (Society of Dyers and Colourists, 1971). According to the Deutsche Forschungsgemeinschaft (DFG, 1955, 1957) this colour was not approved for food use in any of the countries surveyed.

2.2 Occurrence

Sudan brown RR is not known to occur in nature.

2.3 Analysis

See section, "General Remarks on the Substances Considered", p. 28.

3. Biological Data Relevant to the Evaluation of Carcinogenic Risk to Man

A review on azo compounds, including Sudan brown RR, and their carcinogenic properties has been published (Truhaut, 1955).

3.1 Carcinogenicity and related studies in animals

(a) Oral administration

Rat: A group of 20 rats was fed a diet containing Sudan brown RR at a concentration of 1000 mg/kg of diet for life. Seventeen rats survived longer than 1 year and 5 longer than 2 years. One rat dying after 624 days had a spindle-cell sarcoma of the liver with metastases in the pleura and omentum. Other tumours included a carcinoma of the stomach in 1 rat dying after 769 days, a lymphatic leukaemia and a fibroadenoma in 1 rat dying after 656 days and 2 mammary fibroadenomas in 1 rat dying after 719 days.

Although no control data were reported, it was stated that only mammary fibroadenomas occurred in untreated animals (Hackmann, 1951).

3.2 Other relevant biological data

No data were available to the Working Group.

3.3 Observations in man

No data were available to the Working Group.

4. Comments on Data Reported and Evaluation

4.1 Animal data

Sudan brown RR was only tested in rats by the oral route. It produced no evidence of a carcinogenic effect, but the adequacy of the dose level used was not known, and no evaluation could be made.

4.2 Human data

No case reports or epidemiological studies were available to the Working Group.

5. References

DFG (Deutsche Forschungsgemeinschaft) (1955) Kommission zur Bearbeitung des Lebensmittelfarbstoffproblems, *Toxikologische Daten von Farbstoffen und ihre Zulassung für Lebensmittel in verschiedenen Ländern*, Mitt. 6(1), Wiesbaden, Steiner Verlag

DFG (Deutsche Forschungsgemeinschaft) (1957) Farbstoff-Kommission, *Toxikologische Daten von Farbstoffen und ihre Zulassung für Lebensmittel in verschiedenen Ländern*, Mitt. 6(2), Wiesbaden, Steiner Verlag, p. 35

Hackmann, C. (1951) Untersuchungen über die cancerogene Wirkung einiger fettlöslicher Azofarbstoffe. *Z. Krebsforsch.*, $\underline{57}$, 530-541

Society of Dyers and Colourists (1971) *Colour Index*, 3rd ed., Vol. III, Bradford, Yorkshire, Deanhouse Piccadilly, p. 4019

Truhaut, R. (1955) Sur l'action cancérigène de certaines matières colorantes. Importance en hygiène alimentaire, en thérapeutique et en hygiène générale. *Ann. pharm. fr.*, $\underline{13}$, 36-51

SUDAN RED 7B

1. **Chemical and Physical Data**

1.1 **Synonyms and trade names**

Colour Index No.: 26050

Colour Index Name: C.I. Solvent Red 19

Chem. Abstr. Reg. Serial No.: 6368-72-5

Chem. Abstr. Name: N-Ethyl-1-{[4-(phenylazo)phenyl]azo}-2-naphthalenamine

For other names of which the Working Group was aware see index, p. 297.

1.2 **Chemical formula and molecular weight**

$C_{24}H_{21}N_5$ Mol. wt: 379.2

1.3 **Chemical and physical properties of the pure substance**

(a) Melting-point: 128-131.5°C; sublimes above 100-110°C

(b) Solubility: Practically insoluble in water; soluble in ethanol; very soluble in acetone and benzene

1.4 **Technical products and impurities**

No data were available to the Working Group.

2. Production, Use, Occurrence and Analysis

For important background information on this section, see preamble, p. 17.

2.1 Production and use

Sudan red 7B can be synthesized by coupling diazotized aniline with N-ethyl-2-naphthylamine (Henriques, 1884), but it is not known whether this method is used for commercial production.

It is believed that Sudan red 7B has never been produced commercially in the US, but in 1972, about 500 kg were imported through the principal US customs districts (US Tariff Commission, 1973).

There may be as many as six manufacturers of Sudan red 7B in Western Europe, but production is believed to be small. In Japan, one company manufactured approximately 500 kg of Sudan red 7B in 1972; separate data on imports and exports were not available.

It is reportedly used to colour alcoholic, ester and hydrocarbon solvents, vegetable oils, fats and waxes. Another source indicated that it is used to colour printing inks, candles, mineral oils, synthetic resin lacquers and cellulose (Society of Dyers and Colourists, 1971). In Japan, Sudan red 7B is probably used for the colouration of plastics. The Deutsche Forschungsgemeinschaft (DFG, 1955, 1957) reported that this colour was not approved for food use in any of the countries surveyed.

2.2 Occurrence

Sudan red 7B is not known to occur in nature.

2.3 Analysis

See section, "General Remarks on the Substances Considered", p. 28.

3. Biological Data Relevant to the Evaluation of Carcinogenic Risk to Man

A review on azo compounds, including Sudan red 7B, and their carcinogenic properties has been published (Truhaut, 1955).

3.1 Carcinogenicity and related studies in animals

(a) Oral administration

Rat: A group of 75 rats (strain unspecified) was fed a diet containing 1000 mg Sudan red 7B per kg of diet for up to 350 days (daily dose, 10-15 mg/animal; total dose, 3.4 g/animal). The experiment was terminated at the end of exposure, but survival rates were not given. One hepatoma and 1 caecal tumour were found; no control data were reported (Klinke, unpublished study quoted in DFG, 1957).

Of a group of 20 rats fed a diet containing 1000 mg Sudan red 7B per kg of diet for life, 19 rats survived for 1 year and 5 rats survived more than 2 years. No tumours occurred, and no pathological changes were observed in the liver, stomach or intestine. Although controls were used, no data were reported (Hackmann, 1951).

3.2 Other relevant biological data

No data were available to the Working Group.

3.3 Observations in man

No data were available to the Working Group.

4. Comments on Data Reported and Evaluation

4.1 Animal data

Sudan red 7B was tested only by the oral route in rats. Although the available studies did not demonstrate a significant increase in tumour incidence, they were considered inadequate for evaluation.

4.2 Human data

No case reports or epidemiological studies were available to the Working Group.

5. References

DFG (Deutsche Forschungsgemeinschaft) (1955) Kommission zur Bearbeitung des Lebensmittelfarbstoffproblems, Toxikologische Daten von Farbstoffen und ihre Zulassung für Lebensmittel in verschiedenen Ländern, Mitt. 6(1), Wiesbaden, Steiner Verlag

DFG (Deutsche Forschungsgemeinschaft) (1957) Farbstoff-Kommission, Toxikologische Daten von Farbstoffen und ihre Zulassung für Lebensmittel in verschiedenen Ländern, Mitt. 6(2), Wiesbaden, Steiner Verlag, p. 54

Hackmann, C. (1951) Untersuchungen über die cancerogene Wirkung einiger fettlöslicher Azofarbstoffe. Z. Krebsforsch., 57, 530-541

Henriques, R. (1884) Sudan red 7B. Ber. dtsch. chem. Ges., 17, 268

Society of Dyers and Coloursts (1971) Colour Index, 3rd ed., Vol. III, Bradford, Yorkshire, Deanhouse Piccadilly, p. 3592

Truhaut, R. (1955) Sur l'action cancérigène de certaines matières colorantes. Importance en hygiène alimentaire, en thérapeutique et en hygiène générale. Ann. pharm. fr., 13, 36-51

US Tariff Commission (1973) Imports of Benzenoid Chemicals and Products, 1972, TC Publication 601, Washington DC, US Government Printing Office, p. 68

SUNSET YELLOW FCF

1. Chemical and Physical Data

1.1 Synonyms and trade names

Colour Index No.: 15985

Colour Index Name: C.I. Food Yellow 3

Chem. Abstr. Reg. Serial No.: 2783-94-0

Chem. Abstr. Name: 6-Hydroxy-5-[(4-sulphophenyl)azo]-2-naphthalene-sulphonic acid, disodium salt

For other names of which the Working Group was aware see index, p. 297.

1.2 Chemical formula and molecular weight

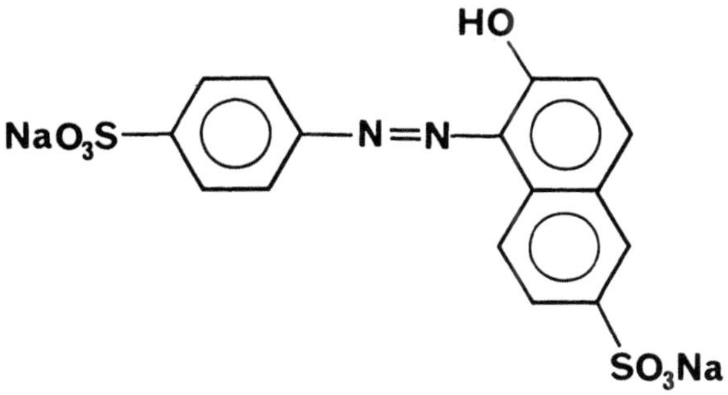

$C_{16}H_{10}N_2Na_2O_7S_2$ Mol. wt: 452.4

1.3 Chemical and physical properties of the pure substance

(a) Description: Orange-red crystals

(b) Absorption spectroscopy: λ_{max} 480 nm (in 0.02N ammonium acetate solution)

(d) Solubility: Soluble in water; very slightly soluble in ethanol

1.4 Technical products and impurities

Specifications for sunset yellow FCF used in foods, drugs or cosmetics require that the product contain a minimum of 85% pure compound (US Code of Federal Regulations, 1974). Specifications for sunset yellow FCF are also given by the British Standards Institution (1960, 1961), together with appropriate analytical methods: the product must contain a minimum of 85% pure colour; the FAO/WHO (1966) standard requires the same minimum. When used as a colour reference standard the product must contain 99.9% pure colour (Inoue *et al.*, 1967).

2. Production, Use, Occurrence and Analysis

For important background information on this section, see preamble, p. 17.

2.1 Production and use

Sunset yellow FCF appears to have been first prepared by coupling diazotized 4-aminobenzenesulphonic acid with 2-naphthol-6-sulphonic acid (Griess, 1878), and it is manufactured commercially by the same procedure (Zuckermann, 1964).

Large-scale production of sunset yellow FCF in the US was first reported in 1929 (US Tariff Commission, 1930). In 1972, six US manufacturers reported a total production of 369,000 kg (US Tariff Commission, 1974); separate data on imports and exports were not available.

In Western Europe, there are believed to be 15 manufacturers of sunset yellow FCF, with a total annual production estimated at several hundred thousand kg. In Japan in 1973, seven producers manufactured about 203,000 kg; about 22,000 kg were exported in 1972 and 8000 kg in 1973.

The Deutsche Forschungsgemeinschaft (DFG, 1955) reported that this material was approved for use as a general food colouring in Australia, Austria, Canada, the Federal Republic of Germany, Greece, Italy, Japan, Mexico, New Zealand, The Netherlands, Norway, Peru, South Africa, Spain, Sweden, Switzerland, the United Kingdom, the US and Yugoslavia. A later edition (DFG, 1957) reported additional approvals in Cuba, Denmark, the Dominican Republic, Egypt, Finland, Guatemala, India, Israel, the Philippines, and Uruguay, but indicated that approval had been withdrawn in Italy and Switzerland.

A recent report indicated that sunset yellow FCF was permitted for food, drug and cosmetic use in a number of EEC countries (Society of Dyers and Colourists, 1971), and according to another source, all Western European countries except Portugal currently permit the use of this colour in foods (DeGiacomi, 1974). It has been estimated that 95% of the sunset yellow FCF consumed in Japan is in food and the remainder in drugs, cosmetics and pens.

Zuckerman (1964) reported that sunset yellow FCF was used in gelatin, frozen desserts, carbonated beverages, dry drink powders, confectionary products, bakery products, cereals, puddings, aqueous drug solutions, tablets, capsules, toothpaste and hair rinses. A US consumption pattern for this colour in foods, drugs and cosmetics for the first nine months of 1967 was reported as follows: sweets and confections, 24,000 kg; beverages, 82,400 kg; dessert powders, 23,500 kg; cereals, 16,100 kg; maraschino cherries, 2200 kg; pet food, 10,500 kg; bakery goods, 19,100 kg; ice cream, sherbet and dairy products, 10,800 kg; sausages, 45,300 kg; snack foods, 5200 kg; and miscellaneous, 13,200 kg; for a total consumption in food of about 250,000 kg. Pharmaceutical consumption was reported to be about 7250 kg and cosmetic consumption about 1000 kg. The maximum quantity of this colour ingested in the US per capita per day per food category during this period was estimated to be as follows: sweets and confections, 1.8 mg; beverages, 4.1 mg; dessert powders, 1.8 mg; cereals, 0.5 mg; maraschino cherries, 0.06 mg; bakery goods, 3.6 mg; ice cream, sherbet and dairy products, 1.3 mg; sausages, 1.8 mg; snack foods, 0.3 mg; and miscellaneous, 0.2 mg (Anon., 1968).

The Joint FAO/WHO Expert Committee on Food Additives, which provides information to those concerned with regulating the use of chemical substances in food, recommends an acceptable human daily intake of sunset yellow FCF of 0-5.0 mg/kg bw (FAO/WHO, 1966).

2.2 Occurrence

Sunset yellow FCF is not known to occur in nature.

2.3 Analysis

See section, "General Remarks on the Substances Considered", p. 28.

3. Biological Data Relevant to the Evaluation of Carcinogenic Risk to Man

Two reviews on azo compounds, including sunset yellow FCF, and their carcinogenic properties have been published (Radomski, 1974; Truhaut, 1955).

3.1 Carcinogenicity and related studies in animals

(a) Oral administration

Mouse: A group of 15 male and 15 female mice (strain unspecified) was administered 0.05% sunset yellow FCF in drinking-water for 52 weeks, providing a weekly intake of 17 mg/animal. Thereafter mice were allowed to survive as long as possible; however, due to a high mortality in the early part of the experiment only 9 males and 10 females survived longer than 20 weeks; no mice survived longer than 89 weeks. Lymphomas occurred in 3/9 males and 6/10 females, and a benign intestinal tumour was observed in 1/5 females examined. An osteogenic sarcoma of the jaw also occurred in 1 female mouse at 74 weeks. Lymphomas were reported to occur in approximately 33% of untreated mice of this strain. In a control group of mice injected with 0.1 ml arachis oil twice weekly for 52 weeks, lymphomas occurred in 1/9 males and 4/9 females surviving longer than 20 weeks; and 1/5 males examined had a benign intestinal tumour (Bonser *et al.*, 1956).

Two-year feeding studies were carried out using C57 black and C3H mice and dietary levels of 10,000 and 20,000 mg sunset yellow FCF per kg of diet. One hundred animals of each strain were fed the colour at both dosage levels, and 200 animals of each strain were fed a control diet. There was no effect on tumour formation (US Food and Drug Administration, unpublished study quoted in FAO/WHO, 1966). [No further details of this study were available.]

Groups of 30 male and 30 female Charles River CD mice were fed 2000, 4000 or 16,000 mg sunset yellow FCF per kg of diet for 80 weeks. A group of 60 males and 60 females was used as controls. About 50-65% of the males and 80% of the females survived longer than 64 weeks. Generalized lymphomas, reticulum-cell neoplasms and lung adenomas occurred in a small number of both control and treated animals. Tumours not occurring in controls included 1 malignant tumour of the Harderian gland and 1 granulosa-cell tumour of the ovary in 2 females fed the highest level of the colour, and 1 mammary carcinoma and 1 haemangiosarcoma of the spleen in 2 females fed the lowest level (Gaunt et al., 1974).

Rat: Mannell et al. (1958) reported no increase as compared to controls in the incidence of tumours in test animals fed 300, 3000 or 15,000 mg sunset yellow FCF per kg of diet. Groups of 15 males and 15 females were used; all animals were sacrificed after 64 weeks. [The Working Group noted the short duration of the experiment.]

Groups of 12 male and 12 female Osborne-Mendel rats were fed diets containing 0, 5000, 10,000, 20,000 or 50,000 mg sunset yellow FCF per kg of diet. There was no statistically significant increase in the number of mammary tumours: 2, 1, 6, 3 and 6 occurred in the different groups, respectively. In a follow-up study, 100 Osborne-Mendel and 100 Sprague-Dawley rats were fed the compound at concentrations of 10,000 or 20,000 mg/kg of diet, respectively. Two hundred animals of each strain served as controls. Gross and microscopic pathology showed no effects on tumour formation (US Food and Drug Administration, unpublished study quoted in FAO/WHO, 1966). [No further details of the experiments were available.]

Groups of 10 male and 10 female Wistar rats were fed 0, 5000, 10,000 or 20,000 mg sunset yellow FCF per kg of diet. Among 14 rats killed at 79 weeks, mammary tumours were found in 4 females at the highest dose level. Of 19 rats at the 10,000 mg/kg level killed at 102 weeks, 9 males had intraperitoneal fibrosarcomas and 1 rat a liver-cell adenoma; 5 control male rats also developed intraperitoneal fibrosarcomas. The authors considered that sunset yellow FCF had no carcinogenic effect in rats (Kanisawa et al., 1967).

(b) Subcutaneous and/or intramuscular injection

Rat: A group of 20 Sprague-Dawley rats (divided approximately equally by sex) was given three twice weekly s.c. injections of 1 ml of a 2% aqueous solution of sunset yellow FCF and, after a break of 1-2 weeks, 52 twice weekly injections of 1 ml of a 1% solution. Thereafter rats were allowed to survive as long as possible, and the average survival times were 16 months in males and 25 months in females. No tumours developed at the injection site; 1 female developed a carcinoma of the uterus. In groups of 20 untreated controls and 20 rats injected with 0.9% saline, average survival times were 19 and 18 months, respectively. Slightly more tumours developed in controls than in treated animals, including malignant tumours of the ovary and mesentery (Oettel et al., 1965).

3.2 Other relevant biological data

(a) Animals

The i.p. LD_{50}'s of sunset yellow FCF in rats and mice ranged from 3.8-5.5 g/kg bw. Orally administered doses of up to 10 g/kg bw in rats and up to 6 g/kg bw in mice were tolerated without ill-effect (Gaunt et al., 1967). Mice fed 2000-16,000 mg of the colour per kg of diet for 80 weeks were not adversely affected (Gaunt et al., 1974). Groups of 15 male and 15 female rats fed 5000, 10,000, 20,000 or 30,000 mg/kg of diet for 90 days grew normally, but the diets containing 20,000 and 30,000 mg/kg caused slight diarrhoea and enlargement of the caecum. There were no effects on blood or liver and kidney function. The no-effect level in this 90-day study was 10,000 mg/kg in the diet, equivalent to 500 mg/kg bw/day (Gaunt et al., 1967).

Two groups of 4 beagle dogs were fed 10,000 and 50,000 mg sunset yellow FCF per kg of diet. Two out of 4 at the higher level and 1/4 at the lower level lost weight progressively and were killed after 2-3 months. Gross and microscopic pathological changes were present but not characteristic (US Food and Drug Administration, unpublished study quoted in FAO/WHO, 1966).

When the colour is given orally to rats, 3% is absorbed and excreted unchanged in urine and in bile: thus little is reduced in the liver. The unabsorbed colour was mainly reduced by intestinal bacteria and excreted as sulphanilic acid and 1-amino-2-hydroxy-6-naphthalenesulphonic acid in the urine (Radomski & Mellinger, 1962). In addition to these two compounds Daniel (1962) also found N-acetylsulphanilic acid as a metabolite in rabbits after oral administration of this colour. After its i.v. injection in rats, 20-30% was excreted in bile (Ryan & Wright, 1961).

Sunset yellow FCF is easily reduced *in vitro* by bacteria present in the intestine and caecum of rats (Roxon et al., 1967; Ryan et al., 1968). It binds with serum proteins (Gangolli et al., 1972).

Sunset yellow FCF (of undefined purity) has been shown to produce dominant lethals (three times over the control) in 4-month old non-inbred laboratory rats treated orally with 55 mg/kg bw (Sysoev & Zhurkov, 1974).

3.3 Observations in man

No data were available to the Working Group.

4. Comments on Data Reported and Evaluation

4.1 Animal data

The Working Group considered tests in which sunset yellow FCF was administered to mice and rats by the oral route and to rats by the subcutaneous route. In the oral experiments in mice there was no evidence of carcinogenicity as compared with controls. Tests in rats by the oral route showed negative results, but the experiments were inadequately reported. Repeated subcutaneous injections in rats led to neither local nor distant tumours.

4.2 Human data

No case reports or epidemiological studies were available to the Working Group.

5. References

Anon. (1968) Guidelines for food manufacturing practice: use of certified FD & C colors. Food Technology, 22, 946-949

Bonser, G.M., Clayson, D.B. & Jull, J.W. (1956) The induction of tumours of the subcutaneous tissues, liver and intestine in the mouse by certain dyestuffs and their intermediates. Brit. J. Cancer, 10, 653-667

British Standards Institution (1960) Methods for the analysis of water-soluble coal-tar dyes permitted for use in foods. BS3210:1960, London

British Standards Institution (1961) Sunset yellow FCF for use in foodstuffs. BS3340:1961, London

Daniel, J.W. (1962) The excretion and metabolism of edible food colors. Toxicol. appl. Pharmacol., 4, 572-594

DeGiacomi, R., ed. (1974) Food Processing and Packaging Directory 1974, 13th ed., London, IPC Consumer Industries Press Ltd, pp. 797-802

DFG (Deutsche Forschungsgemeinschaft) (1955) Kommission zur Bearbeitung des Lebensmittelfarbstoffproblems, Toxikologische Daten von Farbstoffen und ihre Zulassung für Lebensmittel in verschiedenen Ländern, Mitt. 6(1), Wiesbaden, Steiner Verlag

DFG (Deutsche Forschungsgemeinschaft) (1957) Farbstoff-Kommission, Toxikologische Daten von Farbstoffen und ihre Zulassung für Lebensmittel in verschiedenen Ländern, Mitt. 6(2), Wiesbaden, Steiner Verlag, p. 29

FAO/WHO (1966) Joint Expert Committee on Food Additives. Specifications for identity and purity and toxicological evaluation of food colours, FAO Nutr. Mtgs Rep. Ser. No. 38B, WHO/Food Add./66.25, pp. 83-87

Gangolli, S.D., Grasso, P., Golberg, L. & Hooson, J. (1972) Protein binding by food colourings in relation to the production of subcutaneous sarcoma. Fd Cosmet. Toxicol., 10, 449-462

Gaunt, I.F., Farmer, M., Grasso, P. & Gangolli, S.D. (1967) Acute (rat and mouse) and short-term (rat) toxicity studies on sunset yellow FCF. Fd Cosmet. Toxicol., 5, 747-754

Gaunt, I.F., Manson, P.L., Grasso, P. & Kiss, I.S. (1974) Long-term toxicity of sunset yellow FCF in mice. Fd Cosmet. Toxicol., 12, 1-10

Griess, P. (1878) Neue Untersuchungen über Diazoverbindungen. VI. Über die Einwirkung einiger Diazosulfosäuren auf Phenole. Ber. dtsch. chem. Ges., 11, 2191-2199

Inoue, T., Kamikura, M. & Murakami, N. (1967) Dye standards of National Institute of Hygienic Sciences. Bull. Nat. Inst. Hyg. Sci. (Tokyo), 85, 152-154

Kanisawa, M., Okamoto, T., Chujo, T. & Aiso, K. (1967) Chronic oral toxicity of sunset yellow FCF. Ann. Rep. Inst. Food Microbiol. Chiba Univ., 20, 101-110

Mannell, W.A., Grice, H.C., Lu, F.C. & Allmark, M.G. (1958) Chronic toxicity studies on food colours. IV. Observations on the toxicity of tartrazine, amaranth and sunset yellow in rats. J. Pharm. Pharmacol., 10, 625-634

Oettel, H., Frohberg, H., Nothdurft, H. & Wilhelm, G. (1965) Die Prüfung einiger synthetischer Farbstoffe auf ihre Eignung zur Lebensmittelfärbung. Arch. Toxikol., 21, 9-29

Radomski, J.L. (1974) Toxicology of food colors. Ann. Rev. Pharmacol., 14, 127-137

Radomski, J.L. & Mellinger, T.J. (1962) The absorption, fate and excretion in rats of the water-soluble azo dyes, FD & C Red No. 2, FD & C Red No. 4 and FD & C Yellow No. 6. J. Pharmacol. exp. Ther., 136, 259-266

Roxon, J.J., Ryan, A.J. & Wright, S.E. (1967) Reduction of water-soluble azo dyes by intestinal bacteria. Fd Cosmet. Toxicol., 5, 367-369

Ryan, A.J. & Wright, S.E. (1961) The excretion of some azo dyes in the rat bile. J. Pharm. Pharmacol., 13, 492-495

Ryan, A.J., Roxon, J.J. & Sivayavirojana, A. (1968) Bacterial azo reduction: a metabolic reaction in mammals. Nature (Lond.), 219, 854-855

Society of Dyers and Colourists (1971) Colour Index, 3rd ed., Vol. II, Bradford, Yorkshire, Deanhouse Piccadilly, p. 2775

Sysoev, A.B. & Zhurkov, V.S. (1974) A study of the mutagenic activity of synthetic food dyes - sun yellow sunset FCF and its analogous compound - sun yellow K. Gig. i Sanit., 9, 26-30

Truhaut, R. (1955) Sur l'action cancérigène de certaines matières colorantes. Importance en hygiène alimentaire, en thérapeutique et en hygiène générale. Ann. pharm. fr., 13, 36-51

US Code of Federal Regulations (1974) Food and Drugs, Title 21, part 9.41, Washington DC, US Government Printing Office, p. 195

US Tariff Commission (1930) Census of Dyes and Other Synthetic Organic Chemicals, 1929, Tariff Information Series No. 39, Washington DC, US Government Printing Office, p. 71

US Tariff Commission (1974) *Synthetic Organic Chemicals, US Production and Sales, 1972*, TC Publication 681, Washington DC, US Government Printing Office, p. 63

Zuckerman, S. (1964) *Colors for Foods, Drugs and Cosmetics.* In: Kirk, R.E. & Othmer, D.F., eds, *Encyclopedia of Chemical Technology*, 2nd ed., Vol. 5, New York, John Wiley & Sons, p. 867

TRYPAN BLUE

1. Chemical and Physical Data

1.1 Synonyms and trade names

Colour Index No.: 23850

Colour Index Name: C.I. Direct Blue 14

Chem. Abstr. Reg. Serial No.: 72-57-1

Chem. Abstr. Name: 3,3'-{[3,3'-Dimethyl(1,1'-biphenyl)-4,4'-diyl]bis(azo)}bis(5-amino-4-hydroxy)-2,7-naphthalenedisulphonic acid, tetrasodium salt

For other names of which the Working Group was aware see index, p. 297.

1.2 Chemical formula and molecular weight

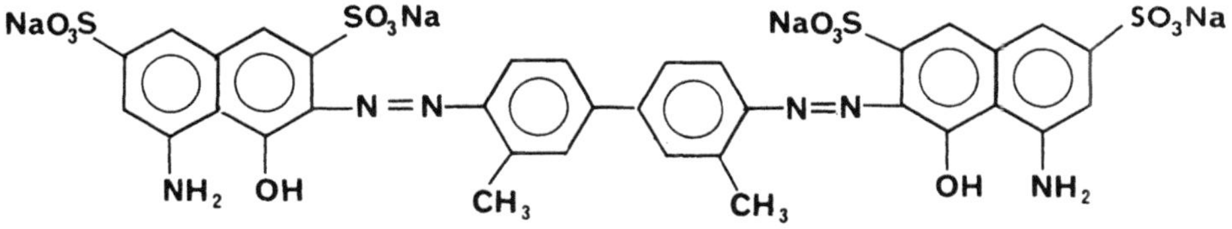

$C_{34}H_{24}N_6Na_4O_{14}S_4$ Mol. wt: 960.8

1.3 Chemical and physical properties of the pure substance

(a) Description: Bluish-grey crystals

(b) Absorption spectroscopy: λ_{max} in aqueous solution varies from 584-617 nm

(c) Identity and purity test: The identification of commercial dyestuffs has been described (Mullikan, 1910).

(d) Solubility: Soluble in water (2% at room temperature); slightly soluble in cellosolve; almost insoluble in ethanol

1.4 Technical products and impurities

According to US industrial sources, trypan blue is not used in foods, drugs or cosmetics; thus, its manufacture and testing do not conform to rigid chemical specifications, and its composition varies in order to meet customer shade and intensity requirements. The relative contributions of various fractions to the optical absorption of a particular sample of trypan blue at 580 nm have been reported by Dijkstra & Gillman (1961): red (violet), 12%; blue, 75%; purple (water fraction) 5%; purple (sodium hydroxide fraction) 7%.

Among the substances identified in various samples of this material were: a red-violet component identified as 8-amino-2-[4'-(3,3'-dimethylbiphenylazo)]-1-naphthol-3,6-disulphonic acid (Lloyd & Field, 1970); 8-amino-2[4'-(3,3'-dimethyl-4-hydroxybiphenylazo)]-1-naphthol-3,6-disulphonic acid; and 8-amino-2-[4'-(3,3'-dimethyl-4-aminobiphenylazo)]-1-naphthol-3,6-disulphonic acid (Dijkstra, 1972). In addition, trypan blue can contain varying amounts of its starting materials, including *ortho*-tolidine (Simpson, 1952) and inorganic salts (Marshall, 1953).

2. Production, Use, Occurrence and Analysis

For important background information on this section, see preamble p. 17.

2.1 Production and use

Trypan blue was first synthesized by M. Hoffmann in 1890 (Society of Dyers and Colourists, 1971). It can be prepared by coupling tetrazotized *ortho*-tolidine with two equivalents of 8-amino-1-naphthol-3,6-disulphonic acid (H acid) in alkaline solution (Richter, 1958), but it is not known whether this is the method used for commercial production.

US production of trypan blue was first reported in 1921 (US Tariff Commission, 1922). In 1972, it was manufactured by four US companies, but separate production data were not reported, and it was included in a group of at least 21 other blue colours with a total production of about 750,000 kg (US Tariff Commission, 1974). Separate data on US imports and exports were not available.

It is believed that there are as many as six manufacturers of trypan blue in Western Europe, with an estimated total annual production of a few hundred thousand kg.

It is reportedly used for dyeing textiles, leather and paper, as a stain in biological investigations and as a therapeutic agent in the treatment of sleeping sickness (Society of Dyers and Colourists, 1971). According to the Deutsche Forschungsgemeinschaft (DFG, 1955, 1957), trypan blue was not approved for food use in any of the countries surveyed.

2.2 Occurrence

Trypan blue is not known to occur in nature.

2.3 Analysis

See section, "General Remarks on the Substances Considered", p. 28.

3. Biological Data Relevant to the Evaluation of Carcinogenic Risk to Man

Several review articles on azo compounds, including trypan blue, and their carcinogenic activity have been published (Druckrey, 1955; Miller & Miller, 1953; Truhaut, 1955).

Trypan blue, like other polysulphonic acids, is difficult to purify, and the commercial product is often a mixture; thus, some of the biological effects described as being caused by trypan blue may have been produced by impurities.

3.1 Carcinogenicity and related studies in animals

(a) Oral administration

Rat: Oral administration of commercial trypan blue to rats for periods up to 1 year induced neither reticulosis nor reticulum-cell sarcomas (Oka et al., 1957).

Of 5 rats given 0.1% commercial trypan blue in drinking-water, 1 died after 213 days and 4 died between 214 and 365 days. No tumours or enlargement of liver, lymph nodes or spleen were seen (Ooneda et al., 1957).

(b) Subcutaneous and/or intramuscular injection

Mouse: A group of 50 Swiss mice received s.c. injections of 0.1 ml of a 1% aqueous solution of commercial trypan blue (composition not stated) at fortnightly intervals and was observed until death; 27 mice survived more than 50 weeks. It was reported that trypan blue "slightly enhanced the incidence and time of appearance of malignant lymphomas", but no figures were reported; 1 local sarcoma was recorded (Tomatis, 1963). In a subsequent experiment the commercial product was purified with ether in a Soxhlet apparatus for 20 hours, at which time there remained a non-measurable amount of reddish deposit. Groups of 19 female and 29 male C57BL mice and 50 female Swiss mice received 20 s.c. injections of 0.1 ml of a 1% aqueous solution of trypan blue every two weeks. More than 50% of mice in each group were alive after 60 weeks. In C57BL mice, tumours occurred sporadically in the same incidence as in the control group; in the 50 female Swiss mice 1 local fibrosarcoma was observed, and malignant lymphomas, lung adenomas, mammary carcinomas and liver angiomas occurred, respectively, in 3, 13, 5 and 2 mice. Although no control was included in this study, it was stated that "no effect on the incidence of lymphomas was recorded" (Tomatis, 1966).

Rat: Since 1948 a series of experiments by Gillman *et al.* (1948a, 1949a, 1949b, 1952, 1973) have shown unequivocally that repeated injections of trypan blue to rats induce sarcomas of the reticulo-endothelial system. Trypan blue was made up in a 1% solution, and 0.5-1.0 ml were given at weekly or fortnightly intervals. The chemical used is referred to either as "trypan blue" (Gillman *et al.*, 1948a, 1952) or as "trypan blue from the original Grübler dye" (Gillman *et al.*, 1949a, b, 1973).

In one of these studies, 193 rats of both sexes each received s.c. injections of 1 ml fortnightly or 0.5 ml weekly of a 1% solution of trypan blue for 14-410 days; 75/133 rats surviving 70-410 days developed tumours of the reticulo-endothelial system, mainly of the hepatic lymph nodes. These tumours were classified as histiocytomas (51%), plasmacytomas (29%), paramonocytomas (7.9%) endotheliomas (10.7%) and haemohistioblastomas (1.4%) (Gillman *et al.*, 1952).

In a recent study, groups of rats of five different strains, 4-8 weeks old, were given s.c. injections of 1 ml of a 1% aqueous solution of trypan blue every second week (total, 60-210 mg/animal). Tumours of the reticuloendothelial system and of the liver developed in rats of three strains: in 2/28 male and female rats of Agricultural Research Council Compton strain, in 4/8 male Harwell Wistar rats and in 19/20 male and female Wistar rats of the Agricultural Research Councils Labs, Babraham. The localization of the tumours was mainly in the liver and hepatic lymph nodes, but they also occurred in mesenteric lymph nodes, thymus, thymic lymph nodes, non-abdominal lymph nodes and kidney. Neither Wistar rats originating from AGUS, Oxfordshire (5 males and 6 females) and from Animal Suppliers Ltd, London (6 males and 2 females) nor 3 control rats in each of the strains showed pathological changes in the reticulo-endothelial system (Gillman et al., 1973).

In an earlier experiment, a single s.c. injection of 10 mg trypan blue was found to produce highly malignant spindle-cell sarcomas in the liver and other organs of a "small percentage of young adult rats" within 134 days (Gillman et al., 1949a).

The production of tumours in rats following repeated s.c. injections of trypan blue (0.5-1.5 ml of a 1% solution at weekly or fortnightly intervals, or 100 mg/kg bw at fortnightly intervals) has been confirmed in several other reports (Brown & Norlind, 1959, 1961; Ito & Farber, 1966; Marshall, 1953; Oka et al., 1957; Ooneda et al., 1957; Simpson, 1952). Tumours were diagnosed as reticulum-cell sarcomas, histiocytic tumours or lymphosarcomas and were located in the liver; involvement of other organs was reported in some studies. Simpson (1952) identified the trypan blue used in his study as BPC; in the other studies, either purity was not indicated or a commercial product was used.

A dose-response study was reported by Brown (1963), using a commercial product. Rats were given injections of trypan blue at doses of 25, 50, 100, 150 or 200 mg/kg bw every two weeks. The numbers of rats dying with histiocytic tumours of the liver over survivors at time of appearance of the first tumour were 7/25, 5/25, 6/24, 7/23 and 2/5, respectively. Subcutaneous tumours were also observed, and the respective incidences were 1/21, 5/17, 9/18, 3/15 and 4/5.

Subcutaneous tumours have also been reported in a further study: of 35 Wistar rats weighing 200 g and given s.c. injections of 1 ml of a 1% solution of commercial trypan blue every 15 days until death (2-15 months) or until the appearance of a subcutaneous tumours (7-18 months), subcutaneous tumours (fibrosarcomas) occurred at the injection site in 22 rats; 4 other rats had liver tumours. A further eight groups of 5 rats/group were given 5-15 s.c. injections of the colour solution. After a minimum of 8 injections, 14/40 rats developed subcutaneous tumours at the injection site; 3 other rats had liver tumours (Driessens et al., 1962).

(c) Intraperitoneal administration

Rat: A group of 20 rats of both sexes weighing 200-250 g received weekly i.p. injections of 1 ml of a 1% aqueous solution of trypan blue, and 3/8 rats surviving 275-430 days developed abdominal spindle-cell sarcomas. No control data were reported (Papacharalampous, 1957).

Thirty male rats weighing 200-300 g were given i.p. injections of 1-1.5 ml of a 1% aqueous solution of trypan blue (composition unspecified) every 2 days. The animals were sacrificed between the 100th and 300th days, and 2 rats developed reticulum-cell sarcomas of the liver at 150 and 240 days after the start of treatment (Papacharalampous, 1966).

3.2 Other relevant biological data

(a) Animals

The s.c. LD_{50} of a 1% trypan blue solution in adult NMRI/Han mice has been reported to be 267 mg/kg bw. The LD_{50} for mouse embryos has been reported to be 67 mg/kg bw (Schlüter, 1970).

Following s.c. or i.p. injections into mice or rats, trypan blue is rapidly absorbed and widely distributed throughout the body. Maximum serum concentrations are reached within 2 hours; it appears bound to serum proteins, with an exponential decay of plasma levels due to rapid excretion in the urine and uptake by the reticulo-endothelial system (Belitskii, 1963; Brown et al., 1963; Dijkstra & Gillman, 1960; Rabinovitch et al., 1961; Thilander, 1963; Uchino & Hosokawa, 1972).

Trypan blue was found to stain transplanted tumours and to inhibit respiration and glycolysis of tumour tissue (Boyland & Boyland, 1939). Injected subcutaneously into rats at 2-week intervals at levels of 200-400 mg/kg bw, trypan blue induced anaemia with leucopenia and thrombocytopenia (Brown et al., 1961).

It is reduced *in vitro* by a rat liver enzyme to *ortho*-tolidine and 2,8-diamino-1-naphthol-3,6-disulphonic acid (Lloyd *et al.*, 1968).

Trypan blue of undefined purity was shown to be teratogenic in mice, rats, guinea-pigs and amphibia (Gillman *et al.*, 1948b). The ethanol extraction residue produced no foetal resorptions while the ether extraction residue produced resorptions but no malformations. Benzopurpurine, a common contaminant, produced no malformations (Tuchmann-Duplessis & Mercier-Parot, 1959). A red impurity isolated by Beck & Lloyd (1963) and Bertini & Sacerdote (1970) caused malformations in mice embryos but not consistently in rats. Neither *ortho*-tolidine nor 1,7-diamino-8-naphthol-3,6-disulphonic acid were teratologically active (Christie, 1965; Wilson, 1955).

Trypan blue of undefined purity exerts direct mutagenic activity, producing deletions in *Aspergillus nidulans* (Cooke *et al.*, 1970; Roper, 1971). No mutagenicity data involving mammalian metabolic systems were available to the Working Group.

(b) Carcinogenicity of metabolites

ortho-Tolidine, a possible metabolite of trypan blue, is carcinogenic in rats (IARC, 1972).

3.3 Observations in man

No data were available to the Working Group.

4. Comments on Data Reported and Evaluation[1]

4.1 Animal data

Trypan blue is carcinogenic in rats following its subcutaneous or intraperitoneal injection, producing reticulum-cell sarcomas, mainly of the liver, as well as fibrosarcomas at the site of injection. Liver spindle-cell sarcomas were also induced in rats by single subcutaneous

---

[1] See also the section, "Animal Data in Relation to the Evaluation of Risk to Man" in the introduction to this volume, p. 15.

injections. Experiments by the oral route in rats and by subcutaneous injection in mice could not be evaluated because of the small number of animals used or because the adequacy of the dose used could not be assessed.

4.2 Human data

No case reports or epidemiological studies were available to the Working Group.

5. References

Beck, F. & Lloyd, J.B. (1963) The preparations and teratogenic properties of pure trypan blue and its common contaminants. J. Embryol. exp. Morphol., 11, 175-184

Belitskii, G.A. (1963) Sex differences in renal excretion of o-aminoazotoluene in the mouse. Byull. exp. Biol. Med., 55, 523-525

Bertini, F. & Sacerdote, F. (1970) Malformations caused in mouse embryos by a red dye contained in commercial trypan blue. Teratology, 3, 371-376

Boyland, E. & Boyland, M.E. (1939) The independence of respiration and glycolysis and the growth rate of tumours. Biochem. J., 33, 618-621

Brown, D.V. (1963) Subcutaneous neoplasms induced by trypan blue. Lab. Invest., 12, 1221-1227

Brown, D.V. & Norlind, L.M. (1959) Trypan blue-induced tumors of rats: morphologic, hematologic and serologic observations. Amer. J. Path., 35, 696-697

Brown, D.V. & Norlind, L.M. (1961) Irradiation and trypan blue treatment. Arch. Path., 72, 251-273

Brown, D.V., Boehni, E.M. & Norlind, L.M. (1961) Anemia with positive direct Coombs' test induced by trypan blue. Blood, 18, 543-560

Brown, D.V., Norlind, L.M., Adamovics, A. & Bowen, A. (1963) Studies on serum protein changes and organ dye concentrations in trypan blue carcinogenesis. Proc. Soc. exp. Biol. (N.Y.), 114, 290-293

Christie, G.A. (1965) Teratogenic effects of synthetic compounds related to trypan blue: the effect of 1,7-diamino-8-naphthol-3,6-disulfonic acid on pregnancy in the rat. Nature (Lond.), 208, 1219-1220

Cooke, P., Roper, J.A. & Watmough, W. (1970) Trypan blue-induced deletions in duplication strains of *Aspergillus nidulans*. Nature (Lond.), 226, 276-277

DFG (Deutsche Forschungsgemeinschaft) (1955) Kommission zur Bearbeitung des Lebensmittelfarbstoffproblems, Toxikologische Daten von Farbstoffen und ihre Zulassung für Lebensmittel in verschiedenen Ländern, Mitt. 6(1), Wiesbaden, Steiner Verlag

DFG (Deutsche Forschungsgemeinschaft) (1957) Farbstoff-Kommission, Toxikologische Daten von Farbstoffen und ihre Zulassung für Lebensmittel in verschiedenen Ländern, Mitt. 6(2), Wiesbaden, Steiner Verlag

Dijkstra, J. (1972) The so-called red impurity of trypan blue. Experientia (Basel), 28, 252-253

Dijkstra, J. & Gillman, J. (1960) Trypan blue concentration and protein composition in sera of rats injected repeatedly with trypan blue in relation to reticulosis and to reticulo-sarcoma. S. Afr. J. med. Sci., 25, 119-131

Dijkstra, J. & Gillman, J. (1961) Chromatographic separation of biologically active components from commercial trypan blue. Nature (Lond.), 191, 803-804

Driessens, J., Clay, A., Vanlerenberghe, J. & Adenis, L. (1962) Sarcomes au lieu d'injection sous-cutanée du bleu trypan chez le rat blanc. I. Etude histologique. C.R. Soc. Biol. (Paris), 156, 1099-1102

Druckrey, H. (1955) Schädliche und unschädliche Farbstoffe für Lebensmittel. Z. Krebsforsch., 60, 344-360

Gillman, J., Gilbert, C., Gillman, T. & Spence, I. (1948a) Experimental production of hepato-splenomegaly, reticulum-cell sarcoma and Hodgkin's disease. S. Afr. med. J., 22, 783-784

Gillman, J., Gilbert, C. & Gillman, T. (1948b) A preliminary report on hydrocephalus, spina bifida and other congenital anomalies in the rat produced by trypan blue. S. Afr. J. med. Sci., 13, 47-90

Gillman, J., Gillman, T. & Gilbert, C. (1949a) Reticulosis and reticulum-cell tumours of the liver produced in rats by trypan blue with reference to hepatic necrosis and fibrosis. S. Afr. J. med. Sci., 14, 21-84

Gillman, J., Gillman, T., Gilbert, C. & Spence, I. (1949b) Lymphomata (including Hodgkin's-like sarcomata). Their experimental production, study of their pathogenesis and aetiology and a comparison with corresponding tumours in man. Clin. Proc., 8, 222-302

Gillman, J., Gillman, T., Gilbert, C. & Spence, I. (1952) The pathogenesis of experimentally produced lymphomata in rats (including Hodgkin's-like sarcoma). Cancer, 5, 792-846

Gillman, T., Kinns, A.M., Hallowes, R.C. & Lloyd, J.B. (1973) Malignant lymphoreticular tumors induced by trypan blue and transplanted in inbred rats. J. nat. Cancer Inst., 50, 1179-1193

IARC (1972) IARC Monographs on the Evaluation of Carcinogenic Risk of Chemicals to Man, 1, Lyon, pp. 87-91

Ito, N. & Farber, E. (1966) Effects of trypan blue on hepatocarcinogenesis in rats given ethionine or N-2-fluorenylacetamide. J. nat. Cancer Inst., 37, 775-785

Lloyd, J.B. & Field, F.E. (1970) The red impurity in trypan blue. Experientia (Basel), 26, 868-869

Lloyd, J.B., Beck, F., Griffiths, A. & Parry, L.M. (1968) The mechanism of action of acid bisazo dyes. In: Campbell, P.N., ed., The Interaction of Drugs and Subcellular Components in Animal Cells, London, J. & A. Churchill Ltd, pp. 171-202

Marshall, A.H.E. (1953) The production of tumours of the reticular tissue by di-azo vital dyes. Acta path. microbiol. scand., 33, 1-9

Miller, J.A. & Miller, E.C. (1953) The carcinogenic aminoazo dyes. Advanc. Cancer Res., 1, 339-396

Mullikan, S.P. (1910) Identification of the Commercial Dyestuffs, Vol. III, New York, John Wiley & Sons, pp. 607, 642

Oka, K., Matsuyama, K., Araki, Y. & Ooneda, G. (1957) Experimental studies on reticulum-cell sarcoma. Gann, 48, 573-575

Ooneda, G., Matsuyama, K., Oka, K., Ninomiya, S., Araki, Y. & Takano, M. (1957) Experimental studies on reticulum-cell sarcoma and reticulosis. Gunma J. med. Sci., 6, 295-317

Papacharalampous, N.X. (1957) Befunde an der Ratte nach langfristigen Versuchen mit intraperitonealen Injektionen von Trypanblau. Beitr. Path. Anat., 117, 85-89

Papacharalampous, N.X. (1966) Die Übertragung von Reticulosarkomen der Ratte nach Trypanblauinjektionen. Frankfurt Z. Path., 75, 74-77

Rabinovitch, M., Brentani, R., Ferreira, S., Fausto, N. & Maack, T. (1961) Alkaline ribonuclease activity increase in rat kidney cortex and liver after trypan blue and other azo dyes administration. J. biophys. biochem. Cytol., 10, 105-112

Richter, F. (1958) Beilsteins Handbuch der Organischen Chemie, Vol. 16, I, Berlin, Springer-Verlag, p. 346

Roper, J.A. (1971) Aspergillus. In: Hollander, A., ed., Chemical Mutagens: Principle and Methods for their Detection, Ch. 12, New York, Plenum Press, pp. 343-363

Schlüter, G. (1970) Embryotoxische Dosis-Wirkungs-Beziehungen von Trypanblau bei Mäusen. Naunyn-Schmiedebergs Arch. Pharmak., 267, 31-40

Simpson, C.L. (1952) Trypan blue-induced tumours of rats. Brit. J. exp. Path., 33, 524-528

Society of Dyers and Colourists (1971) Colour Index, 3rd ed., Vol. II, Bradford, Yorkshire, Deanhouse Piccadilly, p. 2226

Thilander, H. (1963) Disappearance rate of trypan blue in rat plasma after intraperitoneal injection. Acta path. microbiol. scand., 57, 57-59

Tomatis, L. (1963) Studies in subcutaneous carcinogenesis with implants of glass and teflon in mice. Acta Un. int. Cancr, 19, 607-611

Tomatis, L. (1966) Subcutaneous carcinogenesis by implants and by 7,12-dimethylbenz(a)anthracene. Tumori, 52, 1-16

Truhaut, R. (1955) Sur l'action cancérigène de certaines matières colorantes. Importance en hygiène alimentaire, en thérapeutique et en hygiène générale. Ann. pharm. fr., 13, 36-51

Tuchmann-Duplessis, H. & Mercier-Parot, L. (1959) A propos de malformations produites par le bleu trypan. Biol. Méd., 48, 238-251

Uchino, F. & Hosokawa, S. (1972) Pathological study on amyloidosis. A new induction method of amyloidosis by trypan blue. Acta path. jap., 22, 131-140

US Tariff Commission (1922) Census of Dyes and Other Synthetic Organic Chemicals, 1921, Tariff Information Series No. 26, Washington DC, US Government Printing Office, p. 65

US Tariff Commission (1974) Synthetic Organic Chemicals, US Production and Sales, 1972, TC Publication 681, Washington DC, US Government Printing Office, p. 77

Wilson, J.G. (1955) Teratogenic activity of several azo dyes chemically related to trypan blue. Anat. Rec., 123, 313-333

YELLOW AB

1. Chemical and Physical Data

1.1 Synonyms and trade names

   Colour Index No.: 11380

   Colour Index Name: C.I. Solvent Yellow 5

   Chem. Abstr. Reg. Serial No.: 85-84-7

   Chem. Abstr. Name: 1-(Phenylazo)-2-naphthalenamine

   For other names of which the Working Group was aware see index, p. 297.

1.2 Chemical formula and molecular weight

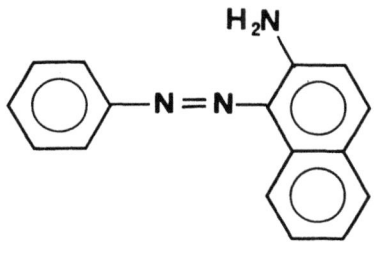

$C_{16}H_{13}N_3$ Mol. wt: 247.3

1.3 Chemical and physical properties of the pure substance

   (a) Description: Orange crystals; orange-red platelets

   (b) Melting-point: 104°C (recrystallized from ethanol)

   (c) Solubility: Soluble in ethanol and acetic acid; insoluble in water

   (d) Absorption spectroscopy: λ_{max} 434 nm (in chloroform)

1.4 Technical products and impurities

One set of specifications for yellow AB require that the product contain a minimum of 99.9% pure colour (Japan Food Hygiene Association, 1974). It has been reported, however, that this colour cannot be produced commercially with any assurance that it does not contain 2-naphthylamine, a known carcinogen (US Code of Federal Regulations, 1974).

2. Production, Use, Occurrence and Analysis

For important background information on this section, see preamble, p. 17.

2.1 Production and use

Yellow AB was first prepared by T.A. Lawson in 1885 (Lawson, 1885). It can be synthesized by coupling diazotized aniline with 2-naphthylamine (Hodgson & Foster, 1942), but it is not known whether this method is used for commercial production.

Large-scale production of yellow AB in the US was first reported in 1921 (US Tariff Commission, 1922). Separate production data were not generally given, although 13,000 kg were manufactured in 1956 (US Tariff Commission, 1957), and no commercial production has been reported since 1960.

In Western Europe there may be as many as four producers of yellow AB, but production is believed to be small. Several companies in Japan probably manufactured it prior to 1967, when production was believed to have been stopped.

Yellow AB was used in the past in the US as a dye, in a cold preparation applied by vaporizer. It is marketed in small quantities by one US company as a stain for use in biological investigations. It is also reported to be used in colouring oil and spirit products (Society of Dyers and Colourists, 1971).

Yellow AB was approved for food use in the US in 1918, and it was subsequently used to colour margarine both in the US and Japan. The Deutsche Forschungsgemeinschaft (DFG, 1955) reported that it had also been approved for use as a general food colouring in Australia, Canada, Greece, Japan, Mexico, New Zealand, Norway, Peru, South Africa and the US. A later edition (DFG, 1957) reported additional approvals in Costa Rica, Cuba, Guatemala and the Philippines, but indicated that approval had been withdrawn in New Zealand and Norway. It was used in France between April 1947 and October 1949 to colour margarine (Truhaut, 1958).

In 1959, yellow AB was removed from the US approved list for use in foods, but was permitted in externally applied drugs and cosmetics; but in 1960 it was removed completely from the approved list (National Research Council, 1971). Approval for its use in food in Japan was withdrawn in 1966, although approval was retained for certain non-food uses (Japan Food Hygiene Association, 1974).

The Joint FAO/WHO Expert Committee on Food Additives, which provides information to those concerned with regulating the use of chemical substances in food, considers yellow AB, on the basis of toxicological evidence, to be unsafe for use in food (FAO/WHO, 1973).

2.2 Occurrence

Yellow AB is not known to occur in nature.

2.3 Analysis

See section, "General Remarks on the Substances Considered", p. 28.

3. Biological Data Relevant to the Evaluation of Carcinogenic Risk to Man

Review articles on azo dyes, including yellow AB, and their carcinogenic activity have been published (Druckrey, 1955; Miller & Miller, 1953; Radomski, 1974; Truhaut, 1955).

3.1 Carcinogenicity and related studies in animals

(a) Oral administration

Rat: A group of 84 Sherman stock rats of both sexes, weighing about 150 g, was fed a diet containing yellow AB (daily intake, 8-12 mg/animal). Two rats died by 50 days and 68 more by 300 days; 14 lived over 300 days. No liver tumours or cirrhosis were detected during 50-528 days of feeding (Sugiura, 1946).

A group of 107 rats received yellow AB orally at the rate of 10 mg/animal/day, for a total dose of 8.9 g/rat; the duration of the experiment was 950 days. Three animals developed tumours, 1 a uterine carcinoma, 1 a pancreatic carcinoma and 1 a renal papilloma. The author suggested that the colour had no carcinogenic activity (Druckrey, 1955).

Yellow AB was fed to groups of 25 male and 25 female rats, 5-6 weeks old, at levels of 300, 15,000 or 30,000 mg per kg of diet for up to 65 weeks. Rats receiving the two higher doses died within 5 weeks, and 10/50 animals receiving the lowest dose were alive at 60 weeks, compared with 27/50 controls. One treated rat developed a reticulum-cell sarcoma of the mesentery and another an adenoma of the adrenal gland (Allmark et al., 1955).

Groups of 12 male and 12 female weanling Osborne-Mendel rats weighing 35-50 g received diets containing levels of 500, 1000 or 2500 mg yellow AB per kg of diet for lifespan. An additional group received 1000 mg/kg of diet, which was increased to 2500 mg/kg of diet at the end of 8 weeks' feeding. At the highest level, no animals survived more than 18 months; at the intermediate level, 16 rats survived up to 18 months and 7 up to 24 months; at the lowest level, 20 animals survived up to 18 months and 15 up to 24 months. The authors stated that there was no significant difference in the distribution of tumours among control and experimental groups (Hansen et al., 1963).

(b) Subcutaneous and/or intramuscular injection

Mouse: A group of 18 Swiss mice was injected subcutaneously with approximately 10 mg yellow AB in 0.1 ml glycerol at 1-2 month intervals for lifespan. Maximum survival time was 18 months. No tumours were reported (Hansen et al., 1963). [No further details were available.]

Rat: A group of 18 Osborne-Mendel rats, 7 weeks of age, received weekly s.c. injections of 1-1.5 mg yellow AB in glycerol as a 1% suspension for lifespan. Thirteen rats survived more than 18 months, and 6 survived for 24 months. An injection site fibrosarcoma occurred in 1 animal; no tumours were observed in 18 control rats injected with glycerol, of which 13 survived 18 months and 5 for 24 months (Hansen et al., 1963).

3.2 Other relevant biological data

(a) Animals

Yellow AB is lethal after its s.c. or oral administration to rabbits in doses of 1 g/kg bw; doses of 250 mg/kg bw are tolerated. The colour accumulates in fatty tissues of the body after its s.c. injection and is eliminated slowly: thus, 250 mg/kg bw of the colour administered to rabbits were excreted 17 days later in the urine (Salant & Bengis, 1916).

Daily doses of 200 and 400 mg/kg bw reduce haemoglobin concentration in male and female rats. When rats were fed a diet containing 300 mg yellow AB per kg of diet, growth inhibition and atrophy and degenerative changes in the testes were observed. A diet containing 9000 mg yellow AB per kg of diet caused decreased red-cell counts and increased reticulocyte counts; higher levels (15,000-30,000 mg/kg of diet) caused changes in the liver, thymus, adrenal pancreas and kidney (Allmark et al., 1955). At a dietary concentration of 5000 mg/kg of diet, yellow AB produced Heinz bodies in rats (Rofe, 1957). In rats fed 2500 mg yellow AB per kg of diet, 100% mortality was observed within 18 months; it caused anaemia, oedema, hypertrophy of the heart and changes in the liver, spleen, bone marrow and testis. Levels of 500 mg/kg of diet produced no toxic effects (Hansen et al., 1963). Rats fed a diet containing 40,000 mg yellow AB per kg of diet lived only a few months (Willheim & Ivy, 1953). This colour exerts a cathartic effect in dogs after oral doses of 100 and 200 mg (Radomski & Deichmann, 1956).

3.3 Observations in man

No data were available to the Working Group.

4. Comments on Data Reported and Evaluation

4.1 Animal data

Yellow AB was tested by the oral route in rats and by subcutaneous injection in mice and rats. The substance was not found to be carcinogenic in these studies.

4.2 Human data

No case reports or epidemiological studies were available to the Working Group.

5. References

Allmark, M.G., Grice, H.C. & Lu, F.C. (1955) Chronic toxicity studies in food colours. I. Observations on the toxicity of FD & C Yellow No. 3 (oil yellow AB) and FD & C Yellow No. 4 (oil yellow OB) in rats. J. Pharm. Pharmacol., 7, 591-603

DFG (Deutsche Forschungsgemeinschaft) (1955) Kommission zur Bearbeitung des Lebensmittelfarbstoffproblems, Toxikologische Daten von Farbstoffen und ihre Zulassung für Lebensmittel in verschiedenen Ländern, Mitt. 6(1), Wiesbaden, Steiner Verlag

DFG (Deutsche Forschungsgemeinschaft) (1957) Farbstoff-Kommission, Toxikologische Daten von Farbstoffen und ihre Zulassung für Lebensmittel in verschiedenen Ländern, Mitt. 6(2), Wiesbaden, Steiner Verlag, p. 4

Druckrey, H. (1955) Schädliche und unschädliche Farbstoffe fur Lebensmittel. Z. Krebsforsch., 60, 344-360

FAO/WHO (1973) List of Additives Evaluated for their Safety-in-Use in Food, First Series, CAC/FAL 1-1973, p. 45

Hansen, W.H., Nelson, A.A. & Fitzhugh, O.G. (1963) Chronic toxicity of yellow AB (1-phenylazo-2-naphthylamine) and yellow OB (1-o-tolylazo-2-naphthylamine). Toxicol. Appl. Pharmacol., 5, 16-35

Hodgson, H.H. & Foster, C.K. (1942) Some reactions of the diazonium salts of certain arylazo-β-naphthylamines. J. chem. Soc., 31, 435-437

Japan Food Hygiene Association (1974) Japanese Standards of Food Additives, 3rd ed., Tokyo, Ministry of Health and Welfare

Lawson, T.A. (1885) Über die Einwirkung von Diazoverbindungen auf β-Naphtylamin. Ber. dtsch. chem. Ges., 18, 796-802

Miller, J.A. & Miller, E.C. (1953) The carcinogenic aminoazo dyes. Advanc. Cancer Res., 1, 339-396

National Research Council (1971) Food Colors, Washington DC, National Academy of Sciences, p. 7

Radomski, J.L. (1974) Toxicology of food colors. Ann. Rev. Pharmacol., 14, 127-137

Radomski, J.L. & Deichmann, W.B. (1956) Cathartic action and metabolism of certain coal-tar food dyes. J. Pharmacol. exp. Ther., 118, 322-327

Rofe, P. (1957) Azo dyes and Heinz bodies. Brit. J. industr. Med., 14, 275-280

Salant, W. & Bengis, R. (1916) Physiological and pharmacological studies on coal-tar colors. I. Experiments with fat-soluble dyes. J. biol. Chem., 27, 403-427

Society of Dyers and Colourists (1971) Colour Index, 3rd ed., Vol. III, Bradford, Yorkshire, Deanhouse Piccadilly, p. 3566

Sugiura, K. (1946) Observations on rats fed with yellow AB. Proc. Soc. exp. Biol. (N.Y.), 61, 301-302

Truhaut, R. (1955) Sur l'action cancérigène de certaines matières colorantes. Importance en hygiène alimentaire, en thérapeutique et en hygiène générale. Ann. pharm. fr., 13, 36-51

Truhaut, R. (1958) Sur l'utilisation de colorants en thérapeutique et les dangers qui peuvent en résulter pour la santé humaine. Chimie moderne, 3, 291-321

US Code of Federal Regulations (1974) Food and Drugs, Title 21, part 8.507, Washington DC, US Government Printing Office, p. 178

US Tariff Commission (1922) Census of Dyes and Other Synthetic Organic Chemicals, 1921, Tariff Information Series No. 26, Washington DC, US Government Printing Office, p. 68

US Tariff Commission (1957) Synthetic Organic Chemicals, US Production and Sales, 1956, Report No. 200, Second Series, Washington DC, US Government Printing Office, p. 19

Willheim, R. & Ivy, A.C. (1953) A preliminary study concerning the possibility of dietary carcinogenesis. Gastroenterology, 23, 1-19

YELLOW OB

1. Chemical and Physical Data

1.1 Synonyms and trade names

Colour Index No.: 11390

Colour Index Name: C.I. Solvent Yellow 6

Chem. Abstr. Reg. Serial No.: 131-79-3

Chem. Abstr. Name: 1-(2-Methylphenyl)azo-2-naphthalenamine

For other names of which the Working Group was aware see index, p. 297.

1.2 Chemical formula and molecular weight

$C_{17}H_{15}N_3$ Mol. wt: 261.3

1.3 Chemical and physical properties of the pure substance

(a) Description: Orange crystals; orange-red platelets

(b) Melting-point: 126°C (recrystallized from ethanol)

(c) Solubility: Soluble in ethanol, ether, benzene and toluene; insoluble in water

(d) Absorption spectroscopy: λ_{max} 436 nm (in chloroform)

1.4 Technical products and impurities

One set of specifications for yellow OB require that the product contain a minimum of 99.9% pure colour (Japan Food Hygiene Association, 1974).

It has been reported, however, that this colour cannot be produced commercially with any assurance that it does not contain 2-naphthylamine, a known carcinogen (US Code of Federal Regulations, 1974).

2. Production, Use, Occurrence and Analysis

For important background information on this section, see preamble, p. 17.

2.1 Production and use

Yellow OB was first prepared by P. Krüss in 1905 (Society of Dyers and Colourists, 1971). It can be made by coupling diazotized *ortho*-toluidine with 2-naphthylamine (Hodgson & Foster, 1942), but it is not known whether this method is used for commercial production.

Large-scale production of yellow OB in the US was first reported in 1921 (US Tariff Commission, 1922). Separate production data were not generally given, although 18,000 kg were manufactured in 1957 (US Tariff Commission, 1958), and no production has been reported since 1960.

In Western Europe there may be one producer of yellow OB, but production is believed to be small. Several companies in Japan probably manufactured this colour prior to 1967, when its production is believed to have been stopped.

Yellow OB was approved for food use in the US in 1918, and it was subsequently used to colour margarine. The Deutsche Forschungsgemeinschaft (DFG, 1955) reported that it had been approved for use as a general food colouring in Australia, Canada, Greece, Japan, Mexico, New Zealand, Norway, Peru, South Africa and the US. A later edition (DFG, 1957) reported additional approvals in Costa Rica, Cuba, Guatemala and the Philippines, but indicated that approval had been withdrawn in New Zealand and Norway. It is believed that yellow OB was also used in foodstuffs in Denmark, Finland and the United Kingdom prior to 1960. It was used in France between April 1947 and October 1958 to colour margarine (Truhaut, 1958).

In 1959, yellow OB was removed from the US approved list for use in foods, but was permitted in externally applied drugs and cosmetics, and in 1960, it was removed entirely from the approved list (National Research Council, 1971). Approval for its use in food in Japan was withdrawn in 1966, although approval was retained for certain non-food uses (Japan Food Hygiene Association, 1974); prior to that time, it had been used to colour margarine, oil products and spirits.

The Joint FAO/WHO Expert Committee on Food Additives, which provides information to those concerned with regulating the use of chemical substances in food, considers yellow OB, on the basis of toxicological evidence, to be unsafe for use in food (FAO/WHO, 1973).

2.2 Occurrence

Yellow OB is not known to occur in nature.

2.3 Analysis

See section, "General Remarks on the Substances Considered", p. 28.

3. Biological Data Relevant to the Evaluation of Carcinogenic Risk to Man

Review articles on azo dyes, including yellow OB, and their carcinogenic activity have been published (Druckrey, 1955; Miller & Miller, 1953; Radomski, 1974; Truhaut, 1955).

3.1 Carcinogenicity and related studies in animals

(a) Oral administration

Rat: A group of 74 rats received yellow OB orally in doses of 9 mg/animal/day, for a total dose of 9.6 g/animal; the duration of the experiment was 950 days. Two rats developed tumours, 1 a carcinoma of the uterus and 1 a pancreatic adenoma. The author suggested that the colour had no carcinogenic activity (Druckrey, 1955).

Yellow OB was fed to groups of 25 male and 25 female rats, 5-6 weeks old, at concentrations of 300, 1500 or 30,000 mg colour per kg of diet for up to 65 weeks. All rats fed the highest level died within 3 weeks, and all those fed the intermediate level, within 10 weeks. At 60 weeks, 26/50 animals fed the lowest level were alive, compared with 27/50 controls.

No tumours were observed in either control or experimental animals (Allmark et al., 1955).

Groups of 12 male and 12 female weanling Osborne-Mendel rats weighing 35-50 g were fed diets containing 500, 1000 or 2500 mg yellow OB per kg of diet for lifespan. An additional group received 1000 mg per kg of diet, which was increased to 2500 mg per kg at the end of 8 weeks' feeding. At the highest level, no animals survived longer than 12 months; at the intermediate level 15 rats survived up to 18 months and 8 up to 24 months; at the lowest level 15 animals survived up to 18 months and 11 up to 24 months. The authors stated that there was no significant difference in the distribution of tumours among the control and experimental groups (Hansen et al., 1963).

(b) Subcutaneous and/or intramuscular administration

Mouse: Groups of 18 Swiss and 18 C57Bl mice were injected subcutaneously with approximately 10 mg yellow OB in 0.1 ml glycerol at 1-2 month intervals for lifespan. Maximum survival time was 18 months. No tumours were found (Hansen et al., 1963). [No further details were available.]

Rat: A group of 18 Osborne-Mendel rats received weekly s.c. injections of 1-1.5 mg yellow OB in glycerol as a 1% suspension for lifespan. Survivors at 18 and 24 months were 10 and 2 rats, respectively, compared with 13 and 5 in controls. Four, or possibly 5, treated animals developed injection site fibrosarcomas; glycerol-injected controls developed no local tumours (Hansen et al., 1963).

3.2 Other relevant biological data

(a) Animals

Yellow OB is lethal to rabbits after its s.c., oral or i.p. administration in doses of 1 g/kg bw; doses of 250 mg/kg bw are tolerated. The colour accumulates in fatty tissues of the body after its s.c. injection and is eliminated slowly; thus, 250 mg/kg bw of the colour administered to rabbits were excreted 16 days later in urine (Salant & Bengis, 1916).

Daily oral dosages of 200 and 400 mg/kg bw yellow OB reduced haemoglobin concentration in male but not in female rats; 400 mg/kg bw/day caused testicular changes (Allmark *et al.*, 1955). When fed continuously to male rats at a dietary level of 5000 mg/kg of diet, the colour induced Heinz bodies (Rofe, 1957). Dietary levels of 15,000 or 30,000 mg yellow OB per kg of diet caused changes in the liver, thymus, adrenal pancreas and kidney (Allmark *et al.*, 1955). Levels of 2500 mg/kg of diet caused anaemia, oedema, hypertrophy of the heart and changes in the liver, spleen, bone marrow and testis, growth inhibition and 100% mortality within 12 months, compared with 4% mortality for controls; levels of 500 mg/kg of diet had no toxic effects (Hansen *et al.*, 1963). Rats fed diets containing 40,000 mg yellow OB per kg of diet lived for only a few months (Willheim & Ivy, 1953).

Yellow OB is converted to an imidazole derivative by reaction with aldehydes in the stomachs of rats or rabbits. Studies with ^{14}C-labelled colour indicated that almost all of the yellow OB was eliminated in 48 hours: the faeces contained 82% and urine 18% of the radioactivity. Bile contained 1-(*ortho*-tolylazo)-6-hydroxy-2-naphthylamine-O-hydrogen sulphate N-glucuronide, 1-(*ortho*-tolylazo)-6-hydroxy-2-sulphonamino-naphthalene-O-glucuronide, 1-(*ortho*-tolylazo)-6-hydroxy-2-naphthylamine-N-glucuronide and 1-(*ortho*-tolylazo)-2-sulphonaminonaphthalene. 1-(*ortho*-Tolylazo)-6-hydroxy-2-sulphonaminonaphthalene-O-glucuronide and 1-(*ortho*-tolylazo)-2-sulphonaminonaphthalene were also present in the urine (Radomski & Harrow, 1966).

3.3 Observations in man

No data were available to the Working Group.

4. Comments on Data Reported and Evaluation

4.1 Animal data

Yellow OB was tested in mice by subcutaneous injection and in rats by oral and subcutaneous administration. Although the feeding experiments in rats and the subcutaneous injection studies in mice were negative, the colour produced local tumours in rats following its subcutaneous administration (see also preamble, p. 21).

4.2 Human data

No case reports or epidemiological studies were available to the Working Group.

5. References

Allmark, M.G., Grice, H.C. & Lu, F.C. (1955) Chronic toxicity studies on food colours. I. Observations on the toxicity of FD & C Yellow No. 3 (oil yellow AB) and FD & C Yellow No. 4 (oil yellow OB) in rats. J. Pharm. Pharmacol., 7, 591-603

DFG (Deutsche Forschungsgemeinschaft) (1955) Kommission zur Bearbeitung des Lebensmittelfarbstoffproblems, Toxikologische Daten von Farbstoffen und ihre Zulassung für Lebensmittel in verschiedenen Ländern, Mitt. 6(1), Wiesbaden, Steiner Verlag

DFG (Deutsche Forschungsgemeinschaft) (1957) Farbstoff-Kommission, Toxikologische Daten von Farbstoffen und ihre Zulassung für Lebensmittel in verschiedenen Ländern, Mitt. 6(2), Wiesbaden, Steiner Verlag, p. 11

Druckrey, H. (1955) Schädliche und unschädliche Farbstoffe fur Lebensmittel. Z. Krebsforsch., 60, 344-360

FAO/WHO (1973) List of Additives Evaluated for their Safety-in-Use in Food, First Series, CAC/FAL 1-1973, p. 45

Hansen, W.H., Nelson, A.A. & Fitzhugh, O.G. (1963) Chronic toxicity of yellow AB (1-phenylazo-2-naphthylamine) and yellow OB (1-o-tolylazo-2-naphthylamine). Toxicol. appl. Pharmacol., 5, 16-35

Hodgson, H.H. & Foster, C.K. (1942) Some reactions of the diazonium salts of certain arylazo-β-naphthylamines. J. chem. Soc., 31, 435-437

Japan Food Hygiene Association (1974) Japanese Standards of Food Additives, 3rd ed., Tokyo, Ministry of Health and Welfare

Miller, J.A. & Miller, E.C. (1953) The carcinogenic aminoazo dyes. Advanc. Cancer Res., 1, 339-396

National Research Council (1971) Food Colors, Washington DC, National Academy of Sciences, p. 7

Radomski, J.L. (1974) Toxicology of food colors. Ann. Rev. Pharmacol., 14, 127-137

Radomski, J.L. & Harrow, L.S. (1966) The metabolism of 1-(o-tolylazo)-2-naphthylamine (yellow OB) in rats. Industr. Med. Surg., 35, 882-888

Rofe, P. (1957) Azo dyes and Heinz bodies. Brit. J. industr. Med., 14, 275-280

Salant, W. & Bengis, R. (1916) Physiological and pharmacological studies on coal-tar colors. I. Experiments with fat-soluble dyes. J. biol. chem., 27, 403-427

Society of Dyers and Colourists (1971) Colour Index, 3rd ed., Vol. III, Bradford, Yorkshire, Deanhouse Piccadilly, p. 3021

Truhaut, R. (1955) Sur l'action cancérigène de certaines matières colorantes. Importance en hygiène alimentaire, en thérapeutique et en hygiène générale. Ann. pharm. fr., 13, 36-51

Truhaut, R. (1958) Sur l'utilisation de colorants en thérapeutique et les dangers qui peuvent en résulter pour la santé humaine. Chimie moderne, 3, 291-321

US Code of Federal Regulations (1974) Food and Drugs, Title 21, part 8.507, Washington DC, US Government Printing Office, p. 178

US Tariff Commission (1922) Census of Dyes and Other Synthetic Organic Chemicals, 1921, Tariff Information Series No. 26, Washington DC, US Government Printing Office, p. 68

US Tariff Commission (1958) Synthetic Organic Chemicals, US Production and Sales, 1957, Report No. 203, Second Series, Washington DC, US Government Printing Office, p. 18

Willheim, R. & Ivy, A.C. (1953) A preliminary study concerning the possibility of dietary carcinogenesis. Gastroenterology, 23, 1-19

INDEX

A

AAB *see para*-Aminoazobenzene	53
AAT *see ortho*-Aminoazotoluene	61
o-AAT *see ortho*-Aminoazotoluene	61
Acetacid red B *see* Carmoisine	83
Acetacid red 2BR *see* Amaranth	41
Acetacid red J *see* Ponceau MX	189
Acetamine yellow CG *see* C.I. Disperse Yellow 3	97
Acetate fast yellow G *see* C.I. Disperse Yellow 3	97
Acetoquinone light yellow *see* C.I. Disperse Yellow 3	97
Acetoquinone light yellow 4JLZ *see* C.I. Disperse Yellow 3	97
N-Acetyl-N-{2-methyl-4-[(2-methylphenyl)azo]phenyl}acetamide *see* Diacetylaminoazotoluene	113
Acidal fast orange *see* Orange G	181
Acidal ponceau G *see* Ponceau MX	189
Acid amaranth *see* Amaranth	41
Acid amaranth I *see* Amaranth	41
Acid amaranth N *see* Amaranth	41
Acid brilliant rubine A2G conc. *see* Carmoisine	83
Acid brilliant rubine 2G *see* Carmoisine	83
Acid brilliant rubine 2GT *see* Carmoisine	83
Acid chrome blue BA *see* Carmoisine	83
Acid chrome blue BA-CF *see* Carmoisine	83
Acid chrome blue FBS *see* Carmoisine	83
Acid chrome blue 2R *see* Carmoisine	83
Acid fast orange EGG *see* Orange G	181
Acid fast orange G *see* Orange G	181
Acid fast red FB *see* Carmoisine	83
Acid leather orange I *see* Orange I	173
Acid leather orange KG *see* Orange G	181
Acid leather orange PGW *see* Orange G	181
Acid leather red 12BW *see* Amaranth	41
Acid leather red KPR *see* Ponceau MX	189
Acid leather red P2R *see* Ponceau MX	189
Acid leather rubine S *see* Amaranth	41

Acid leather scarlet IRW see Ponceau MX	189
Acid light orange G see Orange G	181
Acid light orange 2G see Orange G	181
Acid light orange J see Orange G	181
Acid light orange JA export see Orange G	181
Acid light orange SX see Orange G	181
Acid orange I see Orange I	173
Acid orange 10 see Orange G	181
Acid orange G see Orange G	181
Acid orange 2G see Orange G	181
Acid orange GG see Orange G	181
Acid phosphine CL see Orange I	173
Acid ponceau R see Ponceau MX	189
Acid ponceau 2RL see Ponceau MX	189
Acid ponceau special see Ponceau MX	189
Acid red 14 see Carmoisine	83
Acid red 26 see Ponceau MX	189
Acid red 2C see Carmoisine	83
Acid rubine see Carmoisine	83
Acid rubine extra see Carmoisine	83
Acid scarlet see Ponceau MX	189
Acid scarlet 2B see Ponceau MX	189
Acid scarlet 2BN see Ponceau MX	189
Acid scarlet 2R see Ponceau MX	189
Acid scarlet 2R for lakes see Ponceau MX	189
Acid scarlet 2R for lakes bluish see Ponceau MX	189
Acid scarlet 2RL see Ponceau MX	189
Acid scarlet 2RN see Ponceau MX	189
Acid yellow TRA see Sunset yellow FCF	257
Acilan orange GX see Orange G	181
Acilan ponceau RRL see Ponceau MX	189
Acilan red SE see Amaranth	41
A.F. orange No. 1 see Orange I	173
A.F. orange No. 2 see Oil orange SS	165
A.F. red No. 1 see Ponceau 3R	199

A.F. red No. 5 *see* Sudan II	233
A.F. yellow No. 2 *see* Yellow AB	279
A.F. yellow No. 3 *see* Yellow OB	287
A.F. yellow No. 5 *see* Sunset yellow FCF	257
Ahcocid fast scarlet R *see* Ponceau MX	189
Airedale carmoisine *see* Carmoisine	83
Aizen amaranth *see* Amaranth	41
Aizen food orange No. 1 *see* Orange I	173
Aizen food orange No. 2 *see* Oil orange SS	165
Aizen food red No. 5 *see* Sudan II	233
Aizen food yellow No. 5 *see* Sunset yellow FCF	257
Aizen naphthol orange I *see* Orange I	173
Aizen orange I *see* Orange I	173
Aizen ponceau RH *see* Ponceau MX	189
Alabaster No. 3 *see* Sunset yellow FCF	257
Altco sperse fast yellow GFN new *see* C.I. Disperse Yellow 3	97
Amacel yellow G *see* C.I. Disperse Yellow 3	97
Amacid amaranth *see* Amaranth	41
Amacid carmoisine B *see* Carmoisine	83
Amacid chrome blue R *see* Carmoisine	83
Amacid crystal orange *see* Orange G	181
Amacid lake scarlet 2R *see* Ponceau MX	189
Amacid scarlet 2R *see* Ponceau MX	189
Amanil sky blue *see* Trypan blue	267
Amanil sky blue R *see* Trypan blue	267
Amaranth	41
Amaranth A *see* Amaranth	41
Amaranth B *see* Amaranth	41
Amaranth BPC *see* Amaranth	41
Amaranthe *see* Amaranth	41
Amaranth extra *see* Amaranth	41
Amaranth lake *see* Amaranth	41
Amaranth S *see* Amaranth	41
Amaranth S specially pure *see* Amaranth	41
Amaranth USP *see* Amaranth	41

Amaranth USP (biological stain) *see* Amaranth	41
Amaranth WD *see* Amaranth	41
Amidine blue 4B *see* Trypan blue	267
Aminoazobenzene *see para*-Aminoazobenzene	53
4-Aminoazobenzene *see para*-Aminoazobenzene	53
4-Amino-1,1'-azobenzene *see para*-Aminoazobenzene	53
p-Aminoazobenzene *see para*-Aminoazobenzene	53
para-Aminoazobenzene	53
Aminoazobenzene (indicator) *see para*-Aminoazobenzene	53
4-Aminoazobenzol *see para*-Aminoazobenzene	53
p-Aminoazobenzol *see para*-Aminoazobenzene	53
Aminoazotoluene *see ortho*-Aminoazotoluene	61
Aminoazotoluene (indicator) *see ortho*-Aminoazotoluene	61
2-Amino-5-azotoluene *see ortho*-Aminoazotoluene	61
o-Aminoazotoluene *see ortho*-Aminoazotoluene	61
ortho-Aminoazotoluene	61
p-Aminoazotoluene *see para*-Aminoazobenzene	53
4-Amino-2',3-dimethylazobenzene *see ortho*-Aminoazotoluene	61
4'-Amino-2,3'-dimethylazobenzene *see ortho*-Aminoazotoluene	61
p-Aminodiphenylimide *see para*-Aminoazobenzene	53
Aniline-azo-β-naphthylamine *see* Yellow AB	279
Aniline yellow *see para*-Aminoazobenzene	53
Apocid orange 2G *see* Orange G	181
Artisil yellow G *see* C.I. Disperse Yellow 3	97
Artisil yellow 2GN *see* C.I. Disperse Yellow 3	97
Astra chrysoidine R *see* Chrysoidine	91
o-AT *see ortho*-Aminoazotoluene	61
Atrisil direct yellow G *see* C.I. Disperse Yellow 3	97
Atul acid crystal orange G *see* Orange G	181
Atul acid crystal red *see* Carmoisine	83
Atul brilliant oil yellow G *see* 4-Hydroxyazobenzene	157
Atul crystal red F *see* Carmoisine	83
Atul fast yellow R *see para*-Dimethylaminoazobenzene	125
Atul oil orange T *see* Oil orange SS	165
Atul oil red G *see* Sudan III	241

Atul orange R *see* Sudan I	225
Atul sunset yellow FCF *see* Sunset yellow FCF	257
Azidinblau 3B *see* Trypan blue	267
Azidine blue 3B *see* Trypan blue	267
Azobenzene	75
Azobenzide *see* Azobenzene	75
Azobenzol *see* Azobenzene	75
Azobisbenzene *see* Azobenzene	75
Azodibenzene *see* Azobenzene	75
Azodyne *see* 2,6-Diamino-3-(phenylazo)pyridine (hydrochloride)	117
Azo red R *see* Amaranth	41
Azorubin *see* Carmoisine	83
Azorubine *see* Carmoisine	83
Azo rubine *see* Carmoisine	83
Azo rubine AF *see* Carmoisine	83
Azo rubine (biological stain) *see* Carmoisine	83
Azo rubine extra LC *see* Carmoisine	83
Azo rubine for food *see* Carmoisine	83
Azo rubine LZ *see* Carmoisine	83
Azo rubine S *see* Amaranth	41
and see Carmoisine	83
Azo rubine SF *see* Amaranth	41
Azo rubine S.FQ *see* Amaranth	41
Azo rubine S specially pure *see* Carmoisine	83
Azo rubin extra *see* Carmoisine	83
Azo rubine XX *see* Carmoisine	83
Azorubin S *see* Amaranth	41
and see Carmoisine	83
Azo ruby S *see* Amaranth	41
Azovan blue *see* Evans blue	151
Azovannatrium *see* Evans blue	151
Azovanum coeruleum *see* Evans blue	151
Azurro diretto 3B *see* Trypan blue	267

B

Bay 22555 *see* para-Dimethylaminobenzenediazo sodium sulphonate	147
BAY 22555 *see* para-Dimethylaminobenzenediazo sodium sulphonate	147
Bayer 22555 *see* para-Dimethylaminobenzenediazo sodium sulphonate	147
Bencidal blue 3B *see* Trypan blue	267
Benzaminblau 3B *see* Trypan blue	267
Benzamine blue *see* Trypan blue	267
Benzamine blue 3B *see* Trypan blue	267
Benzanil blue 3BN *see* Trypan blue	267
Benzanil blue R *see* Trypan blue	267
4-Benzeneazoaniline *see* para-Aminoazobenzene	53
Benzeneazobenzene *see* Azobenzene	75
Benzeneazobenzeneazo-β-naphthol *see* Sudan III	241
Benzeneazodimethylaniline *see* para-Dimethylaminoazobenzene	125
Benzeneazo-β-naphthol *see* Sudan I	225
1-Benzeneazo-2-naphthol *see* Sudan I	225
Benzene-1-azo-2-naphthol *see* Sudan I	225
1-Benzeneazo-2-naphthylamine *see* Yellow AB	279
1-Benzeneazo-β-naphthylamine *see* Yellow AB	279
p-Benzeneazophenol *see* 4-Hydroxyazobenzene	157
Benzoblau 3B *see* Trypan blue	267
Benzo blue *see* Trypan blue	267
Benzo blue 3B *see* Trypan blue	267
Benzo blue 3BS *see* Trypan blue	267
Biebrich scarlet BPC *see* Scarlet red	217
Biebrich scarlet red *see* Scarlet red	217
Biebrich scarlet R medicinal *see* Scarlet red	217
4,4'-Bis(1-amino-8-hydroxy-2,4-disulfo-7-naphthylazo)-3,3'-bitolyl, tetrasodium salt *see* Evans blue	151
4,4'-Bis[7-(1-amino-8-hydroxy-2,4-disulfo)naphthylazo]-3,3'-bitolyl, tetrasodium salt *see* Evans blue	151
4,4'-Bis(1-amino-8-hydroxy-2,4-disulpho-7-naphthylazo)-3,3'-bitolyl, tetrasodium salt *see* Evans blue	151
4,4'-Bis[7-(1-amino-8-hydroxy-2,4-disulpho)naphthylazo]-3,3'-bitolyl, tetrasodium salt *see* Evans blue	151
Bisteril *see* 2,6-Diamino-3-(phenylazo)pyridine (hydrochloride)	117

Bleu diamine *see* Trypan blue	267
Bleu diazole N 3B *see* Trypan blue	267
Bleu directe 3B *see* Trypan blue	267
Bleue diretto 3B *see* Trypan blue	267
Bleu trypane N *see* Trypan blue	267
Blue 3B *see* Trypan blue	267
Blue EMB *see* Trypan blue	267
Bordeaux *see* Amaranth	41
Bordeaux S *see* Amaranth	41
Bordeaux S extra conc. A. export *see* Amaranth	41
Bordeaux S extra pure A *see* Amaranth	41
Bordeaux SF *see* Amaranth	41
Brasilamina blue 3B *see* Trypan blue	267
Brasilan azo rubine 2NS *see* Carmoisine	83
Brasilan orange 2G *see* Orange G	181
Brasilazina blue 3B *see* Trypan blue	267
Brasilazina oil orange *see* Sudan I	225
Brasilazina oil red B *see* Scarlet red	217
Brasilazina oil scarlet *see* Sudan III	241
Brasilazina oil scarlet 6G *see* Sudan II	233
Brasilazina oil yellow G *see para*-Aminoazobenzene	53
Brasilazina oil yellow O *see* 4-Hydroxyazobenzene	157
Brasilazina oil yellow R *see ortho*-Aminoazotoluene	61
Brasilazina orange Y *see* Chrysoidine	91
Bright red *see* D & C Red No. 9	107
Brilliant acid rubine M *see* Carmoisine	83
Brilliant carmoisine *see* Carmoisine	83
Brilliant crimson red *see* Carmoisine	83
Brilliant crimson 2R.FQ *see* Carmoisine	83
Brilliant fast oil yellow *see para*-Dimethylaminoazobenzene	125
Brilliant fast spirit yellow *see para*-Dimethylaminoazobenzene	125
Brilliant fast yellow *see para*-Dimethylaminoazobenzene	125
Brilliant oil orange R *see* Sudan I	225
Brilliant oil orange Y base *see* Chrysoidine	91
Brilliant oil scarlet B *see* Sudan II	233

Brilliant oil yellow *see para*-Dimethylaminoazobenzene	125
Brilliant ponceau G *see* Ponceau MX	189
Brilliant red *see* D & C Red No. 9	107
Brilliant scarlet *see* D & C Red No. 9	107
Brilliant toner Z *see* D & C Red No. 9	107
Bronze red RO *see* D & C Red No. 9	107
Bronze red 16913 yellowish *see* D & C Red No. 9	107
Bronze scarlet *see* D & C Red No. 9	107
Bronze scarlet C *see* D & C Red No. 9	107
Bronze scarlet CA *see* D & C Red No. 9	107
Bronze scarlet CBA *see* D & C Red No. 9	107
Bronze scarlet CT *see* D & C Red No. 9	107
Bronze scarlet CTA *see* D & C Red No. 9	107
Bronze scarlet toner *see* D & C Red No. 9	107
Bucacid azo rubine *see* Carmoisine	83
Bucacid fast orange G *see* Orange G	181
Butter or methyl yellow *see para*-Dimethylaminoazobenzene	125
Butter yellow *see ortho*-Aminoazotoluene	61
and *see para*-Dimethylaminoazobenzene	125

C

Calcocid amaranth *see* Amaranth	41
Calcocid fast light orange 2G *see* Orange G	181
Calcocid 2RIL *see* Ponceau MX	189
Calcocid rubine XX *see* Carmoisine	83
Calcocid scarlet 2R *see* Ponceau MX	189
Calcocid scarlet 2RIL *see* Ponceau MX	189
Calcogas M *see* Sudan I	225
Calcogas orange NC *see* Sudan I	225
Calcolake scarlet 2R *see* Ponceau MX	189
Calco oil orange 7078 *see* Sudan I	225
Calco oil orange 7078-Y *see* Sudan I	225
Calco oil orange Z-7078 *see* Sudan I	225
Calco oil red D *see* Scarlet red	217
Calco oil scarlet BL *see* Sudan II	233

Calco oil scarlet ZBL *see* Sudan II	233
Calcosyn yellow GC *see* C.I. Disperse Yellow 3	97
Calcosyn yellow GCN *see* C.I. Disperse Yellow 3	97
Calcozine chrysoidine Y *see* Chrysoidine	91
Calcozine orange YS *see* Chrysoidine	91
Campbelline oil orange *see* Sudan I	225
Canacert amaranth *see* Amaranth	41
Canacert sunset yellow FCF *see* Sunset yellow FCF	257
Candle scarlet B *see* Scarlet red	217
Candle scarlet 2B *see* Scarlet red	217
Candle scarlet G *see* Scarlet red	217
2-Carboxy-4'-(dimethylamino)azobenzene *see* Methyl red	161
Carminaph *see* Sudan I	225
Carmoisine	83
Carmoisine aluminium lake *see* Carmoisine	83
Carmoisine BA *see* Carmoisine	83
Carmoisine BA-CF *see* Carmoisine	83
Carmoisine BSS *see* Carmoisine	83
Carmoisine FU *see* Carmoisine	83
Carmoisine GRN *see* Carmoisine	83
Carmoisine LAS *see* Carmoisine	83
Carmoisine S *see* Carmoisine	83
Carmoisine supra *see* Carmoisine	83
Carmoisine W *see* Carmoisine	83
Carmoisine WS *see* Carmoisine	83
Cellitazol R *see para*-Aminoazobenzene	53
Celliton discharge yellow GL *see* C.I. Disperse Yellow 3	97
Celliton fast yellow G *see* C.I. Disperse Yellow 3	97
Celliton fast yellow GA *see* C.I. Disperse Yellow 3	97
Celliton fast yellow GA-CF *see* C.I. Disperse Yellow 3	97
Celliton yellow G *see* C.I. Disperse Yellow 3	97
Celutate yellow GH *see* C.I. Disperse Yellow 3	97
Centraline blue 3B *see* Trypan blue	267
Cerasine yellow GG *see para*-Dimethylaminoazobenzene	125
Cerasin red *see* Sudan III	241

Cerasinrot *see* Sudan III	241
Ceres orange R *see* Sudan I	225
Ceres orange RR *see* Sudan II	233
Ceres red 7B *see* Sudan red 7B	253
Ceres red BB *see* Scarlet red	217
Ceres yellow R *see para*-Aminoazobenzene	53
Cerisol scarlet G *see* Sudan II	233
Cerisol yellow AB *see* Yellow AB	279
Cerisol yellow TB *see* Yellow OB	287
Cerotine ponceau 3B *see* Scarlet red	217
Cerotinorange G *see* Sudan I	225
Cerotinscharlach G *see* Sudan II	233
Cerotinscharlach R *see* Sudan III	241
Certicol amaranth S *see* Amaranth	41
Certicol carmoisine S *see* Carmoisine	83
Certicol orange GS *see* Orange G	181
Certicol ponceau MXS *see* Ponceau MX	189
Certicol ponceau SXS *see* Ponceau SX	207
Certicol sunset yellow CFS *see* Sunset yellow FCF	257
Certiqual oil red *see* Sudan III	241
Certiqual orange I *see* Orange I	173
Certolake sunset yellow *see* Sunset yellow FCF	257
Cetil light orange GG *see* Orange G	181
Chloramiblau 3B *see* Trypan blue	267
Chloramine blue *see* Trypan blue	267
Chloramine blue 3B *see* Trypan blue	267
Chlorazol blue 3B *see* Trypan blue	267
Chlorazol sky blue FF *see* Evans blue	151
5-Chloro-2-[(2-hydroxy-1-naphthalenyl)azo]-4-methylbenzene-sulfonic acid, barium salt *see* D & C Red No. 9	107
5-Chloro-2-[(2-hydroxy-1-naphthalenyl)azo]-4-methylbenzene-sulfonic acid, barium salt (2:1) *see* D & C Red No. 9	107
5-Chloro-2-[(2-hydroxy-1-naphthalenyl)azo]-4-methylbenzene-sulphonic acid, barium salt *see* D & C Red No. 9	107
5-Chloro-2-[(2-hydroxy-1-naphthalenyl)azo]-4-methylbenzene-sulphonic acid, barium salt (2:1) *see* D & C Red No. 9	107

5-Chloro-2-[(2-hydroxy-1-naphthyl)azo]-p-toluenesulfonic acid, barium salt see D & C Red No. 9	107
5-Chloro-2-[(2-hydroxy-1-naphthyl)azo]-p-toluenesulphonic acid, barium salt see D & C Red No. 9	107
1-(4-Chloro-o-sulfo-5-tolylazo)-2-naphthol, barium salt see D & C Red No. 9	107
1-(4-Chloro-o-sulpho-5-tolylazo)-2-naphthol, barium salt see D & C Red No. 9	107
Chrome fast blue 2R see Carmoisine	83
Chrome leather blue 3B see Trypan blue	267
Chromotrope FB see Carmoisine	83
Chromotrop FB see Carmoisine	83
Chrysoidin see Chrysoidine	91
Chrysoidine	91
Chrysoidine (II) see Chrysoidine	91
Chrysoidine A see Chrysoidine	91
Chrysoidine B see Chrysoidine	91
Chrysoidine C crystals see Chrysoidine	91
Chrysoidine crystals see Chrysoidine	91
Chrysoidine G see Chrysoidine	91
Chrysoidine GN see Chrysoidine	91
Chrysoidine GS see Chrysoidine	91
Chrysoidine HR see Chrysoidine	91
Chrysoidine J see Chrysoidine	91
Chrysoidine M see Chrysoidine	91
Chrysoidine orange see Chrysoidine	91
Chrysoidine PRL see Chrysoidine	91
Chrysoidine PRR see Chrysoidine	91
Chrysoidine SL see Chrysoidine	91
Chrysoidine special (biological stain and indicator) see Chrysoidine	91
Chrysoidine SS see Chrysoidine	91
Chrysoidine Y see Chrysoidine	91
Chrysoidine Y base new see Chrysoidine	91
Chrysoidine Y crystals see Chrysoidine	91
Chrysoidine Y ex see Chrysoidine	91

Chrysoidine YGH *see* Chrysoidine	91
Chrysoidine YL *see* Chrysoidine	91
Chrysoidine Y special *see* Chrysoidine	91
Chrysoidin FB *see* Chrysoidine	91
Chrysoidin YN *see* Chrysoidine	91
C.I. 3/11855 *see* C.I. Disperse Yellow 3	97
C.I. 16045 *see* Ponceau SX	207
C.I. acid orange 10 *see* Orange G	181
C.I. acid orange 10, disodium salt *see* Orange G	181
C.I. acid orange 20 *see* Orange I	173
C.I. acid orange 20, monosodium salt *see* Orange I	173
C.I. acid red 2 *see* Methyl red	161
C.I. acid red 14 *see* Carmoisine	83
C.I. acid red 26 *see* Ponceau MX	189
C.I. acid red 27 *see* Amaranth	41
C.I. acid red 14, disodium salt *see* Carmoisine	83
C.I. acid red 26, disodium salt *see* Ponceau MX	189
C.I. acid red 27, trisodium salt *see* Amaranth	41
C.I. 11160B *see* *ortho*-Aminoazotoluene	61
Cibacete yellow GBA *see* C.I. Disperse Yellow 3	97
Cibacet yellow 2GC *see* C.I. Disperse Yellow 3	97
Cibacet yellow GBA *see* C.I. Disperse Yellow 3	97
C.I. basic orange 2 *see* Chrysoidine	91
C.I. basic orange 2, monohydrochloride *see* Chrysoidine	91
C.I. direct blue 14 *see* Trypan blue	267
C.I. direct blue 53 *see* Evans blue	151
C.I. direct blue 14, tetrasodium salt *see* Trypan blue	267
C.I. direct blue 53, tetrasodium salt *see* Evans blue	151
C.I. Disperse Yellow 3	97
C.I. food orange 4 *see* Orange G	181
C.I. food red 1 *see* Ponceau SX	207
C.I. food red 3 *see* Carmoisine	83
C.I. food red 5 *see* Ponceau MX	189
C.I. food red 6 *see* Ponceau 3R	199
C.I. food red 9 *see* Amaranth	41

C.I. food red 1, disodium salt *see* Ponceau SX	207
C.I. food red 6, disodium salt *see* Ponceau 3R	199
C.I. food yellow 3 *see* Sunset yellow FCF	257
C.I. food yellow 10 *see* Yellow AB	279
C.I. food yellow 11 *see* Yellow OB	287
C.I. food yellow 3, disodium salt *see* Sunset yellow FCF	257
Cilefa orange S *see* Sunset yellow FCF	257
Cilefa rubine 2B *see* Amaranth	41
Cilefa rubine R *see* Carmoisine	83
Cilla fast yellow G *see* C.I. Disperse Yellow 3	97
C.I. pigment red *see* D & C Red No. 9	107
C.I. pigment red 53:1 *see* D & C Red No. 9	107
C.I. pigment red 53, barium salt *see* D & C Red No. 9	107
C.I. solvent brown I *see* Sudan brown RR	249
C.I. solvent brown RR *see* Sudan brown RR	249
C.I. solvent orange 2 *see* Oil orange SS	165
C.I. solvent orange 3 *see* Chrysoidine	91
C.I. solvent orange 7 *see* Sudan II	233
C.I. solvent red 19 *see* Sudan red 7B	253
C.I. solvent red 23 *see* Sudan III	241
C.I. solvent red 24 *see* Scarlet red	217
C.I. solvent red 80 *see* Citrus red No. 2	101
C.I. solvent yellow 1 *see* *para*-Aminoazobenzene	53
C.I. solvent yellow 2 *see* *para*-Dimethylaminoazobenzene	125
C.I. solvent yellow 3 *see* *ortho*-Aminoazotoluene	61
C.I. solvent yellow 5 *see* Yellow AB	279
C.I. solvent yellow 6 *see* Yellow OB	287
C.I. solvent yellow 7 *see* 4-Hydroxyazobenzene	157
C.I. solvent yellow 14 *see* Sudan I	225
Citrus red 2 *see* Citrus red No. 2	101
Citrus red No. 2	101
Colacid orange G *see* Orange G	181
Colacid ponceau special *see* Ponceau MX	189
Comacid scarlet 2R *see* Ponceau MX	189
Congoblau 3B *see* Trypan blue	267

Congo blue *see* Trypan blue	267
Congo blue 3B *see* Trypan blue	267
Cosmetic coral red KO bluish *see* D & C Red No. 9	107
Cosmetic coral red KO yellowish *see* D & C Red No. 9	107
Cosmetic DVR *see* D & C Red No. 9	107
Cosmetic pigment yellow red DVR *see* D & C Red No. 9	107
Cresotine blue 3B *see* Trypan blue	267
Crimson EMBL *see* Carmoisine	83
Crimson 2EMBL *see* Carmoisine	83
Crystal orange 2G *see* Orange G	181

D

DAB *see* para-Dimethylaminoazobenzene	125
Dainichi lake red C *see* D & C Red No. 9	107
Daishiki amaranth *see* Amaranth	41
D & C orange No. 1 *see* Orange I	173
D & C orange No. 2 *see* Oil orange SS	165
D & C orange No. 3 *see* Orange G	173
D & C red No. 5 *see* Ponceau MX	189
D & C red No. 9	107
D & C red No. 17 *see* Sudan III	241
DAS *see* para-Dimethylaminobenzenediazo sodium sulphonate	147
Deksonal *see* para-Dimethylaminobenzenediazo sodium sulphonate	147
Dermagan *see* Diacetylaminoazotoluene	113
Dermagen *see* Diacetylaminoazotoluene	113
Desert red *see* D & C Red No. 9	107
Dexon *see* para-Dimethylaminobenzenediazo sodium sulphonate	147
Dexoxon *see* para-Dimethylaminobenzenediazo sodium sulphonate	147
Diacelliton fast yellow G *see* C.I. Disperse Yellow 3	97
Diacetazotol *see* Diacetylaminoazotoluene	113
Diacetotoluide *see* Diacetylaminoazotoluene	113
Diacetylaminoazotoluene	113
N,N-Diacetyl-*o*-tolylazo-*o*-toluidine *see* Diacetylaminoazotoluene	113
Diadem chrome blue G *see* Carmoisine	83
Diadem chrome blue R *see* Carmoisine	83

Diaminblau 3B *see* Trypan blue	267
Diamineblue *see* Trypan blue	267
Diamine blue *see* Trypan blue	267
Diamine blue 3B *see* Trypan blue	267
Diamine sky blue FF *see* Evans blue	151
2,4-Diaminoazobenzene hydrochloride *see* Chrysoidine	91
Diaminobenzidine *see* *para*-Dimethylaminoazobenzene	125
p,p'-Diamino-m,m'-dimethyldiphenyl-disazo-bis(1-amino-8-naphthol-3,6-disulfonic acid), tetrasodium salt *see* Trypan blue	267
p,p'-Diamino-m,m'-dimethyldiphenyl-disazo-bis(1-amino-8-naphthol-3,6-disulphonic acid), tetrasodium salt *see* Trypan blue	267
2,6-Diamino-3-(phenylazo)pyridine	117
2,6-Diamino-3-phenylazopyridine *see* 2,6-Diamino-3-(phenylazo)-pyridine	117
2,6-Diamino-3-(phenylazo)pyridine (hydrochloride)	117
2,6-Diamino-3-phenylazopyridine hydrochloride *see* 2,6-Diamino-3-(phenylazo)pyridine hydrochloride	117
Dianilblau *see* Trypan blue	267
Dianilblau H3G *see* Trypan blue	267
Dianil blue *see* Trypan blue	267
Dianil blue H3G *see* Trypan blue	267
Diaphtamine blue TH *see* Trypan blue	267
Diazine blue 3B *see* Trypan blue	267
Diazobenzene *see* Azobenzene	75
Diazobleu *see* Evans blue	151
Diazocard chrysoidine G *see* Chrysoidine	91
p-Diazodimethylaniline sodium sulfonate *see* *para*-Dimethylaminobenzenediazo sodium sulphonate	147
p-Diazodimethylaniline sodium sulphonate *see* *para*-Dimethylaminobenzenediazo sodium sulphonate	147
Diazol blue 3B *see* Trypan blue	267
Diazol pure blue BF *see* Evans blue	151
Dimazon *see* Diacetylaminoazotoluene	113
2,5-Dimethoxybenzeneazo-β-naphthol *see* Citrus red No. 2	101
1-[(2,5-Dimethoxyphenyl)azo]-2-naphthalenol *see* Citrus red No. 2	101
1-(2,5-Dimethoxyphenylazo)-2-naphthol *see* Citrus red No. 2	101

1-[1-(2,5-Dimethoxyphenyl)azo]-2-naphthol *see* Citrus red No. 2	101
Dimethylaminoazobenzene *see para*-Dimethylaminoazobenzene	125
2',3-Dimethyl-4-aminoazobenzene *see ortho*-Aminoazotoluene	61
4-Dimethylaminoazobenzene *see para*-Dimethylaminoazobenzene	125
4-(Dimethylamino)azobenzene *see para*-Dimethylaminoazobenzene	125
N-Dimethylaminoazobenzene *see para*-Dimethylaminoazobenzene	125
N,N-Dimethylaminoazobenzene *see para*-Dimethylaminoazobenzene	125
N,N-Dimethyl-4-aminoazobenzene *see para*-Dimethylaminoazobenzene	125
4-(N,N-Dimethylamino)azobenzene *see para*-Dimethylaminoazobenzene	125
N,N-Dimethyl-*p*-aminoazobenzene *see para*-Dimethylaminoazobenzene	125
p-Dimethylaminoazobenzene *see para*-Dimethylaminoazobenzene	125
para-Dimethylaminoazobenzene	125
p-(Dimethylamino)azobenzene *see para*-Dimethylaminoazobenzene	125
4'-Dimethylaminoazobenzene-2-carboxylic acid *see* Methyl red	161
p-(Dimethylamino)azobenzene-*o*-carboxylic acid *see* Methyl red	161
4-Dimethylaminoazobenzol *see para*-Dimethylaminoazobenzene	125
p-Dimethylaminobenzenediazosodium sulfonate *see para*-Dimethylaminobenzenediazo sodium sulphonate	147
p-Dimethylaminobenzenediazo sodium sulfonate *see para*-Dimethylaminobenzenediazo sodium sulphonate	147
p-(Dimethylamino)benzenediazo sodium sulfonate *see para*-Dimethylaminobenzenediazo sodium sulphonate	147
p-Dimethylaminobenzenediazosodium sulphonate *see para*-Dimethylaminobenzenediazo sodium sulphonate	147
p-Dimethylaminobenzenediazo sodium sulphonate *see para*-Dimethylaminobenzenediazo sodium sulphonate	147
para-Dimethylaminobenzenediazo sodium sulphonate	147
p-(Dimethylamino)benzenediazo sodium sulphonate *see para*-Dimethylaminobenzenediazo sodium sulphonate	147
p-(Dimethylamino)benzenediazosulfonate *see para*-Dimethylaminobenzenediazo sodium sulphonate	147
4-Dimethylaminobenzenediazosulfonic acid, sodium salt *see para*-Dimethylaminobenzenediazo sodium sulphonate	147
p-(Dimethylamino)benzenediazosulfonic acid, sodium salt *see para*-Dimethylaminobenzenediazo sodium sulphonate	147
p-Dimethylaminobenzenediazosulfonic acid, sodium salt *see para*-Dimethylaminobenzenediazo sodium sulphonate	147

p-(Dimethylamino)benzenediazosulphonate *see para*-Dimethyl-aminobenzenediazo sodium sulphonate	147
4-Dimethylaminobenzenediazosulphonic acid, sodium salt *see para*-Dimethylaminobenzenediazo sodium sulphonate	147
p-(Dimethylamino)benzenediazosulphonic acid, sodium salt *see para*-Dimethylaminobenzenediazo sodium sulphonate	147
p-Dimethylaminobenzenediazosulphonic acid, sodium salt *see para*-Dimethylaminobenzenediazo sodium sulphonate	147
4-Dimethylaminoethylbenzene *see para*-Dimethylaminoazobenzene	125
4-Dimethylaminophenylazobenzene *see para*-Dimethylaminoazobenzene	125
2-[(4-Dimethylamino)phenylazo]benzoic acid *see* Methyl red	161
o-{[*p*-(Dimethylamino)phenyl]azo}benzoic acid *see* Methyl red	161
[4-(Dimethylamino)phenyl]diazenesulfonic acid, sodium salt *see para*-Dimethylaminobenzenediazo sodium sulphonate	147
4-[(Dimethylamino)phenyl]diazene sulfonic acid, sodium salt *see para*-Dimethylaminobenzenediazo sodium sulphonate	147
[4-(Dimethylamino)phenyl]diazenesulphonic acid, sodium salt *see para*-Dimethylaminobenzenediazo sodium sulphonate	147
4-[(Dimethylamino)phenyl]diazene sulphonic acid, sodium salt *see para*-Dimethylaminobenzenediazo sodium sulphonate	147
N,N-Dimethyl-*p*-azoaniline *see para*-Dimethylaminoazobenzene	125
6,6'-{[3,3'-Dimethyl(1,1'-biphenyl)-4,4'-diyl]bis(azo)}bis-(4-amino-5-hydroxy)-1,3-naphthalenedisulfonic acid, tetrasodium salt *see* Evans blue	151
3,3'-{[3,3'-Dimethyl(1,1'-biphenyl)-4,4'-diyl]bis(azo)}bis-(5-amino-4-hydroxy)-2,7-naphthalenedisulfonic acid, tetrasodium salt *see* Trypan blue	267
6,6'-{[3,3'-Dimethyl(1,1'-biphenyl)-4,4'-diyl]bis(azo)}bis-(4-amino-5-hydroxy)-1,3-naphthalenedisulphonic acid, tetrasodium salt *see* Evans blue	151
3,3'-{[3,3'-Dimethyl(1,1'-biphenyl)-4,4'-diyl]bis(azo)}bis-(5-amino-4-hydroxy)-2,7-naphthalenedisulphonic acid, tetrasodium salt *see* Trypan blue	267
3,3'-[(3,3'-Dimethyl-4,4'-biphenylene)bis(azo)]bis(5-amino-4-hydroxy)-2,7-naphthalenedisulfonic acid, tetrasodium salt *see* Trypan blue	267
3,3'-[(3,3'-Dimethyl-4,4'-biphenylene)bis(azo)]bis(5-amino-4-hydroxy)-2,7-naphthalenedisulphonic acid, tetrasodium salt *see* Trypan blue	267
2,2'-[(3,3'-Dimethyl-4,4'-biphenylylene)bis(azo)]bis(8-amino-1-hydroxy-3,6-naphthalenedisulfonic acid), tetrasodium salt *see* Trypan blue	267

6,6'-[(3,3'-Dimethyl-4,4'-biphenylylene)bis(azo)] bis(4-amino-5-hydroxy-1,3-naphthalenedisulfonic acid), tetrasodium salt
  see Evans blue   151

2,2'-[(3,3'-Dimethyl-4,4'-biphenylylene)bis(azo)] bis(8-amino-1-hydroxy-3,6-naphthalenedisulphonic acid), tetrasodium salt
  see Trypan blue   267

6,6'-[(3,3'-Dimethyl-4,4'-biphenylylene)bis(azo)]bis(4-amino-5-hydroxy-1,3-naphthalenedisulphonic acid), tetrasodium salt
  see Evans blue   151

2,2'-[(3,3'-Dimethyl-4,4'-biphenylylene)]bis(azo)bis(8-amino-1-naphthol-5,7-disulfonic acid), tetrasodium salt see Evans blue   151

2,2'-[(3,3'-Dimethyl-4,4'-biphenylylene)]bis(azo)bis(8-amino-1-naphthol-5,7-disulphonic acid), tetrasodium salt see Evans blue   151

2',3-Dimethyl-4-(2-hydroxynaphthylazo)azobenzene see Scarlet red   217

N,N-Dimethyl-*p*-phenylazoaniline see *para*-Dimethylaminoazobenzene   125

N,N-Dimethyl-*p*-(phenylazo)aniline see *para*-Dimethylaminoazobenzene   125

N,N-Dimethyl-4-(phenylazo)benzamine see *para*-Dimethylaminoazobenzene   125

N,N-Dimethyl-4-(phenylazo)benzenamine see *para*-Dimethylaminoazobenzene   125

4-[(2,4-Dimethylphenyl)azo]-3-hydroxy-2,7-naphthalenedisulfonic acid, disodium salt see Ponceau MX   189

4-[(2,4-Dimethylphenyl)azo]-3-hydroxy-2,7-naphthalenedisulphonic acid, disodium salt see Ponceau MX   189

1-[(2,4-Dimethylphenyl)azo]-2-naphthalenol see Sudan II   233

3-[(2,4-Dimethyl-5-sulfophenyl)azo]-4-hydroxy-1-naphthalenesulfonic acid, disodium salt see Ponceau SX   207

3-[(2,4-Dimethyl-5-sulphophenyl)azo]-4-hydroxy-1-naphthalenesulphonic acid, disodium salt see Ponceau SX   207

Dimethyl yellow see *para*-Dimethylaminoazobenzene   125

Dimethyl yellow N,N-dimethylaniline see *para*-Dimethylaminoazobenzene   125

Diphenyl blue 3B see Trypan blue   267

Diphenyldiazene see Azobenzene   75

Diphenyldiimide see Azobenzene   75

Directblau 3B see Trypan blue   267

Direct blue 3B see Trypan blue   267

Direct blue 3BX see Trypan blue   267

Direct blue D3B see Trypan blue   267

Direct blue FFN see Trypan blue   267

Direct blue H3G *see* Trypan blue	267
Direct blue M3B *see* Trypan blue	267
Directakol blue 3BL *see* Trypan blue	267
Diridone *see* 2,6-Diamino-3-(phenylazo)pyridine (hydrochloride)	117
Disodium (2,4-dimethylphenylazo)-2-hydroxynaphthalene-3,6-disulfonate *see* Ponceau MX	189
Disodium (2,4-dimethylphenylazo)-2-hydroxynaphthalene-3,6-disulphonate *see* Ponceau MX	189
Disodium 3-hydroxy-4-[(2,4,5-trimethylphenyl)azo]-2,7-naphthalenedisulfonate *see* Ponceau 3R	199
Disodium 3-hydroxy-4-[(2,4,5-trimethylphenyl)azo]-2,7-naphthalenedisulfonic acid *see* Ponceau 3R	199
Disodium 3-hydroxy-4-[(2,4,5-trimethylphenyl)azo]-2,7-naphthalenedisulphonate *see* Ponceau 3R	199
Disodium 3-hydroxy-4-[(2,4,5-trimethylphenyl)azo]-2,7-naphthalenedisulphonic acid *see* Ponceau 3R	199
Disodium salt of 1-(2,4-xylylazo)-2-naphthol-3,6-disulfonic acid *see* Ponceau MX	189
Disodium salt of 1-(2,4-xylylazo)-2-naphthol-3,6-disulphonic acid *see* Ponceau MX	189
Disodium 2-(4-sulfo-1-naphthylazo)-1-naphthol-4-sulfonate *see* Carmoisine	83
Disodium 2-(4-sulpho-1-naphthylazo)-1-naphthol-4-sulphonate *see* Carmoisine	83
Dispersed orange 11348 *see* Sunset yellow FCF	257
Dispersed yellow 12116 *see* Sunset yellow FCF	257
Disperse yellow 3 *see* C.I. Disperse Yellow 3	97
Disperse yellow G *see* C.I. Disperse Yellow 3	97
Disperse yellow Z *see* C.I. Disperse Yellow 3	97
Dispersol fast yellow G *see* C.I. Disperse Yellow 3	97
Dispersol printing yellow G *see* C.I. Disperse Yellow 3	97
Dispersol red PP *see* Scarlet red	217
Dispersol yellow PP *see* Sudan I	225
DMAB *see* *para*-Dimethylaminoazobenzene	125
Dolkwal amaranth *see* Amaranth	41
Dolkwal orange G *see* Orange G	181
Dolkwal orange SS *see* Oil orange SS	165
Dolkwal ponceau 3R *see* Ponceau 3R	199

Dolkwal sunset yellow *see* Sunset yellow FCF	257
Dolkwal yellow AB *see* Yellow AB	279
Dolkwal yellow OB *see* Yellow OB	287
DPP *see* 2,6-Diamino-3-(phenylazo)pyridine	117
Dunkelgelb *see* Sudan I	225
Duplex red lake C20-5925 *see* D & C Red No. 9	107
Durgacet yellow G *see* C.I. Disperse Yellow 3	97
Durosperse yellow G *see* C.I. Disperse Yellow 3	97
Dye Evans blue *see* Evans blue	151
Dye FD & C red 2 *see* Amaranth	41
Dye FD & C red No. 4 *see* Ponceau SX	207
Dye FD and C red No. 4 *see* Ponceau SX	207
Dye FD & C yellow lake 6 *see* Sunset yellow FCF	257
Dye FD & C yellow No. 6 *see* Sunset yellow FCF	257
Dye FDC red 2 *see* Amaranth	41
Dye FDC yellow lake 6 *see* Sunset yellow FCF	257
Dye FDC yellow No. 6 *see* Sunset yellow FCF	257
Dye orange No. 1 *see* Orange I	173
Dye sunset yellow *see* Sunset yellow FCF	257

E

Eastone yellow GN *see* C.I. Disperse Yellow 3	97
Eboliblau 4B *see* Trypan blue	267
Edicol amaranth *see* Amaranth	41
Edicol supra amaranth A *see* Amaranth	41
Edicol supra carmoisine W *see* Carmoisine	83
Edicol supra carmoisine WS *see* Carmoisine	83
Edicol supra ponceau R *see* Ponceau MX	189
Edicol supra ponceau SX *see* Ponceau SX	207
Edicol supra yellow FC *see* Sunset yellow FCF	257
Egacid orange GG *see* Orange G	181
Elcozine chrysoidine Y *see* Chrysoidine	91
Elgacid orange 2G *see* Orange G	181
Eljon lake red C *see* D & C Red No. 9	107
Eniacid brilliant rubine 3B *see* Carmoisine	83

Eniacid light orange G *see* Orange G	181
Eniacid orange I *see* Orange I	173
Eniacid sunset yellow *see* Sunset yellow FCF	257
Enial orange I *see* Sudan I	225
Enial red IV *see* Scarlet red	217
Enial yellow 2G *see* para-Dimethylaminoazobenzene	125
Eniamethyl orange *see* para-Dimethylaminobenzenediazo sodium sulphonate	**147**
Erio fast orange AS *see* Orange G	181
Erio rubine B *see* Carmoisine	83
Esteroquinone light yellow 4JL *see* C.I. Disperse Yellow 3	97
N-Ethyl-1-{[p-(phenylazo)phenyl]azo}-2-naphthalenamine *see* Sudan red 7B	253
N-Ethyl-1-{[4-(phenylazo)phenyl]azo}-2-naphthylamine *see* Sudan red 7B	253
Eurocert amaranth *see* Amaranth	41
Eurocert azorubine *see* Carmoisine	83
Eurocert orange FCF *see* Sunset yellow FCF	257
Evablin *see* Evans blue	151
Evans blue	151
Evans blue dye *see* Evans blue	151
Evans blue, sodium salt *see* Evans blue	151
Ext. D & C orange No. 3 *see* Orange I	173
Ext. D & C orange No. 4 *see* Oil orange SS	165
Ext. D & C red No. 10 *see* Carmoisine	83
Ext. D & C red No. 14 *see* Sudan II	233
Ext. D & C red No. 15 *see* Ponceau 3R	199
Ext. D & C yellow No. 9 *see* Yellow AB	279
Ext. D & C yellow No. 10 *see* Yellow OB	287
External D and C orange No. 3 *see* Orange I	173
External D and C red No. 15 *see* Ponceau 3R	199
Extract D and C orange No. 3 *see* Orange I	173
Extract D and C orange No. 4 *see* Oil orange SS	165
Extract D and C red No. 10 *see* Carmoisine	83
Extract D and C red No. 14 *see* Sudan II	233
Extract D and C red No. 15 *see* Ponceau 3R	199

F

Fast garnet GBC base	*see ortho*-Aminoazotoluene	61
Fast light orange G	*see* Orange G	181
Fast light orange GA	*see* Orange G	181
Fast light orange GA-CF	*see* Orange G	181
Fast oil orange	*see* Sudan I	225
Fast oil orange I	*see* Sudan I	225
Fast oil orange II	*see* Sudan II	233
Fast oil red B	*see* Scarlet red	217
Fast oil scarlet III	*see* Sudan III	241
Fast oil yellow	*see ortho*-Aminoazotoluene	61
Fast oil yellow B	*see para*-Dimethylaminoazobenzene	125
Fast oil yellow 2G	*see* 4-Hydroxyazobenzene	157
Fast orange	*see* Sudan I	225
Fast orange G	*see* Orange G	181
Fast red	*see* Amaranth	41
Fast red BB	*see* Scarlet red	217
Fast red R	*see* Sudan III	241
Fast spirit yellow	*see para*-Aminoazobenzene	53
	and see ortho-Aminoazotoluene	61
Fast spirit yellow AAB	*see para*-Aminoazobenzene	53
Fast yellow	*see para*-Dimethylaminoazobenzene	125
Fast yellow AT	*see ortho*-Aminoazotoluene	61
Fat brown 2G	*see* Sudan brown RR	249
Fat brown 2R	*see* Sudan brown RR	249
Fat brown RR	*see* Sudan brown RR	249
Fat orange I	*see* Sudan I	225
Fat orange II	*see* Oil orange SS	165
Fat orange 4A	*see* Sudan I	225
Fat orange G	*see* Sudan I	225
Fat orange R	*see* Sudan I	225
	and see Sudan II	233
Fat orange RR	*see* Oil orange SS	165
Fat orange RS	*see* Sudan I	225

Fat ponceau see Scarlet red	217
and see Sudan II	233
Fat ponceau G see Sudan III	241
Fat ponceau R see Scarlet red	217
Fat red see Sudan II	233
and see Sudan III	241
Fat red B see Scarlet red	217
Fat red 2B see Scarlet red	217
Fat red 7B see Sudan red 7B	253
Fat red BB see Scarlet red	217
and see Sudan III	241
Fat red (bluish) see Sudan III	241
Fat red BS see Scarlet red	217
Fat red G see Sudan III	241
Fat red HRR see Sudan III	241
Fat red R see Sudan III	241
Fat red RS see Sudan III	241
Fat red TS see Scarlet red	217
Fat red (yellowish) see Sudan II	233
Fat scarlet 2G see Sudan II	233
Fat scarlet LB see Sudan III	241
Fat soluble red Zh see Sudan III	241
Fat yellow A see para-Dimethylaminoazobenzene	125
Fat yellow AAB see para-Aminoazobenzene	53
Fat yellow AD OO see para-Dimethylaminoazobenzene	125
Fat yellow B see ortho-Aminoazotoluene	61
Fat yellow ES see para-Dimethylaminoazobenzene	125
Fat yellow ES extra see para-Dimethylaminoazobenzene	125
Fat yellow extra conc. see para-Dimethylaminoazobenzene	125
Fat yellow R see para-Dimethylaminoazobenzene	125
Fat yellow R (8186) see para-Dimethylaminoazobenzene	125
FD & C No. 6 see Sunset yellow FCF	257
FD & C orange 2 see Oil orange SS	165
FD & C orange No. 1 see Orange I	173
FD & C orange No. 2 see Oil orange SS	165

FD & C red 32 *see* Sudan II	233
FD & C red No. 1 *see* Ponceau 3R	199
FD & C red No. 2 *see* Amaranth	41
FD & C red No. 4 *see* Ponceau SX	207
FD & C red No. 32 *see* Sudan II	233
FD & C red No. 2 - aluminium lake *see* Amaranth	41
FD & C red No. 2 - alumnum lake *see* Amaranth	41
FD & C red No. 4 - aluminium lake *see* Ponceau SX	207
FD & C yellow 3 *see* Yellow AB	279
FD & C yellow 4 *see* Yellow OB	287
FD & C yellow 6 *see* Sunset yellow FCF	257
FD & C yellow lake No. 6 *see* Sunset yellow FCF	257
FD & C yellow No. 3 *see* Yellow AB	279
FD & C yellow No. 4 *see* Yellow OB	287
FD & C yellow No. 6 *see* Sunset yellow FCF	257
FD & C yellow No. 6 aluminium lake *see* Sunset yellow FCF	257
FDC orange I *see* Orange I	173
FDC red No. 2 *see* Amaranth	41
FDC yellow No. 6 *see* Sunset yellow FCF	257
Fenacet fast yellow G *see* C.I. Disperse Yellow 3	97
Fenacet yellow G *see* C.I. Disperse Yellow 3	97
Fenazo light orange 2G *see* Orange G	181
Fenazo red C *see* Carmoisine	83
Fenazo scarlet 2R *see* Ponceau MX	189
Fettorange 4A *see* Sudan I	225
Fettorange B *see* Sudan II	233
Fettorange LG *see* Sudan I	225
Fettorange R *see* Sudan I	225
Fettponceau G *see* Sudan III	241
Fettrot *see* Sudan III	241
Fettscharlach *see* Sudan III	241
Fettscharlach LB *see* Sudan III	241
Foodcol sunset yellow FCF *see* Sunset yellow FCF	257
Food orange GG *see* Orange G	181
Food red 2 *see* Amaranth	41

Food red 3 *see* Carmoisine	83
Food red 4 *see* Ponceau SX	207
Food red 5 *see* Carmoisine	83
Food red 9 *see* Amaranth	41
Food yellow 3 *see* Sunset yellow FCF	257
Food yellow 6 *see* Sunset yellow FCF	257
Fruit red A extra yellowish Geigy *see* Carmoisine	83
Fruit red A Geigy *see* Amaranth	41

G

Gastracid *see* 2,6-Diamino-3-(phenylazo)pyridine	117
Geigy-blau 536 *see* Evans blue	151
Geigy blue 536, med *see* Evans blue	151
Genacron yellow G *see* C.I. Disperse Yellow 3	97
Gold orange MP *see* *para*-Dimethylaminobenzenediazo sodium sulphonate	147
Grasal brilliant red B *see* Scarlet red	217
Grasal brilliant red G *see* Sudan III	241
Grasal brilliant yellow *see* *para*-Dimethylaminoazobenzene	125
Grasal orange *see* Sudan I	225
Grasal yellow *see* Yellow AB	279
Grasán brilliant red B *see* Scarlet red	217
Grasán brilliant red G *see* Sudan III	241
Grasán brown DT new *see* Sudan brown RR	249
Grasán orange R *see* Sudan I	225
Grasán orange 3R *see* Sudan II	233

H

Hamilton red *see* D & C Red No. 9	107
HD amaranth B *see* Amaranth	41
HD amaranth supra *see* Amaranth	41
HD carmoisine *see* Carmoisine	83
HD carmoisine supra *see* Carmoisine	83
HD sunset yellow FCF *see* Sunset yellow FCF	257
HD sunset yellow FCF supra *see* Sunset yellow FCF	257

Helianthin see *para*-Dimethylaminobenzenediazo sodium sulphonate	147
Helio red toner LCLL see D & C Red No. 9	107
Hexacert red No. 2 see Amaranth	41
Hexacol amaranth B extra see Amaranth	41
Hexacol carmoisine see Carmoisine	83
Hexacol carmoisine conc. see Carmoisine	83
Hexacol oil orange SS see Oil orange SS	165
Hexacol orange G see Orange G	181
Hexacol orange GG crystals see Orange G	181
Hexacol ponceau MX see Ponceau MX	189
Hexacol ponceau 2R see Ponceau MX	189
Hexacol ponceau SX see Ponceau SX	207
Hexacol sunset yellow F & F supra see Sunset yellow FCF	257
Hexacol sunset yellow FCF see Sunset yellow FCF	257
Hexacol sunset yellow FCF supra see Sunset yellow FCF	257
Hexacol sunset yellow FCP see Sunset yellow FCF	257
Hexatype brown N see Sudan brown RR	249
Hexatype carmine B see Sudan red 7B	253
Hidacid amaranth see Amaranth	41
Hidacid azo rubine see Carmoisine	83
Hidacid fast orange G see Orange G	181
Hidacid fast orange 2G see Orange G	181
Hidacid scarlet 2R see Ponceau MX	189
Hidaco oil orange see Sudan I	225
Hidaco oil red see Scarlet red	217
Hidaco oil yellow see *ortho*-Aminoazotoluene	61
Hispacet fast yellow G see C.I. Disperse Yellow 3	97
Hispacid fast orange 2G see Orange G	181
Hispacid orange 1 see Orange I	173
Hispacid ponceau R see Ponceau MX	189
Hispacid red AM see Amaranth	41
Hispacid rubine F see Carmoisine	83
Hispamin blue 3BX see Trypan blue	267
Hisperse yellow G see C.I. Disperse Yellow 3	97
Hydroxyazobenzene see 4-Hydroxyazobenzene	157

4-Hydroxyazobenzene	157
p-Hydroxyazobenzene see 4-Hydroxyazobenzene	157
4-Hydroxy-3,4'-azodi-1-naphthalenesulfonic acid, disodium salt see Carmoisine	83
4-Hydroxy-3,4'-azodi-1-naphthalenesulphonic acid, disodium salt see Carmoisine	83
2-Hydroxy-1,1'-azonaphthalene-3,6,4'-trisulfonic acid, trisodium salt see Amaranth	41
2-Hydroxy-1,1'-azonaphthalene-3,6,4'-trisulphonic acid, trisodium salt see Amaranth	41
N-{4-[(2-Hydroxy-5-methylphenyl)azo]phenyl}acetamide see C.I. Disperse Yellow 3	97
4-[(4-Hydroxy-1-naphthalenyl)azo]benzenesulfonic acid, monosodium salt see Orange I	173
4-[(4-Hydroxy-1-naphthalenyl)azo]benzenesulphonic acid, monosodium salt see Orange I	173
p-[(4-Hydroxy-1-naphthyl)azo]benzenesulfonic acid, monosodium salt see Orange I	173
p-[(4-Hydroxy-1-naphthyl)azo]benzenesulfonic acid, sodium salt see Orange I	173
p-[(4-Hydroxy-1-naphthyl)azo]benzenesulphonic acid, monosodium salt see Orange I	173
p-[(4-Hydroxy-1-naphthyl)azo]benzenesulphonic acid, sodium salt see Orange I	173
7-Hydroxy-8-(phenylazo)-1,3-naphthalenedisulfonic acid, disodium salt see Orange G	181
7-Hydroxy-8-(phenylazo)-1,3-naphthalenedisulphonic acid, disodium salt see Orange G	181
3-Hydroxy-4-[(4-sulfo-1-naphthalenyl)azo]-2,7-naphthalenedisulfonic acid, trisodium salt see Amaranth	41
4-Hydroxy-3-[(4-sulfo-1-naphthalenyl)azo]-1-naphthalenesulfonic acid, disodium salt see Carmoisine	83
3-Hydroxy-4-[(4-sulfo-1-naphthyl)azo]-2,7-naphthalenedisulfonic acid, trisodium salt see Amaranth	41
6-Hydroxy-5-[(4-sulfophenyl)azo]-2-naphthalenesulfonic acid, disodium salt see Sunset yellow FCF	257
6-Hydroxy-5-[(*p*-sulfophenyl)azo]-2-naphthalenesulfonic acid, disodium salt see Sunset yellow FCF	257
4-Hydroxy-3-[(5-sulfo-2,4-xylyl)azo]-1-naphthalenesulfonic acid, disodium salt see Ponceau SX	207
3-Hydroxy-4-[(4-sulpho-1-naphthalenyl)azo]-2,7-naphthalenedisulphonic acid, trisodium salt see Amaranth	41

4-Hydroxy-3-[(4-sulpho-1-naphthalenyl)azo]-1-naphthalene-sulphonic acid, disodium salt *see* Carmoisine	83
3-Hydroxy-4-[(4-sulpho-1-naphthyl)azo]-2,7-naphthalenedisulphonic acid, trisodium salt *see* Amaranth	41
6-Hydroxy-5-[(4-sulphophenyl)azo]-2-naphthalenesulphonic acid, disodium salt *see* Sunset yellow FCF	257
6-Hydroxy-5-[(*p*-sulphophenyl)azo]-2-naphthalenesulphonic acid, disodium salt *see* Sunset yellow FCF	257
4-Hydroxy-3-[(5-sulpho-2,4-xylyl)azo]-1-naphthalenesulphonic acid, disodium salt *see* Ponceau SX	207
4'-[(6-Hydroxy-*m*-tolyl)azo]acetanilide *see* C.I. Disperse Yellow 3	97
3-Hydroxy-4-[(2,4,5-trimethylphenyl)azo]-2,7-naphthalenedisulfonic acid, disodium salt *see* Ponceau 3R	199
3-Hydroxy-4-[(2,4,5-trimethylphenyl)azo]-2,7-naphthalenedisulphonic acid, disodium salt *see* Ponceau 3R	199
3-Hydroxy-4-(2,4-xylylazo)-3,7-naphthalenedisulfonic acid, disodium salt *see* Ponceau MX	189
3-Hydroxy-4-(2,4-xylylazo)-3,7-naphthalenedisulphonic acid, disodium salt *see* Ponceau MX	189

I

Induline R *see para*-Aminoazobenzene	53
Ink orange JSN *see* Orange G	181
Interchem acetate yellow G *see* C.I. Disperse Yellow 3	97
Interchem hisperse yellow GH *see* C.I. Disperse Yellow 3	97
Intracid fast orange G *see* Orange G	181
Intrasperse yellow GBA *see* C.I. Disperse Yellow 3	97
Irgalite red CBN *see* D & C Red No. 9	107
Irgalite red CBR *see* D & C Red No. 9	107
Irgalite red CBT *see* D & C Red No. 9	107
Irgalite red MBC *see* D & C Red No. 9	107
Isol lake red LCS 12527 *see* D & C Red No. 9	107
Isol red LCR 2517 *see* D & C Red No. 9	107

J

Jaune AB *see* Yellow AB	279
Jaune OB *see* Yellow OB	287

Java amaranth *see* Amaranth	41
Java orange I *see* Orange I	173
Java orange 2G *see* Orange G	181
Java ponceau 2R *see* Ponceau MX	189
Java rubine N *see* Carmoisine	83

K

Karmesin *see* Carmoisine	83
Kayaku amaranth *see* Amaranth	41
Kayaku food colour red No. 2 *see* Amaranth	41
Kayalon fast yellow G *see* C.I. Disperse Yellow 3	97
KCA acetate fast yellow G *see* C.I. Disperse Yellow 3	97
KCA foodcol amaranth A *see* Amaranth	41
KCA foodcol sunset yellow FCF *see* Sunset yellow FCF	257
Kenachrome blue 2R *see* Carmoisine	83
Kiton crimson 2R *see* Carmoisine	83
Kiton fast orange G *see* Orange G	181
Kiton ponceau R *see* Ponceau MX	189
Kiton ponceau 2R *see* Ponceau MX	189
Kiton rubine R *see* Carmoisine	83
Kiton rubine S *see* Amaranth	41
Kiton scarlet 2RC *see* Ponceau MX	189

L

Lacquer orange V *see* Oil orange SS	165
Lacquer orange VG *see* Sudan I	225
Lacquer orange VR *see* Sudan II	233
Lacquer red V *see* Scarlet red	217
Lacquer red V3B *see* Sudan red 7B	253
Lacquer red VS *see* Scarlet red	217
Lake ponceau *see* Ponceau MX	189
Lake red 1520 *see* D & C Red No. 9	107
Lake red C *see* D & C Red No. 9	107
Lake red C 18287 *see* D & C Red No. 9	107
Lake red C 18958 *see* D & C Red No. 9	107

Lake red C 21245 *see* D & C Red No. 9	107
Lake red C 27200 *see* D & C Red No. 9	107
Lake red C 27217 *see* D & C Red No. 9	107
Lake red C 27218 *see* D & C Red No. 9	107
Lake red C barium toner *see* D & C Red No. 9	107
Lake red CC *see* D & C Red No. 9	107
Lake red CCT *see* D & C Red No. 9	107
Lake red CR *see* D & C Red No. 9	107
Lake red CRLC-232 (barium) *see* D & C Red No. 9	107
Lake red C toner 8195 *see* D & C Red No. 9	107
Lake red C toner 8366 *see* D & C Red No. 9	107
Lake red GB barium salt *see* D & C Red No. 9	107
Lake red RRG *see* D & C Red No. 9	107
Lake red toner C *see* D & C Red No. 9	107
Lake red toner LCLL *see* D & C Red No. 9	107
Lake scarlet R *see* Ponceau MX	189
Lake scarlet 2RBN *see* Ponceau MX	189
Latexol scarlet R *see* D & C Red No. 9	107
Latexol scarlet R solupowder *see* D & C Red No. 9	107
LD rubber red 16913 *see* D & C Red No. 9	107
Leather orange GG *see* Orange G	181
Leather orange HR *see* Chrysoidine	91
Lighthouse chrome blue 2R *see* Carmoisine	83
Light orange G *see* Orange G	181
Lipid crimson *see* Scarlet red	217
Lissamine amaranth AC *see* Amaranth	41
Lithofor brown A *see* Sudan brown RR	249
L-orange 2 *see* Sunset yellow FCF	257
L. orange Z2010 *see* Sunset yellow FCF	257
L-red 3 *see* Amaranth	41
L. red Z 3040 *see* Carmoisine	83
Lutetia red CLN *see* D & C Red No. 9	107
Lutetia red CLN-ST *see* D & C Red No. 9	107

M

Mallophene *see* 2,6-Diamino-3-(phenylazo)pyridine (hydrochloride)	117
Maple amaranth *see* Amaranth	41
Maple ponceau 3R *see* Ponceau 3R	199
Maple ponceau SX *see* Ponceau SX	207
Maple sunset yellow FCF *see* Sunset yellow FCF	257
2-Methyl-4-[(2-methylphenyl)azo]benzenamine *see* ortho-Aminoazotoluene	61
1-{{2-Methyl-4-[(2-methylphenyl)azo]phenyl}azo}-2-naphthalene *see* Scarlet red	217
1-{{2-Methyl-4-[(2-methylphenyl)azo]phenyl}azo}-2-naphthalenol *see* Scarlet red	217
Methyl orange *see* para-Dimethylaminobenzenediazo sodium sulphonate	147
1-(2-Methylphenyl)azo-2-naphthalenamine *see* Yellow OB	287
1-[(2-Methylphenyl)azo]-2-naphthalenamine *see* Yellow OB	287
1-[(2-Methylphenyl)azo]-2-naphthalenol *see* Oil orange SS	165
1-(2-Methylphenyl)azo-2-naphthylamine *see* Yellow OB	287
Methyl red	161
Methyl yellow *see* para-Dimethylaminoazobenzene	125
Microsetile yellow GR *see* C.I. Disperse Yellow 3	97
Microtex lake red CR *see* D & C Red No. 9	107
Miketon fast yellow G *see* C.I. Disperse Yellow 3	97
Mohican red A-8008 *see* D & C Red No. 9	107
Motiorange R *see* Sudan I	225
Motirot G *see* Sudan II	233
Motirot 2R *see* Sudan III	241

N

Nacarat *see* Carmoisine	83
Nacarat A-CE *see* Carmoisine	83
Nacarat A export *see* Carmoisine	83
Nacarat extra pure A *see* Carmoisine	83
Nacelan fast yellow CG *see* C.I. Disperse Yellow 3	97
Nankai acid orange I *see* Orange I	173
Naphtamine blue 2B *see* Trypan blue	267
Naphtamine blue 3BX *see* Trypan blue	267

1-Naphthalenazo-2',4'-diaminobenzene see Sudan brown RR	249
Naphthalene fast orange 2G see Orange G	181
Naphthalene fast orange 2GS see Orange G	181
Naphthalene lake scarlet R see Ponceau MX	189
Naphthalene orange I see Orange I	173
Naphthalene scarlet R see Ponceau MX	189
2-Naphthalenesulfonic acid, 6-hydroxy-5-, disodium salt see Sunset yellow FCF	257
2-Naphthalenesulphonic acid, 6-hydroxy-5-, disodium salt see Sunset yellow FCF	257
4-(1-Naphthalenylazo)-1,3-phenylenediamine see Sudan brown RR	249
Naphthaminblau 3BX see Trypan blue	267
Naphthamine blue 3BX see Trypan blue	267
Naphthazine scarlet 2R see Ponceau MX	189
Naphthol orange see Orange I	173
α-Naphthol orange see Orange I	173
Naphthol red B see Amaranth	41
Naphthol red C see Amaranth	41
Naphthol red LZS see Amaranth	41
Naphthol red O see Amaranth	41
Naphthol red S see Amaranth	41
Naphthol red S conc. specially pure see Amaranth	41
Naphthol red SI see Amaranth	41
Naphthol red S specially pure see Amaranth	41
Naphthylamine blue see Trypan blue	267
4-(1-Naphthylazo)-m-phenylenediamine see Sudan brown RR	249
4-(1-Naphthylazo-m-phenylenediamine) see Sudan brown RR	249
NC 150 see 2,6-Diamino-3-(phenylazo)pyridine (hydrochloride)	117
Neklacid azorubine W see Carmoisine	83
Neklacid fast light orange GG see Orange G	181
Neklacid fast orange 2G see Orange G	181
Neklacid orange 1 see Orange I	173
Neklacid red A see Amaranth	41
Neklacid red RR see Ponceau MX	189
Neklacid rubine W see Carmoisine	83

New ponceau 4R *see* Ponceau MX	189
Niagara blue *see* Trypan blue	267
Niagara blue 3B *see* Trypan blue	267
Nippon Kagaku chrysoidine *see* Chrysoidine	91
No. 3 conc. bronze scarlet *see* D & C Red No. 9	107
No. 3 conc. scarlet *see* D & C Red No. 9	107
Novalon yellow 2GN *see* C.I. Disperse Yellow 3	97
Nylomine acid red P4B *see* Carmoisine	83
Nyloquinone light yellow 4JL *see* C.I. Disperse Yellow 3	97
Nyloquinone yellow 4J *see* C.I. Disperse Yellow 3	97

O

OAAT *see* *ortho*-Aminoazotoluene	61
Oil orange *see* Sudan I	225
Oil orange 31 *see* Sudan I	225
Oil orange 2311 *see* Sudan I	225
Oil orange 2B *see* Sudan I	225
Oil orange E *see* Sudan I	225
Oil orange EP *see* Sudan I	225
Oil orange G *see* Sudan I	225
Oil orange KB *see* Sudan II	233
Oil orange N extra *see* Sudan II	233
Oil orange O'PEL *see* Oil orange SS	165
Oil orange OPEL *see* Oil orange SS	165
Oil orange PEL *see* Sudan I	225
Oil orange R *see* Sudan I	225
and see Sudan II	233
Oil orange 2R *see* Sudan II	233
Oil orange R-14 *see* Sudan I	225
Oil orange SS	165
Oil orange TX *see* Oil orange SS	165
Oil orange 7078-V *see* Sudan I	225
Oil orange X *see* Sudan II	233
Oil orange XO *see* Oil orange SS	165
and see Sudan II	233

Oil orange Z-7078 *see* Sudan I	225
Oil red *see* Sudan III	241
Oil red 3 *see* Scarlet red	217
Oil red IV *see* Scarlet red	217
Oil red 7 *see* Scarlet red	217
Oil red 47 *see* Scarlet red	217
Oil red 282 *see* Scarlet red	217
Oil red 6566 *see* Sudan III	241
Oil red A *see* Scarlet red	217
Oil red APT *see* Scarlet red	217
Oil red AS *see* Sudan III	241
Oil red B *see* Sudan III	241
Oil red 2B *see* Scarlet red	217
Oil red 3B *see* Scarlet red	217
and see Sudan III	241
Oil red 4B *see* Scarlet red	217
Oil red BB *see* Scarlet red	217
Oil red BS *see* Scarlet red	217
Oil red D *see* Scarlet red	217
Oil red ED *see* Scarlet red	217
Oil red F *see* Scarlet red	217
Oil red G *see* Sudan III	241
Oil red 3G *see* Sudan III	241
Oil red GO *see* Scarlet red	217
Oil red GRO *see* Sudan II	233
Oil red O *see* Sudan II	233
and see Sudan III	241
Oil red PEL *see* Scarlet red	217
Oil red RC *see* Scarlet red	217
Oil red RO *see* Sudan II	233
Oil red RR *see* Scarlet red	217
Oil red S *see* Scarlet red	217
Oil red TAX *see* Scarlet red	217
Oil red XO *see* Sudan II	233
Oil red ZD *see* Scarlet red	217

Oil scarlet *see* Scarlet red	217
and see Sudan II	233
and see Sudan III	241
Oil scarlet 48 *see* Scarlet red	217
Oil scarlet 371 *see* Sudan II	233
Oil scarlet APYO *see* Sudan II	233
Oil scarlet AS *see* Sudan III	241
Oil scarlet BL *see* Sudan II	233
Oil scarlet G *see* Sudan III	241
Oil scarlet 6G *see* Sudan II	233
Oil scarlet L *see* Sudan II	233
Oil scarlet Y *see* Sudan II	233
Oil scarlet YS *see* Sudan II	233
Oil-sol. aniline yellow *see para*-Aminoazobenzene	53
Oil violet *see* Sudan red 7B	253
Oil yellow *see ortho*-Aminoazotoluene	61
and see para-Dimethylaminoazobenzene	125
Oil yellow I *see ortho*-Aminoazotoluene	61
Oil yellow II *see para*-Dimethylaminoazobenzene	125
Oil yellow 20 *see para*-Dimethylaminoazobenzene	125
Oil yellow 21 *see ortho*-Aminoazotoluene	61
Oil yellow 2625 *see para*-Dimethylaminoazobenzene	125
Oil yellow 2681 *see ortho*-Aminoazotoluene	61
Oil yellow 7463 *see para*-Dimethylaminoazobenzene	125
Oil yellow A *see ortho*-Aminoazotoluene	61
and see Yellow AB	279
Oil yellow AAB *see para*-Aminoazobenzene	53
Oil yellow AB *see* Yellow AB	279
Oil yellow AB pure *see* Yellow AB	279
Oil yellow AN *see para*-Aminoazobenzene	53
Oil yellow AT *see ortho*-Aminoazotoluene	61
Oil yellow B *see para*-Aminoazobenzene	53
Oil yellow BB *see para*-Dimethylaminoazobenzene	125
Oil yellow C *see ortho*-Aminoazotoluene	61
Oil yellow D *see para*-Dimethylaminoazobenzene	125

Oil yellow DN *see para*-Dimethylaminoazobenzene	125
Oil yellow FF *see para*-Dimethylaminoazobenzene	125
Oil yellow FN *see para*-Dimethylaminoazobenzene	125
Oil yellow G *see para*-Dimethylaminoazobenzene	125
Oil yellow G-2 *see para*-Dimethylaminoazobenzene	125
Oil yellow 2G *see para*-Aminoazobenzene	53
and see para-Dimethylaminoazobenzene	125
Oil yellow GG *see para*-Dimethylaminoazobenzene	125
Oil yellow GR *see para*-Dimethylaminoazobenzene	125
Oil yellow N *see para*-Dimethylaminoazobenzene	125
Oil yellow OB *see* Yellow OB	287
Oil yellow OB pure *see* Yellow OB	287
Oil yellow PEL *see para*-Dimethylaminoazobenzene	125
Oil yellow R *see para*-Aminoazobenzene	53
Oil yellow 2R *see ortho*-Aminoazotoluene	61
Oil yellow T *see ortho*-Aminoazotoluene	61
Oleal orange R *see* Sudan I	225
Oleal orange SS *see* Oil orange SS	165
Oleal red BB *see* Scarlet red	217
Oleal yellow 2G *see para*-Dimethylaminoazobenzene	125
Omega chrome blue FB *see* Carmoisine	83
1333 Orange *see* Orange I	173
1370 Orange *see* Orange G	181
Orange I	173
Orange III *see para*-Dimethylaminobenzenediazo sodium sulphonate	147
Orange à l'huile *see* Sudan I	225
Orange BN *see* Oil orange SS	165
Orange BPC *see* Orange G	181
Orange I extra conc. A export *see* Orange I	173
Orange G	181
Orange 2G *see* Orange G	181
Orange G (biological stain) *see* Orange G	181
Orange G BPC *see* Orange G	181
Orange G dye *see* Orange G	181
Orange GG *see* Orange G	181

Orange G (indicator) *see* Orange G	181
Orange GMP *see* Orange G	181
Orange IM *see* Orange I	173
Orange 2 insoluble *see* Sudan I	225
Orange insoluble OLG *see* Sudan I	225
and see Sudan II	233
Orange insoluble RR *see* Sudan II	233
Orange oil KB *see* Sudan II	233
Orange OT *see* Oil orange SS	165
Orange PAL *see* Sunset yellow FCF	257
Orange PEL *see* Sudan I	225
Orange II R *see* Sunset yellow FCF	257
Orange 3R soluble in grease *see* Oil orange SS	165
Orange 3RA soluble in grease *see* Sudan I	225
Orange resénole No. 3 *see* Sudan I	225
Orange R fat soluble *see* Sudan I	225
Orange RGL conc. specially pure *see* Sunset yellow FCF	257
Orange RR *see* Sudan II	233
Orange S *see* Orange I	173
Orange I, sodium salt *see* Orange I	173
Orange soluble à l'huile *see* Sudan I	225
Orange SS *see* Oil orange SS	165
Orange yellow S *see* Sunset yellow FCF	257
Orange yellow S.AF *see* Sunset yellow FCF	257
Orange yellow S.FQ *see* Sunset yellow FCF	257
Organol bordeaux B *see* Sudan red 7B	253
Organol brown 2R *see* Sudan brown RR	249
Organol orange *see* Sudan I	225
Organol orange 2R *see* Oil orange SS	165
Organol 2R *see* Sudan brown RR	249
Organol red B *see* Scarlet red	217
Organol red BS *see* Sudan III	241
Organol scarlet *see* Sudan III	241
Organol yellow *see* *para*-Aminoazobenzene	53
Organol yellow 2A *see* *para*-Aminoazobenzene	53

Organol yellow ADM *see* *para*-Dimethylaminoazobenzene	125
Organol yellow AP *see* 4-Hydroxyazobenzene	157
Organol yellow 2T *see* *ortho*-Aminoazotoluene	61
Orient oil orange PS *see* Sudan I	225
Orient oil red RR *see* Scarlet red	217
Orient oil yellow GG *see* *para*-Dimethylaminoazobenzene	125
Orion blue 3B *see* Trypan blue	267
Ostacet yellow P2G *see* C.I. Disperse Yellow 3	97

P

Palacet yellow GN *see* C.I. Disperse Yellow 3	97
Palanil yellow G *see* C.I. Disperse Yellow 3	97
Pamacel yellow G-3 *see* C.I. Disperse Yellow 3	97
PAP *see* 2,6-Diamino-3-(phenylazo)pyridine (hydrochloride)	117
Paper red HRR *see* Ponceau MX	189
Paramine blue 3B *see* Trypan blue	267
Para orange *see* Sunset yellow FCF	257
Paraphenolazo aniline *see* *para*-Aminoazobenzene	53
Paridine red LCL *see* D & C Red No. 9	107
Parkibleu *see* Trypan blue	267
Parkipan *see* Trypan blue	267
Pellidol *see* Diacetylaminoazotoluene	113
Pellidole *see* Diacetylaminoazotoluene	113
Periphermin *see* Diacetylaminoazotoluene	113
Perliton yellow G *see* C.I. Disperse Yellow 3	97
Petrol orange Y *see* Sudan I	225
Petrol yellow WT *see* *para*-Dimethylaminoazobenzene	125
Phenazodine *see* 2,6-Diamino-3-(phenylazo)pyridine (hydrochloride)	117
Phenazopyridine *see* 2,6-Diamino-3-(phenylazo)pyridine	117
Phenoplaste organol red B *see* Scarlet red	217
p-(Phenylazo)aniline *see* *para*-Aminoazobenzene	53
4-(Phenylazo)benzenamine *see* *para*-Aminoazobenzene	53
4-(Phenylazo)-1,3-benzenediamine, monohydrochloride *see* Chrysoidine	91

3-Phenylazo-2,6-diaminopyridine, hydrochloride see 2,6-Diamino-3-(phenylazo)pyridine (hydrochloride)	117
β-Phenylazo-α,α'-diaminopyridine, hydrochloride see 2,6-Diamino-3-(phenylazo)pyridine (hydrochloride)	117
Phenylazo-α,α'-diaminopyridine, monohydrochloride see 2,6-Diamino-3-(phenylazo)pyridine (hydrochloride)	117
1-Phenylazo-2-naphthalenamine see Yellow AB	279
1-(Phenylazo)-2-naphthalenamine see Yellow AB	279
1-(Phenylazo)-2-naphthalenol see Sudan I	225
1-Phenylazo-2-naphthol see Sudan I	225
1-(Phenylazo)-2-naphthol see Sudan I	225
1-Phenylazo-β-naphthol see Sudan I	225
1-Phenylazo-2-naphthol-6,8-disulfonic acid, disodium salt see Orange G	181
1-Phenylazo-2-naphthol-6,8-disulphonic acid, disodium salt see Orange G	181
1-Phenylazo-2-naphthylamine see Yellow AB	279
1-(Phenylazo)-2-naphthylamine see Yellow AB	279
4-(Phenylazo)-phenol see 4-Hydroxyazobenzene	157
p-Phenylazophenol see 4-Hydroxyazobenzene	157
p-(Phenylazo)phenol see 4-Hydroxyazobenzene	157
p-Phenylazophenylamine see para-Aminoazobenzene	53
(Phenylazo-4-phenylazo)-1-ethylamino-2-naphthalene see Sudan red 7B	253
1-(4-Phenylazo-phenylazo)-2-ethylaminonaphthalene see Sudan red 7B	253
1-{[4-(Phenylazo)phenyl]azo}-2-naphthalenol see Sudan III	241
1-(p-Phenylazophenylazo)-2-naphthol see Sudan III	241
1-[(p-Phenylazo)phenyl]azo-2-naphthol see Sudan III	241
4-(Phenylazo)-m-phenylenediamine, hydrochloride see Chrysoidine	91
4-(Phenylazo)-m-phenylenediamine, monohydrochloride see Chrysoidine	91
3-(Phenylazo)-2,6-pyridinediamine see 2,6-Diamino-3-(phenylazo)-pyridine	117
3-(Phenylazo)-2,6-pyridinediamine, hydrochloride see 2,6-Diamino-3-(phenylazo)pyridine (hydrochloride)	117
Phenylazo tablet see 2,6-Diamino-3-(phenylazo)pyridine (hydrochloride)	117
Pigment lake red BFC see D & C Red No. 9	107

Pigment lake red CD *see* D & C Red No. 9	107
Pigment lake red LC *see* D & C Red No. 9	107
Pigment ponceau R *see* Ponceau MX	189
Pigment red CD *see* D & C Red No. 9	107
Pirid *see* 2,6-Diamino-3-(phenylazo)pyridine (hydrochloride)	117
Pirocard green 491 *see* 4-Hydroxyazobenzene	157
Plastoresin orange F4A *see* Sudan I	225
Plastoresin red F *see* Scarlet red	217
Poloxal red 2B *see* Carmoisine	83
Ponceau à l'huile *see* Sudan II	233
Ponceau BNA *see* Ponceau MX	189
Ponceau de xylidine *see* Ponceau MX	189
Ponceau FR *see* Ponceau MX	189
Ponceau G *see* Ponceau MX	189
Ponceau GR *see* Ponceau MX	189
Ponceau insoluble OLG *see* Sudan II	233
and see Sudan III	241
Ponceau J *see* Ponceau MX	189
Ponceau MX	189
Ponceau NR *see* Ponceau MX	189
Ponceau PXM *see* Ponceau MX	189
Ponceau R *see* Ponceau MX	189
Ponceau 2R *see* Ponceau MX	189
Ponceau 3R *see* Ponceau MX	189
and see Ponceau 3R	199
Ponceau 4R *see* Ponceau MX	189
Ponceau R (biological stain) *see* Ponceau MX	189
Ponceau 2R (biological stain) *see* Ponceau MX	189
Ponceau 2RE *see* Ponceau MX	189
Ponceau red *see* Ponceau MX	189
Ponceau red R *see* Ponceau MX	189
Ponceau 2R extra A export *see* Ponceau MX	189
Ponceau RG *see* Ponceau MX	189
Ponceau 2RL *see* Ponceau MX	189
Ponceau 3R lake *see* Ponceau 3R	199

Ponceau RN see Ponceau 3R	199
Ponceau 3RN see Ponceau 3R	199
Ponceau RR see Ponceau MX	189
Ponceau RR type 8019 see Ponceau MX	189
Ponceau RS see Ponceau MX	189
Ponceau 3R sodium salt see Ponceau 3R	199
Ponceau 2RX see Ponceau MX	189
Ponceau SX	207
Ponceau SX lake see Ponceau SX	207
Ponceau xylidine see Ponceau MX	189
Ponceau xylidine (biological stain) see Ponceau MX	189
Pontacyl rubine R see Carmoisine	83
Pontamine blue 3BX see Trypan blue	267
Potomac red see D & C Red No. 9	107
Pure chrysoidine YBH see Chrysoidine	91
Pure chrysoidine YD see Chrysoidine	91
Pyracryl orange Y see Chrysoidine	91
Pyrazofen see 2,6-Diamino-3-(phenylazo)pyridine (hydrochloride)	117
Pyrazol blue 3B see Trypan blue	267
Pyridacil see 2,6-Diamino-3-(phenylazo)pyridine (hydrochloride)	117
Pyridium see 2,6-Diamino-3-(phenylazo)pyridine (hydrochloride)	117
Pyripyridium see 2,6-Diamino-3-(phenylazo)pyridine (hydrochloride)	117
Pyronalorange see Sudan I	225
Pyronalrot B see Sudan III	241
Pyronalrot R see Sudan II	233
Pyrotropblau see Trypan blue	267

R

Rakuto amaranth see Amaranth	41
Raspberry red for jellies see Amaranth	41
Recolite red lake C see D & C Red No. 9	107
Recolite red lake CR see D & C Red No. 9	107
1302 Red see Amaranth	41
1306 Red see Ponceau SX	207
1508 Red see Amaranth	41

1695 Red	*see* Ponceau MX	189
1860 Red	*see* D & C Red No. 9	107
Red 1860	*see* D & C Red No. 9	107
Red 11938	*see* D & C Red No. 9	107
11954 Red	*see* Carmoisine	83
11959 Red	*see* Carmoisine	83
12101 Red	*see* Ponceau SX	207
111440 Red	*see* Sudan III	241
Red B	*see* Sudan II	233
Red for lake C	*see* D & C Red No. 9	107
Red for lake C toner RA-5190	*see* D & C Red No. 9	107
Red for lakes J	*see* Ponceau MX	189
Red for lake toner RA-5190	*see* D & C Red No. 9	107
Red 16913H	*see* D & C Red No. 9	107
Red lake CM 20-5650	*see* D & C Red No. 9	107
Red lake CR-1	*see* D & C Red No. 9	107
Red lake C toner	*see* D & C Red No. 9	107
Red lake C toner 20-5650	*see* D & C Red No. 9	107
Red lake C toner RA-5190	*see* D & C Red No. 9	107
Red lake 89865N	*see* Ponceau SX	207
Red lake R-91	*see* D & C Red No. 9	107
Red No. 1	*see* Ponceau SX	207
Red No. 2	*see* Amaranth	41
Red No. 4	*see* Ponceau SX	207
Red No. 5	*see* Sudan II	233
Red R	*see* Ponceau MX	189
Red 3R soluble in grease	*see* Scarlet red	217
Red scarlet	*see* D & C Red No. 9	107
Red toner Z	*see* D & C Red No. 9	107
Red Zh	*see* Sudan III	241
Reliton yellow C	*see* C.I. Disperse Yellow 3	97
Renolblau 3B	*see* Trypan blue	267
Resinol brown RRN	*see* Sudan brown RR	249
Resinol orange R	*see* Sudan I	225
Resinol yellow GR	*see para*-Dimethylaminoazobenzene	125

Resinol red 2B *see* Scarlet red	217
Resinol RRN *see* Sudan brown RR	249
Resin scarlet 2R *see* Sudan II	233
Resoform orange G *see* Sudan I	225
Resoform orange R *see* Sudan II	233
Resoform red G *see* Scarlet red	217
Resoform yellow GGA *see* para-Dimethylaminoazobenzene	125
Rot B *see* Sudan II	233
Rot C *see* Sudan III	241
Rot G *see* Sudan III	241
Rot GG fettlöslich *see* Sudan II	233
Rouge cérasine *see* Sudan III	241
Rubber red 16913R *see* D & C Red No. 9	107
Rubrum scarlatinum *see* Scarlet red	217

S

Safaritone yellow G *see* C.I. Disperse Yellow 3	97
Samaron yellow PA3 *see* C.I. Disperse Yellow 3	97
San-ei amaranth *see* Amaranth	41
Sansei orange G *see* Sudan I	225
Sanyo lake red C *see* D & C Red No. 9	107
S-azo rubine *see* Amaranth	41
Scarlet B fat soluble *see* Sudan III	241
Scarlet R *see* Ponceau MX	189
and *see* Scarlet red	217
Scarlet 2R *see* Ponceau MX	189
Scarlet 2RB *see* Ponceau MX	189
Scarlet red	217
Scarlet red, Biebrich *see* Scarlet red	217
Scarlet 2RL *see* Ponceau MX	189
Scarlet 2RL bluish *see* Ponceau MX	189
Scarlet R (michaelis) *see* Scarlet red	217
Scarlet RRA *see* Ponceau MX	189
Scarlet toner Y *see* D & C Red No. 9	107
Scharlach B *see* Sudan I	225

Scharlachrot see Scarlet red	217
Sedural see 2,6-Diamino-3-(phenylazo)pyridine (hydrochloride)	117
Segnale red LC see D & C Red No. 9	107
Segnale red LCG see D & C Red No. 9	107
Segnale red LCL see D & C Red No. 9	107
Serinyl hosiery yellow GD see C.I. Disperse Yellow 3	97
Serisol fast yellow GD see C.I. Disperse Yellow 3	97
Setacyl yellow G see C.I. Disperse Yellow 3	97
Setacyl yellow 2GN see C.I. Disperse Yellow 3	97
Setacyl yellow P-2GL see C.I. Disperse Yellow 3	97
Shikiso amaranth see Amaranth	41
Sico lake red 2L see D & C Red No. 9	107
Silotras brown TRN see Sudan brown RR	249
Silotras orange TR see Sudan I	225
Silotras red T3B see Scarlet red	217
Silotras scarlet TB see Sudan III	241
Silotras yellow T2G see para-Dimethylaminoazobenzene	125
Silotras yellow TSG see C.I. Disperse Yellow 3	97
Sodium azo-α-naphtholsulfanilate see Orange I	173
Sodium azo-α-naphtholsulphanilate see Orange I	173
Sodium cumeneazo-β-naphthol disulfonate see Ponceau 3R	199
Sodium cumeneazo-β-naphthol disulphonate see Ponceau 3R	199
Sodium 4-(dimethylamino)benzenediazosulfonate see para-Dimethyl-aminobenzenediazo sodium sulphonate	147
Sodium p-(dimethylamino)benzenediazosulfonate see para-Dimethyl-aminobenzenediazo sodium sulphonate	147
Sodium 4-(dimethylamino)benzenediazosulphonate see para-Dimethyl-aminobenzenediazo sodium sulphonate	147
Sodium p-(dimethylamino)benzenediazosulphonate see para-Dimethyl-aminobenzenediazo sodium sulphonate	147
Sodium ditolyldisazobis-8-amino-1-naphthol-3,6-disulfonate see Trypan blue	267
Sodium ditolyldisazobis-8-amino-1-naphthol-3,6-disulphonate see Trypan blue	267
Solar light orange GX see Orange G	181
Solar red O see Amaranth	41
Solar rubine see Carmoisine	83

Solochrome blue FB *see* Carmoisine	83
Solvent yellow 14 *see* Sudan I	225
Somalia orange I *see* Sudan I	225
Somalia orange A2R *see* Sudan II	233
Somalia orange 2R *see* Sudan II	233
Somalia red III *see* Sudan III	241
Somalia red IV *see* Scarlet red	217
Somalia yellow A *see* *para*-Dimethylaminoazobenzene	125
Somalia yellow 2G *see* *para*-Aminoazobenzene	53
Somalia yellow R *see* *ortho*-Aminoazotoluene	61
Soudan I *see* Sudan I	225
Soudan II *see* Sudan II	233
Soudan III *see* Sudan III	241
Spiritorange *see* Sudan I	225
Spirit orange *see* Sudan I	225
Spirit yellow I *see* Sudan I	225
Standacol carmoisine *see* Carmoisine	83
Standacol orange G *see* Orange G	181
Standacol sunset yellow FCF *see* Sunset yellow FCF	257
Stéarix brown 4R *see* *para*-Aminoazobenzene	53
Stéarix orange *see* Sudan I	225
Stéarix red 4B *see* Scarlet red	217
Stéarix red 4S *see* Scarlet red	217
Stéarix scarlet *see* Sudan III	241
Stéar yellow JB *see* *para*-Dimethylaminoazobenzene	125
Straight orange G *see* Orange G	181
Sudan I	225
Sudan II	233
Sudan III	241
Sudan IV *see* Scarlet red	217
Sudan AX *see* Sudan II	233
Sudan brown RR	249
Sudan brown YR *see* Sudan brown RR	249
Sudan G *see* Sudan III	241
Sudan G III *see* Sudan III	241

Sudan III (G) see Sudan III	241
Sudan J see Sudan I	225
Sudan orange see Sudan II	233
Sudan orange R see Sudan I	225
Sudan orange RA see Sudan I	225
Sudan orange RA new see Sudan I	225
Sudan orange RPA see Sudan II	233
Sudan orange RR see Sudan II	233
Sudan orange RRA see Sudan II	233
Sudan P see Scarlet red	217
Sudan P III see Sudan III	241
Sudan red see Sudan II	233
Sudan red III see Sudan III	241
Sudan red IV see Scarlet red	217
Sudan red 7B	253
Sudan red 4BA see Scarlet red	217
Sudan red BB see Scarlet red	217
Sudan red BBA see Scarlet red	217
Sudanrot 7B see Sudan red 7B	253
Sudan scarlet 6G see Sudan II	233
Sudan X see Sudan II	233
Sudan yellow see para-Dimethylaminoazobenzene	125
and see Sudan I	225
and see Sudan III	241
Sudan yellow GG see para-Dimethylaminoazobenzene	125
Sudan yellow GGA see para-Dimethylaminoazobenzene	125
Sudan yellow R see para-Aminoazobenzene	53
Sudan yellow RA see para-Aminoazobenzene	53
Sudan yellow RRA see ortho-Aminoazotoluene	61
Sugai chrysoidine see Chrysoidine	91
Sulfacid light orange J see Orange G	181
1-(4-Sulfo-1-naphthylazo)-2-naphthol-3,6-disulfonic acid, trisodium salt see Amaranth	41
2-(4-Sulfo-1-naphthylazo)-1-naphthol-4-sulfonic acid, disodium salt see Carmoisine	83

1-*p*-Sulfophenylazo-2-hydroxynaphthalene-6-sulfonate, disodium salt *see* Sunset yellow FCF	257
4-*p*-Sulfophenylazo-1-naphthol, monosodium salt *see* Orange I	173
1-*p*-Sulfophenylazo-2-naphthol-6-sulfonic acid, disodium salt *see* Sunset yellow FCF	257
2-(6-Sulfo-2,4-xylylazo)-1-naphthol-4-sulfonic acid, disodium salt *see* Ponceau SX	207
1-(4-Sulpho-1-naphthylazo)-2-naphthol-3,6-disulphonic acid, trisodium salt *see* Amaranth	41
2-(4-Sulpho-1-naphthylazo)-1-naphthol-4-sulphonic acid, disodium salt *see* Carmoisine	83
1-*p*-Sulphophenylazo-2-hydroxynaphthalene-6-sulphonate, disodium salt *see* Sunset yellow FCF	257
4-*p*-Sulphophenylazo-1-naphthol, monosodium salt *see* Orange I	173
1-*p*-Sulphophenylazo-2-naphthol-6-sulphonic acid, disodium salt *see* Sunset yellow FCF	257
2-(6-Sulpho-2,4-xylylazo)-1-naphthol-4-sulphonic acid, disodium salt *see* Ponceau SX	207
Sun orange A Geigy *see* Sunset yellow FCF	257
Sunset yellow *see* Sunset yellow FCF	257
Sunset yellow BSS *see* Sunset yellow FCF	257
Sunset yellow FCF	257
Sunset yellow FCF supra *see* Sunset yellow FCF	257
Sunset yellow FU *see* Sunset yellow FCF	257
Sunset yellow FU supra *see* Sunset yellow FCF	257
Sunset yellow lake *see* Sunset yellow FCF	257
Sun yellow *see* Sunset yellow FCF	257
Sun yellow A-CE *see* Sunset yellow FCF	257
Sun yellow A-FDC *see* Sunset yellow FCF	257
Sun yellow extra conc. A export *see* Sunset yellow FCF	257
Sun yellow extra pure A *see* Sunset yellow FCF	257
Sun yellow FCF *see* Sunset yellow FCF	257
Superol red C RT-265 *see* D & C Red No. 9	107
Supracet fast yellow G *see* C.I. Disperse Yellow 3	97
Symuler lake red C *see* D & C Red No. 9	107
Synten yellow 2G *see* C.I. Disperse Yellow 3	97
Synton yellow 2G *see* C.I. Disperse Yellow 3	97

T

T 1824 *see* Evans blue	151
Takaoka amaranth *see* Amaranth	41
Terasil yellow GBA extra *see* C.I. Disperse Yellow 3	97
Terasil yellow 2GC *see* C.I. Disperse Yellow 3	97
Termosolido red LCG *see* D & C Red No. 9	107
Tertracid light orange G *see* Orange G	181
Tertracid orange I *see* Orange I	173
Tertracid ponceau 2R *see* Ponceau MX	189
Tertracid red A *see* Amaranth	41
Tertracid red CA *see* Carmoisine	83
Tertranese yellow N-2GL *see* C.I. Disperse Yellow 3	97
Tertrochrome blue FB *see* Carmoisine	83
Tertrogas red N *see* Scarlet red	217
Tertrogras orange SV *see* Sudan I	225
Tertrophene brown CG *see* Chrysoidine	91
Tetrasodium-2,2'-[(3,3'-dimethyl-4,4'-biphenylylene)bis(azo)]-bis(5-amino-4-hydroxy-3,6-naphthalenedisulfonate) *see* Trypan blue	267
Tetrasodium-3,3'-[(3,3'-dimethyl-4,4'-biphenylylene)bis(azo)]-bis(5-amino-4-hydroxy-2,7-naphthalenedisulfonate) *see* Trypan blue	267
Tetrasodium-6,6'-[(3,3'-dimethyl-4,4'-biphenylylene)bis(azo)]-bis(4-amino-5-hydroxy-1,3-naphthalenedisulfonate) *see* Evans blue	151
Tetrasodium-2,2'-[(3,3'-dimethyl-4,4'-biphenylylene)bis(azo)]-bis(5-amino-4-hydroxy-3,6-naphthalenedisulphonate) *see* Trypan blue	267
Tetrasodium-3,3'-[(3,3'-dimethyl-4,4'-biphenylylene)bis(azo)]-bis(5-amino-4-hydroxy-2,7-naphthalenedisulphonate) *see* Trypan blue	267
Tetrasodium-6,6'-[(3,3'-dimethyl-4,4'-biphenylylene)bis(azo)]-bis(4-amino-5-hydroxy-1,3-naphthalenedisulphonate) *see* Evans blue	151
Tetrasodium-2,2'-(3,3'-dimethyl-4,4'-biphenylylene)bis(azo)-bis(8-amino-1-naphthol-5,7-disulfonate) *see* Evans blue	151
Tetrasodium-2,2'-(3,3'-dimethyl-4,4'-biphenylylene)bis(azo)-bis(8-amino-1-naphthol-5,7-disulphonate) *see* Evans blue	151
Tetrazobenzene-β-naphthol *see* Sudan III	241
Texan red toner D *see* D & C Red No. 9	107

Toluazotoluidine *see* *ortho*-Aminoazotoluene	61
Toluene-2-azonaphthol-2 *see* Oil orange SS	165
o-Toluene-1-azo-2-naphthylamine *see* Yellow OB	287
o-Tolueneazo-*o*-tolueneazo-β-naphthol *see* Scarlet red	217
o-Tolueneazo-*o*-toluene-β-naphthol *see* Scarlet red	217
o-Tolueneazo-*o*-toluidine *see* *ortho*-Aminoazotoluene	61
5-(*o*-Tolylazo)-2-aminotoluene *see* *ortho*-Aminoazotoluene	61
4-*o*-Tolylazo-*o*-diacetotoluide *see* Diacetylaminoazotoluene	113
4'-(*o*-Tolylazo)-*o*-diacetotoluidide *see* Diacetylaminoazotoluene	113
1-*o*-Tolylazo-2-naphthol *see* Oil orange SS	165
1-(*o*-Tolylazo)-β-naphthol *see* Oil orange SS	165
1-*o*-Tolylazo-2-naphthylamine *see* Yellow OB	287
1-(*o*-Tolylazo)-2-naphthylamine *see* Yellow OB	287
4-*o*-Tolylazo-*o*-toluidine *see* *ortho*-Aminoazotoluene	61
4-(*o*-Tolylazo)-*o*-toluidine *see* *ortho*-Aminoazotoluene	61
1-[4-(*o*-Tolylazo)-*o*-tolylazo]-2-naphthol *see* Scarlet red	217
1-{[4-(*o*-Tolylazo)-*o*-tolyl]azo}-2-naphthol *see* Scarlet red	217
o-Tolylazo-*o*-tolylazo-2-naphthol *see* Scarlet red	217
o-Tolylazo-*o*-tolylazo-β-naphthol *see* Scarlet red	217
Toner lake red C *see* D & C Red No. 9	107
Toney red *see* Sudan III	241
Tony red *see* Sudan III	241
Toyo amaranth *see* Amaranth	41
Toyo oil orange *see* Sudan I	225
Toyo oil red BB *see* Scarlet red	217
Toyo oil yellow G *see* *para*-Dimethylaminoazobenzene	125
Transparent bronze scarlet *see* D & C Red No. 9	107
Trianol direct blue 3B *see* Trypan blue	267
Triazolblau 3BX *see* Trypan blue	267
Tripan blue *see* Trypan blue	267
Trisodium salt of 1-(4-sulfo-1-naphthylazo)-2-naphthol-3,6-disulfonic acid *see* Amaranth	41
Trisodium salt of 1-(4-sulpho-1-naphthylazo)-2-naphthol-3,6-disulphonic acid *see* Amaranth	41
Tropaeolin 1 *see* Orange I	173

Tropaeolin D *see para*-Dimethylaminobenzenediazo sodium sulphonate	147
Tropaeolin G *see* Orange I	173
Tropaeolin OOO No. 1 *see* Orange I	173
Trypanblau *see* Trypan blue	267
Trypan blue	267
Trypan blue BPC *see* Trypan blue	267
Trypan blue sodium salt *see* Trypan blue	267
Trypane blue *see* Trypan blue	267
Tulabase fast garnet GB *see ortho*-Aminoazotoluene	61
Tulabase fast garnet GBC *see ortho*-Aminoazotoluene	61
Tuladisperse fast yellow 2G *see* C.I. Disperse Yellow 3	97
Typogen brown N *see* Sudan brown RR	249
Typogen carmine *see* Sudan red 7B	253

U

Unitertracid light orange G *see* Orange G	181
Uridinal *see* 2,6-Diamino-3-(phenylazo)pyridine (hydrochloride)	117
Urodine *see* 2,6-Diamino-3-(phenylazo)pyridine (hydrochloride)	117
Usacert FD & C red No. 4 *see* Ponceau SX	207
Usacert FD & C yellow No. 6 *see* Sunset yellow FCF	257
Usacert red No. 1 *see* Ponceau 3R	199
Usacert red No. 2 *see* Amaranth	41
Usacert red No. 4 *see* Ponceau SX	207
Usacert yellow No. 6 *see* Sunset yellow FCF	257
Usalake FD & C yellow No. 6 lake *see* Sunset yellow FCF	257

V

Victoria rubine O *see* Amaranth	41
Victoria rubine O for food *see* Amaranth	41
Vondacid light orange 2G *see* Orange G	181
Vonteryl yellow G *see* C.I. Disperse Yellow 3	97
Vonteryl yellow R *see* C.I. Disperse Yellow 3	97
Vulcafix scarlet R *see* D & C Red No. 9	107
Vulcafix scarlet R-D Masse *see* D & C Red No. 9	107
Vulcafor red 2R *see* D & C Red No. 9	107

Vulcan red LC *see* D & C Red No. 9	107
Vulcol fast red L *see* D & C Red No. 9	107

W

W 1655 *see* 2,6-Diamino-3-(phenylazo)pyridine (hydrochloride)	117
Waxakol orange GL *see* Sudan I	225
Waxakol red BL *see* Scarlet red	217
Waxakol vermilion L *see* Sudan II	233
Waxakol yellow NL *see* *ortho*-Aminoazotoluene	61
Waxoline red O *see* Scarlet red	217
Waxoline red OM *see* Scarlet red	217
Waxoline red OS *see* Scarlet red	217
Waxoline yellow AD *see* *para*-Dimethylaminoazobenzene	125
Waxoline yellow ADS *see* *para*-Dimethylaminoazobenzene	125
Waxoline yellow I *see* Sudan I	225
Waxoline yellow IM *see* Sudan I	225
Waxoline yellow IP *see* Sudan I	225
Waxoline yellow IS *see* Sudan I	225
Wayne red X-2486 *see* D & C Red No. 9	107
Whortleberry red *see* Amaranth	41
Wool bordeaux 6RK *see* Amaranth	41
Wool orange G *see* Orange G	181
Wool orange 2G *see* Orange G	181
Wool red *see* Amaranth	41
Wool red 40F *see* Amaranth	41

X

Xylene fast orange G *see* Orange G	181
Xylidine ponceau *see* Ponceau MX	189
Xylidine ponceau 3RS *see* Ponceau MX	189
Xylidine red *see* Ponceau MX	189
1-Xylylazo-2-naphthol *see* Sudan II	233
1-(2,4-Xylylazo)-2-naphthol *see* Sudan II	233
1-(*o*-Xylylazo)-2-naphthol *see* Sudan II	233

1-(2,4-Xylylazo)-2-naphthol-3,6-disulfonic acid, disodium salt *see* Ponceau MX	189
1-Xylylazo-2-naphthol-3,6-disulfonic acid, disodium salt *see* Ponceau MX	189
1-(2,4-Xylylazo)-2-naphthol-3,6-disulphonic acid, disodium salt *see* Ponceau MX	189
1-Xylylazo-2-naphthol-3,6-disulphonic acid, disodium salt *see* Ponceau MX	189

Y

1351 Yellow *see* Sunset yellow FCF	257
1899 Yellow *see* Sunset yellow FCF	257
Yellow AB	279
Yellow OB	287
Yellow G soluble in grease *see para*-Dimethylaminoazobenzene	125
Yellow No. 2 *see* Yellow AB	279
Yellow No. 6 *see* Sunset yellow FCF	257
Yellow orange S *see* Sunset yellow FCF	257
Yellow orange S specially pure *see* Sunset yellow FCF	257
Yellow orange specially pure 85 *see* Sunset yellow FCF	257
Yellow Reliton G *see* C.I. Disperse Yellow 3	97
Yellow SF for food *see* Sunset yellow FCF	257
Yellow sun *see* Sunset yellow FCF	257
Yellow SY for food *see* Sunset yellow FCF	257
Yellow Z *see* C.I. Disperse Yellow 3	97

SUPPLEMENTARY CORRIGENDA TO VOLUMES 1 - 7

A corrigenda covering Volumes 1 - 6 appeared in Volume 7. The present one covers further errors which have since been brought to our attention.

Volume 1

p. 48	reference 8	*replace* 213 *by* 313
p. 153	line 4	*replace* µg/kg bw per **day** *by* ng/kg bw per day

Volume 4

p. 93	3.3(b)	*delete first two lines and put reference* (**Case** *et al.*, 1954) *at end of paragraph*

CUMULATIVE INDEX TO IARC MONOGRAPHS ON THE EVALUATION OF CARCINOGENIC RISK OF CHEMICALS TO MAN

Numbers underlined indicate volume, and numbers in italics indicate page. References to corrigenda are given in parentheses.

Acetamide	7,*197*
Aflatoxins	1,*145* (corr. 8, *349*)
Aflatoxin B1	1,*145*
Aflatoxin B2	1,*145*
Aflatoxin G1	1,*145* (corr. 7,*319*)
Aflatoxin G2	1,*145*
Aldrin	5,*25*
Amaranth	8,*41*
para-Aminoazobenzene	8,*53*
ortho-Aminoazotoluene	8,*61*
4-Aminobiphenyl	1,*74*
2-Amino-5-(5-nitro-2-furyl)-1,3,4-thiadiazole	7,*143*
Amitrole	7,*31*
Amosite	2,*17*
Aniline	4,*27* (corr. 7,*320*)
Anthophyllite	2,*17*
Aramite^R	5,*39*
Arsenic (inorganic)	2,*48*
Arsenic pentoxide	2,*48*
Arsenic trioxide	2,*48*
Asbestos (mixed)	2,*17* (corr. 7,*319*)
Auramine	1,*69* (corr. 7,*319*)
Azobenzene	8,*75*
Barium chromate	2,*102*
Benz(c)acridine	3,*241*
Benz(a)anthracene	3,*45*
Benzene	7,*203*
Benzidine	1,*80*

Benzo(b)fluoranthene	3,69
Benzo(j)fluoranthene	3,82
Benzo(a)pyrene	3,91
Benzo(e)pyrene	3,137
Beryl ore	1,18
Beryllium	1,17
Beryllium oxide	1,17
Beryllium phosphate	1,25
Beryllium sulphate	1,18
BHC (technical grades)	5,47
N,N'-Bis(2-chloroethyl)-2-naphthylamine	4,119
Bis(chloromethyl)ether	4,231
1,4-Butanediol dimethanesulphonate	4,247
Cadmium acetate	2,92
Cadmium powder	2,74
Cadmium carbonate	2,74
Cadmium chloride	2,74
Cadmium oxide	2,74
Cadmium sulphate	2,74
Cadmium sulphide	2,74
Calcium arsenate	2,48
Calcium arsenite	2,48
Calcium chromate	2,100
Carbon tetrachloride	1,53
Carmoisine	8,83
Chlormadinone acetate	6,149
Chlorobenzilate	5,75
Chloroform	1,61
Chloromethyl methyl ether	4,239
Chromic chromate	2,119
Chromic oxide	2,100
Chromium	2,100
Chromium acetate	2,102
Chromium carbonate	2,102
Chromium dioxide	2,101

Chromium phosphate	2,102
Chromium trioxide	2,101
Chrysene	3,159
Chrysoidine	8,91
Chrysotile	2,17
C.I. Disperse Yellow 3	8,97
Citrus Red No. 2	8,101
Crocidolite	2,17
Cycasin	1,157 (corr. 7,319)
D & C Red No. 9	8,107
DDD (TDE)	5,83 (corr. 7,320)
DDE	5,83
DDT	5,83
Diacetylaminoazotoluene	8,113
2,6-Diamino-3-(phenylazo)pyridine (hydrochloride)	8,117
Diazomethane	7,223
Dibenz(*a,h*)acridine	3,247
Dibenz(*a,j*)acridine	3,254
Dibenz(*a,h*)anthracene	3,178
7H-Dibenzo(*c,g*)carbazole	3,260
Dibenzo(*h,rst*)pentaphene	3,197
Dibenzo(*a,e*)pyrene	3,201
Dibenzo(*a,h*)pyrene	3,207
Dibenzo(*a,i*)pyrene	3,215
Dibenzo(*a,l*)pyrene	3,224
ortho-Dichlorobenzene	7,231
para-Dichlorobenzene	7,231
3,3'-Dichlorobenzidine	4,49
Dieldrin	5,125
1,2-Diethylhydrazine	4,153
Diethylstilboestrol	6,55
Diethyl sulphate	4,277
Dihydrosafrole	1,170
Dimethisterone	6,167
3,3'-Dimethoxybenzidine (*o*-Dianisidine)	4,41

para-Dimethylaminoazobenzene	8,*125*
para-Dimethylaminobenzenediazo sodium sulphonate	8,*147*
trans-2[(Dimethylamino)methylimino]-5-[2-(5-nitro-2-furyl)vinyl]-1,3,4-oxadiazole	7,*147*
3,3'-Dimethylbenzidine (*o*-Tolidine)	1,*87*
1,1-Dimethylhydrazine	4,*137*
1,2-Dimethylhydrazine	4,*145* (corr. 7,*320*)
Dimethyl sulphate	4,*271*
Endrin	5,*157*
Ethinyloestradiol	6,*77*
Ethylenethiourea	7,*45*
Ethyl methanesulphonate	7,*245*
Ethynodiol diacetate	6,*173*
Evans blue	8,*151*
2-(2-Formylhydrazino)-4-(5-nitro-2-furyl)thiazole	7,*151*
Haematite	1,*29*
Heptachlor and its epoxide	5,*173*
Hydrazine	4,*127*
4-Hydroxyazobenzene	8,*157*
Indeno(1,2,3-*cd*)pyrene	3,*229*
Iron-dextran complex	2,*161*
Iron-dextrin complex	2,*161* (corr. 7,*319*)
Iron oxide	1,*29*
Iron-sorbitol-citric acid complex	2,*161*
Isonicotinic acid hydrazide	4,*159*
Isosafrole	1,*169*
Lead acetate	1,*40*
Lead arsenate	1,*41*
Lead carbonate	1,*41*
Lead chromate	2,*101*
Lead phosphate	1,*48*
Lead salts	1,*40* (corr. 7,*319*, 8,*349*
Lead subacetate	1,*40*
Lindane	5,*47*
Magenta	4,*57* (corr. 7,*320*)

Maleic hydrazide	*4*,173
Medroxyprogesterone acetate	*6*,157
Mestranol	*6*,87
Methoxychlor	*5*,193
Methylazoxymethanol acetate	*1*,164
N-Methyl-N,4-dinitrosoaniline	*1*,141
4,4'-Methylene bis (2-chloroaniline)	*4*,65
4,4'-Methylene bis (2-methylaniline)	*4*,73
4,4'-Methylenedianiline	*4*,79 (corr. *7*,320)
Methyl methanesulphonate	*7*,253
N-Methyl-N'-nitro-N-nitrosoguanidine	*4*,183
Methyl red	*8*,
Methylthiouracil	*7*,53
Mirex	*5*,203
5-(Morpholinomethyl)-3-[(5-nitrofurfurylidene)amino]-2-oxazolidinone	*7*,161
1-Naphthylamine	*4*,87 (corr. *8*,349)
2-Naphthylamine	*4*,97
Nickel	*2*,126
Nickel acetate	*2*,126
Nickel carbonate	*2*,126
Nickel carbonyl	*2*,126 (corr. *7*,319)
Nickelocene	*2*,126
Nickel oxide	*2*,126
Nickel powder	*2*,145
Nickel subsulphide	*2*,126
Nickel sulphate	*2*,127
4-Nitrobiphenyl	*4*,113
5-Nitro-2-furaldehyde semicarbazone	*7*,171
1[(5-Nitrofurfurylidene)amino]-2-imidazolidinone	*7*,181
N-[4-(5-Nitro-2-furyl)-2-thiazolyl]acetamide	*1*,181 & *7*,185
N-Nitroso-di-n-butylamine	*4*,197
N-Nitrosodiethylamine	*1*,107
N-Nitrosodimethylamine	*1*,95
Nitrosoethylurea	*1*,135

Nitrosomethylurea	<u>1</u>,125
N-Nitroso-N-methylurethane	<u>4</u>,211
Norethisterone	<u>6</u>,179
Norethisterone acetate	<u>6</u>,179
Norethynodrel	<u>6</u>,191
Norgestrel	<u>6</u>,201
Oestradiol-17β	<u>6</u>,99
Oestriol	<u>6</u>,117
Oestrone	<u>6</u>,123
Oil orange SS	<u>8</u>,165
Orange I	<u>8</u>,173
Orange G	<u>8</u>,181
Polychlorinated biphenyls	<u>7</u>,261
Ponceau MX	<u>8</u>,189
Ponceau 3R	<u>8</u>,199
Ponceau SX	<u>8</u>,207
Potassium arsenate	<u>2</u>,48
Potassium arsenite	<u>2</u>,49
Potassium chromate	<u>2</u>,102
Potassium dichromate	<u>2</u>,101
Progesterone	<u>6</u>,135
1,3-Propane sultone	<u>4</u>,253
β-Propiolactone	<u>4</u>,259
Propylthiouracil	<u>7</u>,67
Quintozene (Pentachloronitrobenzene)	<u>5</u>,211
Saccharated iron oxide	<u>2</u>,161
Safrole	<u>1</u>,169
Scarlet red	<u>8</u>,217
Sodium arsenate	<u>2</u>,49
Sodium arsenite	<u>2</u>,49
Sodium chromate	<u>2</u>,102
Sodium dichromate	<u>2</u>,102
Soot, tars and shale oils	<u>3</u>,22
Sterigmatocystin	<u>1</u>,175
Streptozotocin	<u>4</u>,221

Strontium chromate	2,102
Sudan I	8,225
Sudan II	8,233
Sudan III	8,241
Sudan brown RR	8,249
Sudan red 7B	8,253
Sunset yellow FCF	8,257
Terpene polychlorinates (Strobane^R)	5,219
Testosterone	6,209
Tetraethyllead	2,150
Tetramethyllead	2,150
Thioacetamide	7,77
Thiouracil	7,85
Thiourea	7,95
Trypan blue	8,267
Urethane	7,111
Vinyl chloride	7,291
Yellow AB	8,279
Yellow OB	8,287
Zinc chromate hydroxide	2,102

www.ingramcontent.com/pod-product-compliance
Ingram Content Group UK Ltd.
Pitfield, Milton Keynes, MK11 3LW, UK
UKHW051258180426
11947UKWH00020B/1781